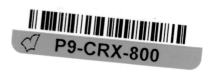

The **TRANSPLANT PATIENT**

Biological, psychiatric, and ethical issues
in organ transplantation

Organ transplantation is now an essential element of treatment for a
wide range of diseases. However, alongside surgical success rates
there are many other issues affecting selection of patients and clinical
outcome with which clinicians and patients themselves must be
familiar.

This book:

- reviews psychosocial, psychiatric and ethical aspects of organ
  transplantation in a uniquely authoritative way;
- draws heavily on the pioneering work of the Pittsburgh transplant
  team;
- surveys the essentials of transplantation biology;
- engages with a range of topics fundamental to the success of the
  procedure and the quality of life of recipients and donors alike.

Its interdisciplinary approach and the authority of the contribu-
tors will commend this book to a wide audience including those who
select, support and advise transplant patients and their families, and
to clinicians performing the procedures.

Paula Trzepacz is Senior Clinical Research Physician, Neurosciences,
Eli Lilly and Company, and Adjunct Professor of Psychiatry and
Neurology, University of Mississippi Medical Center.

Andrea DiMartini is Assistant Professor of Psychiatry at the University
of Pittsburgh Western Psychiatric Institute, which is a pioneer in the
area of transplant psychiatry.

Both authors are widely published in the field of neuropsychiatry and
neuro-science. Dr DiMartini is widely published in issues of transplantation and psychiatry and Dr Trzepacz in neuropsychiatry.

The TRANSPLANT PATIENT

Biological, psychiatric, and ethical issues in organ transplantation

Edited by

Paula T. Trzepacz

Eli Lilly and Company, Indianapolis, and
University of Mississippi Medical Center

and

Andrea F. DiMartini

Psychiatric Consultation – Liaison Program,
University of Pittsburgh Medical Center,
Western Psychiatric Institute and Clinic

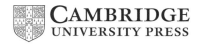
CAMBRIDGE
UNIVERSITY PRESS

PUBLISHED BY THE PRESS SYNDICATE OF THE UNIVERSITY OF CAMBRIDGE
The Pitt Building, Trumpington Street, Cambridge, United Kingdom

CAMBRIDGE UNIVERSITY PRESS
The Edinburgh Building, Cambridge CB2 2RU, UK   http://www.cup.cam.ac.uk
40 West 20th Street, New York, NY 10011-4211, USA   http://www.cup.org
19 Stamford Road, Oakleigh, Melbourne 3166, Australia
Ruiz de Alarcón 13, 28014 Madrid, Spain

First published 2000

Printed in the United Kingdom at the University Press, Cambridge

Typeset in Minion 10/12 pt [vn]

A catalogue record for this book is available from the British Library

Library of Congress Cataloguing in Publications data

The transplant patient: biological, psychiatric, and ethical issues in organ transplantation /
edited by Paula T. Trzepacz and Andrea F. DiMartini.
        p.   cm.
    Includes index.
    ISBN 0 521 55354 7 (hb)
        1. Transplantation of organs, tissues, etc. – Physiological aspects.   2. Transplantation of
    organs, tissues, etc. – Psychological aspects.   3. Transplantation of organs, tissues, etc. –
    Moral and ethical aspects.   I. Trzepacz, Paula T.   II. DiMartini, Andrea F.
        [DNLM: 1. Organ Transplantation – psychology.   2. Ethics, Medical.   3. Organ
    Transplantation – physiology.   WO 690 T772 2000]
    RD120.7.T657   2000
    617.9'5 – dc21
    DNLM/DLC
    for Library of Congress   99-25872 CIP

ISBN 0 521 553547 hardback

Contents

Contributors

Aishe S. Allen, B.S.
Western Psychiatric Institute and Clinic
Iroquois Building, Suite 502
3600 Forbes Avenue
Pittsburgh, PA 15213
USA

Julio Bobes, M.D., Ph.D.
Department of Medicine
University of Oviedo
Julian Claveria, 6
33006 Oviedo
Spain

Robert D. Canning, Ph.D.
Department of Psychiatry
UC Davis Medical Center
2315 Stockton Boulevard
Sacramento, CA 95817
USA

Mary Amanda Dew, Ph.D.
Western Psychiatric Institute and Clinic
3811 O'Hara Street
Pittsburgh, PA 15213-2593
USA

Andrea F. DiMartini, M.D.
Western Psychiatric Institute and Clinic
Psychiatric Consultation-Liaison
Program
3811 O'Hara Street
Pittsburgh, PA 15213-2593
USA

Grant Gillett, D. Phil.
Dunedin Hospital
University of Otago
201 Great King Street
Dunedin
New Zealand

Maria Paz González, M.D., Ph.D.
Department of Medicine
University of Oviedo
Julián Calvería, 6
33006 Oviedo
Spain

Jean Goycoolea, B.A.
Western Psychiatric Institute and Clinic
Iroquois Building, Suite 502
3600 Forbes Avenue
Pittsburgh, PA 15213
USA

Babu Gupta, M.D.
1008 Deer Ridge Drive
Baltimore, MD 21210
USA

Richard Kradin, M.D.
Harvard Medical School
Harvard University
15 Parkman Street – WAAC 817
Boston, MA 02114
USA

James L. Levenson, M.D.
Medical College of Virginia Hospitals
Virgina Commonwealth University
Box 268 MCV
Richmond, VA 23298-0268
USA

Maureen Martin, M.D., F.R.C.S. (C)
Iowa Methodist Medical Center
1215 Pleasant Street
Suite 300A
Des Moines, IA 50309
USA

Ellen Olbrisch, Ph.D.
Department of Psychiatry
Medical College of Virginia Hospitals
Virginia Commonwealth University
PO Box 980268
Richmond, VA 23298-0268
USA

Thomas E. Starzl, M.D., Ph.D.
Thomas E. Starzl Transplant Institute
University of Pittsburgh School of
Medicine
3601 Fifth Avenue
Pittsburgh, PA 15213
USA

Margaret Stuber, M.D.
UCLA Neuropsychiatric Institute
Division of Child and Adolescent
Psychiatry
760 Westwood Plaza
Los Angeles, CA 90024-1759
USA

Abraham Sudilovsky, M.D.
10 Huston Road
Oakmont, PA 15139-1913
USA

Owen S. Surman, M.D.
Massachusetts General Hospital
Harvard Medical School
15 Parkman Street – WAAC 812
Boston, MA 02114
USA

JoAnn Switala, M.P.A.
Western Psychiatric Institute and Clinic
Center for Education and Drug Abuse
Research
3501 Forbes Avenue
Suite 830
Pittsburgh, PA 15213
USA

Galen E. Switzer, Ph.D.
Western Psychiatric Institute and Clinic
Department of Psychiatry
Iroqois Building, Suite 502
3811 O'Hara Street
Pittsburgh, PA 15213-2593
USA

Ralph E. Tarter, Ph.D.
Western Psychiatric Institute and Clinic
3811 O'Hara Street
Pittsburgh, PA 15213-2593
USA

Paula T. Trzepacz,, M.D.
Lilly Corporate Center
Drop code 4133
Indianapolis
IN 46285
USA

Robert K. Twillman, Ph.D.
School of Medicine
University of Kansas Cancer Center
3901 Rainbow Boulevard
Kansas City, MO 66160-7820
USA

Preface

The transplant patient faces extraordinary challenges in their emotional and social lives as they undergo the physical transformations associated with the transplantation process. The need for an organ transplant may occur acutely or as a consequence of chronic organ insufficiency, each with its own set of biopsychosocial consequences. The interrelationships between physiology and psychological health are important for bodily health. Even immunological functions show links between brain and other body areas that may bridge emotional and physical states in complex and heretofore poorly understood ways. Pharmacological interventions often cross the blood–brain barrier, causing psychiatric side effects – for example, during uremia or hypocholesterolemia combined with cyclosporine treatment.

Our book opens with a chapter, "The mystique of transplantation: biologic and psychiatric considerations", by Thomas Starzl, the distinguished pioneer of liver transplantation from the laboratory to the human situation. Starzl traces the history of immunological barriers that were overcome in order to allow orthotopic organ transplantation, including engraftments of kidney, liver, lung, heart, pancreas, intestine and multiple abdominal viscera. He describes bidirectional immunologic confrontation between graft and host and the important discovery of donor leukocyte chimerism in solid organ transplantation, contrasting it with bone marrow transplantation, where host cells are deliberately cytoablated.

The closing chapter, by Maureen Martin, "Current trends and new developments in transplantation", addresses new approaches to clinical immunosuppression, based on the concept of chimerism, which use bone marrow and stem cell-derived factors combined with solid organ transplantation. She describes the feat of liver xenotransplantation from baboon to human, as well as the introduction of novel immunosuppressive agents that allow for enhanced allograft survival, including tacrolimus, mycophenolate mofetil, rapamycin, Brequinar sodium and 15-deoxyspergualin. Martin describes newer ventures such as intestinal transplantation, the use of bone marrow transplantation to prolong solid organ survival, and the potential clinical application of chimerism.

Bridging these two chapters by transplant surgeons is a chapter by Richard

Kradin, and Owen Surman, "Psychoneuroimmunology and organ transplantation: theory and practice". These authors explore the multiple interfaces between the immune system and the brain because psychoneuroimmunology is the science of neural, endocrine and immune interactions. They address psychosomatic issues relating to graft survival, and immunity and the mind – noting the many parallels between neural and immune tissues in discrimination of "self" and "non-self" and learning. The brain is the organ of psychiatry. They describe in detail the bidirectional transfer and processing of information between the neural and immune systems, as well as the different mechanisms that achieve parallel functions of recognition, memory, and response. They review stress and immunity and how it may impact on transplant patients, including the effects of psychiatric disorders on immune function. Finally, they review effects of psychotropic medications on immune function.

Chapter 7, "Pharmacologic issues in organ transplantation: psychopharmacology and neuropsychiatric medicine side effects", by Paula T. Trzepacz, Babu Gupta, and Andrea DiMartini, is also a bridging chapter between biological and behavioral systems. They begin with a review of physiological issues during organ insufficiency that affect drug metabolism and clearance (hepatic, renal, and cardiovascular systems). Differences in phase I and II hepatic drug metabolism during organ insufficiency states are described, along with examples of handling of drugs with different pharmacological characteristics. Advances in the understanding of hepatic cytochrome P_{450} isozymes for drug metabolism and potential drug interactions are discussed and highlighted by tables of information and psychotropic medications as well as other medications commonly used in transplant patients. Detailed sections describe reports of neuropsychiatric side effects of each major immunosuppressive agent (cyclosporine, tacrolimus, OKT3, corticosteroids, azathioprine, mycophenolate mofetil) and antiviral, antifungal and antibacterial drugs commonly used in transplant patients.

Three chapters address specialty populations – pediatric and geriatric age groups, and patients with alcoholism. "Pediatric transplantation" (Chapter 11), by Robert D. Canning, and Margaret L. Stuber, focuses on a relatively sparse literature, as compared to adults, about children and adolescents undergoing transplantation. They discuss unique issues affecting pediatric patients including epidemiology, family role, development and medical caregiver responses. Psychiatric assessment and management of transplant patients is complicated by dealing with the family including axis II pathology in the parents and legal issues. Adolescents have a greater capacity to comprehend and make decisions, but have other developmental transitional issues that make them a high-risk population. Psychiatric problems include delirium and depression, as well as noncompliance, similar to adults.

Chapter 5, "Quality of life of geriatric patients following transplantation:

short- and long term outcomes", by Maria Paz Gonzáles, Abraham Sudilousky, Julio Bobes, and Andrea F. DiMartini, focuses on controversies in transplantation of aging patients. A larger literature exists in geriatrics than for pediatrics. Donor organ shortages combined with problems of aging bodies bring up economic and ethical issues, mandating objective review of outcome data. Maintenance of a high functional level and independence is considered an appropriate outcome measure in the elderly. These authors carefully review numerous studies of survival and quality of life of geriatric transplant patients for a variety of types of organs, with positive results attainable especially for well-selected patients.

Chapter 8, "Alcoholism and organ transplantation", by Andrea F. DiMartini and Paula T. Trzepacz, provides an overview of the history and policies related to performing transplants on patients with alcoholism, a special population associated with many controversies. Most literature describes alcoholic cirhosis and liver transplantation, though there is a smaller body of information on transplantation for alcoholic cardiomyopathy. The authors review screening and monitoring procedures for alcoholic transplant patients and medical sequelae, compliance, and resumption of drinking following transplantation.

Two chapters describe assessment of psychiatric characteristics of transplant patients. Chapter 6, "Cognitive assessment in organ transplantation", by Ralph Tarter and JoAnn Switala, describes neuropsychological approaches to types of cognitive deficits that appear in pre- and post-transplantation populations. These authors point out the multifactorial etiologies that can produce cognitive impairments, including and beyond the obvious physiological effects of organ failure on the brain. Patterns of deficits may assist in delineation of possible causes. Specific neuropsychological tests are suggested for screening, comprehensive, and modality-specific assessments. Chapter 12, "Psychosocial screening and selection of candidates for organ transplantation", by James Levenson and Mary Ellen Olbrisch describes two psychosocial screening instruments, the PACT and the TERS, as used in transplant patients. They discuss the rationale for such screening, as part of a thorough and multispecialty evaluation of candidates, and note that these are not conducted to determine social worthiness to be transplanted. Nearly all US transplant programs utilize some form of psychosocial evaluation of candidates, while about half of non-US programs do. These authors also compare US and non-US transplant programs' attitudes relative to and absolute psychosocial and psychiatric contraindications to transplantation.

Grant Gillett wrote Chapter 9, "Ethics and images in organ transplantation", which stretches the reader beyond the usual medical and psychiatric thinking about transplantation. He delves into difficult ethical questions about donation: economics, autonomy, coercion and discrimination. The author proposes that the most accessible ethical justification for organ transplantation is a utilitarian argument. Transplantation also is discussed as an incentive for death itself among young, healthy incompetent or vulnerable patients. Patients who are anencephalic or in persistent vegetative states and are potential donors pose particular dilemmas. Living healthy donors bring up other ethical concerns, including relatives of the transplant candidate and strangers paid for their organs in an organ market. Symbolic concerns (imagistic) affect societal attitudes as much as scientific ones. Finally, the idea of a donation as a gift is argued.

Chapter 3 and 4 address organ donors and organ recipients, respectively. In "Psychosocial issues in organ donation", Galen F. Switzer, Mary Amanda Dew, and Robert K. Twillman introduce an organ or bone marrow donation as a gift, though without an expectation for reciprocity and with significant discomfort and sacrifice. Issues affect donors both pre- and post-donation. Motives differ between related and unrelated donors. Decision-making may be a moral as well as rational process, may not always be spontaneous, may differ between donors and non-donors, and may be fraught with ambivalence. Studies of post-donation outcomes reveal two categories – psychological reactions and donor perceptions of physical status – among kidney and bone marrow donors.

Chapter 4, "Quality of life in organ transplantation: effects on adult recipients and their families", by Mary Amanda Dew, Jean M. Goycoolea, Glen Switzer, and Aishe S. Allen, reviews 144 studies from 19 countries covering six types of transplants. Quality of life post-transplantation is increasingly appreciated as an important outcome, along with survival, though it is multidimensional and is often measured in different ways – generic, broad measures, and illness-specific measures. Several domains of quality of life are reviewed – physical function, mental health/cognitive, social, and overall. Extensive tables summarize numerous variables of the studies. Overall, physical and global quality of life improves pre- to post-transplantation. However, mental health/cognitive and social domains are less certain to improve. The authors also review 15 studies about how transplantation affects recipients' families' quality of life.

The Transplant Patient provides a comprehensive scientific and scholarly review of the psychiatric, psychosocial, and biologic aspects of organ and bone marrow transplantation, it is essential reading for all involved in organ transplantation, whether the reader's interest is clinical or research. From the history to the future, special issues and special populations, it will provide valuable insights to all physicians, psychiatrists, psychologists, nurses, transplant coordinators and related health care professionals involved in the care of transplant patients.

Paula T. Trzepacz
Andrea F. DiMartini

The mystique of transplantation: biologic and psychiatric considerations

Thomas E. Starzl M.D., Ph.D.

Most major advances in medicine spring from discoveries in basic science and are therefore predictable, or at least logical. Organ transplantation was the supreme exception to the rule. Although the potential benefit of whole-organ replacement in the absence of an immune barrier was dramatically demonstrated with the identical-twin kidney transplantation performed, in December 1954, by Joseph E. Murray (Nobel Laureate, 1990; Merrill et al. 1956), this achievement only confirmed what already was known to be possible with identical-twin skin grafts (Padgett 1932; Brown 1937). In 1961, two months after receiving the 1960 Nobel Prize for research in immunology, Macfarland Burnet wrote in the *New England Journal of Medicine* that "much thought has been given to ways by which tissues or organs not genetically and antigenetically identical with the patient might be made to survive and function in the alien environment. On the whole, the present outlook is highly unfavorable to success..." (Burnet 1961).

This grim prospect, only a third of a century ago, faced the pioneer organ recipients whose courage in offering themselves up for human experimentation made it possible to crack the immunologic barrier (Starzl 1992). For three decades after this was done, there was no explanation for what had been accomplished. The resulting mystique of transplantation as well as the unpredictable outcome of these procedures created a fertile emotional soil for psychiatric complications. Consequently, when the light of understanding was finally switched on in 1992, it was as much a spiritual as a scientific awakening. The acquisition of this insight exposed a seminal principle of allograft acceptance that is the same with all kinds of whole organs.

The immunologic barrier: the one-way paradigm

What was the immunologic barrier described in such pessimistic terms by Burnet, who saw no way that a transplanted histoincompatible organ could pass through the seemingly inviolate barrier of immunologic reactivity? In the identical-twin kidney transplantations, the problem was by-passed, but in all other cases, it was necessary to reckon with two potential complications, either separately or together: rejection and graft-versus-host disease (GVHD).

Rejection

Although the details remain incomplete today, there was little mystery about the general meaning of rejection, following its elucidation in 1944 by Medawar (Nobel co-Laureate with Burnet 1960) as an immunologic event (Medawar 1944). This great contribution created the indelible image that transplantation involved a one-way immune reaction. Thus, a tissue (or organ) allograft was a defenseless island in a hostile recipient sea (Figure 1.1(a)).

Tolerance

In this context, an unsolved mystery of biology for nearly 40 years was how allografts could escape rejection without the recipient being crippled with immunosuppression. The description of acquired tolerance by Billingham, Brent, and Medawar (1953, 1956) did not provide an answer. In their experimental model, immunocompetent adult spleen cells were injected in utero or perinatally into mice that had not yet evolved the necessary immunologic maturity to reject them. The engrafted cells flourished and were thought to have in effect endowed the recipient with the donor immune system (donor leukocyte chimerism) (Figure 1.1(b)).

Thereafter, the mice failed to recognize donor strain skin grafts or other tissues as alien (i.e. they had acquired tolerance). The switch in immunologic apparatus was consistent with the definition of transplantation immunology in terms of a unidirectional immune reaction (the "one-way paradigm"). Main and Prehn (1955) demonstrated the same tolerance outcome as Billingham et al. in irradiated adult mice, whose cytoablated hematolymphopoietic cells were reconstituted with bone marrow instead of spleen cells. Thousands of subsequent tolerance induction experiments in animals, and eventually clinical bone marrow transplantation, seemingly depended upon a similar natural, or iatrogenically imposed, defenseless recipient state (Figure 1.1(b)).

Graft-versus-host disease

It was recognized as early as 1957 in mouse (Billingham and Brent 1957) and chicken (Simonsen 1957) models that an immunologically active graft had a genetically controlled repertoire of immune reactivity comparable to that of the recipient, and could therefore turn the tables and reject the recipient. This was called graft-versus-host disease (GVHD), or alternatively "runt disease". The risk if the host was immunologically defenseless was roughly propor-

tional to the extent of the major histocompatibility complex (MHC) difference between donor and recipient. Such disparities became measurable
serologically in humans after identification of the human leukocyte antigens
(HLAs) by Dausset (1990; Nobel Laureate 1980), Terasaki, and others whose
reminiscences have been collected (Terasaki 1990). The complication of
GVHD in rodent (Trentin 1957) and large animal irradiation chimera
models (Mannick et al. 1959; Hume et al. 1960; Rapaport et al. 1979; Thomas
1991) forestalled for many years the clinical use of HLA mismatched bone
marrow cells or other mature immunocytes, either for immunologic reconstitution with purely hematologic objectives or as a means of facilitating
whole-organ graft acceptance.

Clinical bone marrow transplantation

The strategy that made possible the first successful clinical bone marrow
transplantations in 1968 was an extension of the rodent experiments, with
similar histocompatibility-imposed restrictions (Mathe et al. 1963; Bach
1968; Gatti et al. 1968). After recipient cytoablation with total body irradiation (TBI) or cytotoxic drugs (Figure 1.1(b)), stable chimerism could be
induced in humans by the infusion of donor bone marrow, but only if there
was a good HLA match. Otherwise there was an intolerable incidence of
lethal GVHD. Maintenance immunosuppression could frequently be stopped in these patients, mimicking the kind of acquired immunologic tolerance
originally described by Billingham et al. (1953, 1956), and by Main and Prehn
(1955).

Clinical organ transplantation

Ironically, surgeons and physicians had recorded thousands of successful
human whole-organ transplantations (mostly kidneys) by the time bone
marrow transplantation was finally accomplished. However, the conditions
were dramatically different. First, continuous immunosuppression was
needed, presumably for life. Second, success did not depend on HLA matching. Third, the complication of GVHD was rare. Most immunologists were
dumbfounded by these results. The inability to explain them detached
workers in the whole-organ field from the scientific base enjoyed by bone
marrow transplanters. Thus, further steps in the improvement of whole-
organ transplantation were largely the product of trial and error. To comprehend how this occurred requires a historical perspective.

With total body irradiation

Host preconditioning played an important role in the first six successful renal

(a) One-Way Paradigm (Organ)

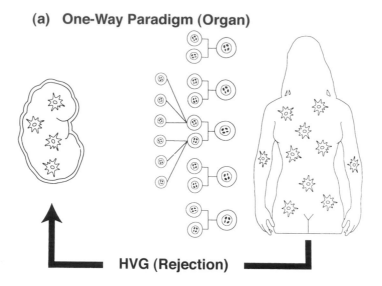

HVG (Rejection)

(c) Two-way Paradigm (Organ)

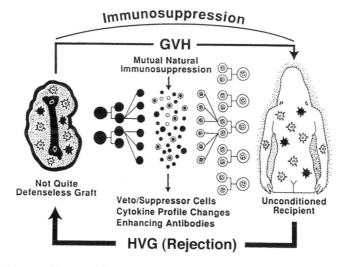

Immunosuppression

GVH

Mutual Natural
Immunosuppression

Not Quite
Defenseless Graft

Veto/Suppressor Cells
Cytokine Profile Changes
Enhancing Antibodies

Unconditioned
Recipient

HVG (Rejection)

Figure 1.1. Upper panels: One-way paradigm in which transplantation is conceived as involving a unidirectional immune reaction: host-versus-graft (HVG) with whole organs (a) and graft-versus-host (GVH) with bone marrow or other lymphopoietic transplants (b). Lower panels: Two-way paradigm with which transplantation is seen as a bidirectional and mutually cancelling immune reaction that is predominantly HVG with whole-organ grafts (c), and predominantly GVH with bone marrow grafts and (d).

(b) One-Way Paradigm (Bone Marrow)

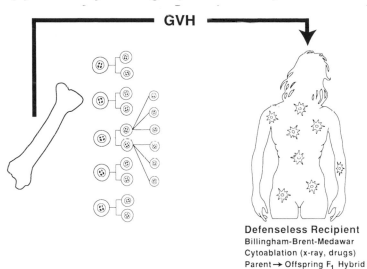

Defenseless Recipient
Billingham-Brent-Medawar
Cytoablation (x-ray, drugs)
Parent → Offspring F$_1$ Hybrid

(d) Two-way Paradigm (Bone Marrow)

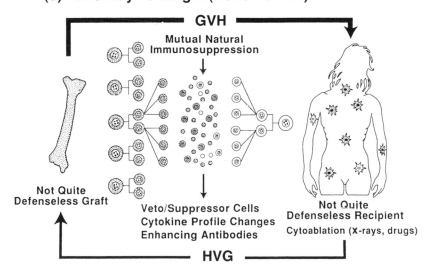

Not Quite
Defenseless Graft

Veto/Suppressor Cells
Cytokine Profile Changes
Enhancing Antibodies

Not Quite
Defenseless Recipient
Cytoablation (X-rays, drugs)

transplantations (defined as survival to more than one year) between 1959 and 1962, one in Boston (Merrill et al. 1960) and five in France (Hamburger et al. 1962; Kuss et al. 1962). The recipients were prepared for operation with sublethal TBI, but without donor bone marrow; their own bone marrow recovered and one of these patients (in Paris) survived for 26 years. However, these were isolated successes in a sea of failures, and pessimism set in worldwide about the prospects of moving forward.

Chemical immunosuppression

The introduction, for human renal transplantation, of 6-mercaptopurine (6-MP) and its analogue azathioprine did not at first relieve the frustration. The clinical use of these drugs followed the demonstration of their immunosuppressive effects in extensive experimental studies, first with rodent skin transplantation (Meeker et al. 1959; Schwartz and Dameshek, 1960) and then with the canine kidney transplant models (Calne 1960, 1961; Zukoski, Lee, and Hume 1960; Murray et al. 1962). The drugs had been developed originally for their antileukemic effect by Elion and Hitchings (Nobel Laureates, 1988; Elion, Bieber, and Hitchings 1955) and were first demonstrated to be immunosuppressive by Schwartz and Dameshek (1959). Although the kidney of the sixth patient treated by Murray with one of these myelotoxic drugs had the function of a non-related renal allograft for 17 months, the clinical results with chemical immunosuppression were generally poor at first (Murray et al. 1962, 1963), similar to those with TBI.

The drug cocktail breakthrough

The tidal wave of whole-organ cases began in earnest in 1962–3, when a characteristic cycle of convalescence was identified in which kidney rejection could be reversed surprisingly easily when prednisone was added to azathioprine (double-drug therapy) (Starzl, Marchioro, and Waddell 1963). More importantly, the need later on for maintenance immunosuppression often declined as if the immune barrier had been lowered (Figure 1.2), and in occasional cases therapy could be stopped. Since then, the same sequence has been seen with all other organs transplanted and with all of the two-drug and more complex multiple agent immunosuppressive regimens. Drugs introduced later were more potent and reliable in chaperoning the desired chain of events: antilymphocyte globulin (ALG) (Starzl et al. 1967), cyclosporine (Calne et al. 1979), and FK506 (Starzl et al. 1989). Notwithstanding their diversity, all seemed in a fundamentally similar way to have allowed something to change in the host, the graft or both. But what?

Deficiencies of the one-way paradigm

Although the one-way paradigm did not provide the answer, this false

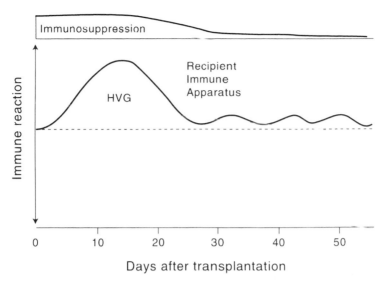

Figure 1.2. Pattern of postoperative events with whole-organ allograft acceptance, in the framework of the one-way paradigm. HVG, host-versus-graft.

conceptualization of graft acceptance as a product of a unidirectional reaction was reinforced with the introduction in 1963 of the one-way mixed lymphocyte reaction (Bach and Hirschhorn 1964; Bain, Vas, and Lowenstein 1964). Although these and other in vitro techniques (the so-called minitransplant models) generated increasingly sophisticated cellular and ultimately molecular studies of one-way immunologic reactions, the resulting plethora of new information resembled an exponentially expanding telephone directory. Most seriously, the flawed context lured successive generations of investigators into the trap of believing that tolerance induction for whole-organ recipients (the "holy grail") lay in variations on the HLA-limiting strategy used for bone marrow transplantation. The strategy always included host preconditioning in preparation for a variety of donor leukocyte preparations.

Cell-mediated immunity

The inability of clinicians to explain what was going on with their patients did not dissuade them from developing their own voluminous literature which, was largely phenomenologic. An increasing number of transplant surgeons and physicians began to regard basic immunology as an interesting hobby, but one that was irrelevant to their practice. Meanwhile, most virologists and the majority of basic immunologists trying to understand rejection had shifted their efforts by the early 1970s from whole-animal studies to T

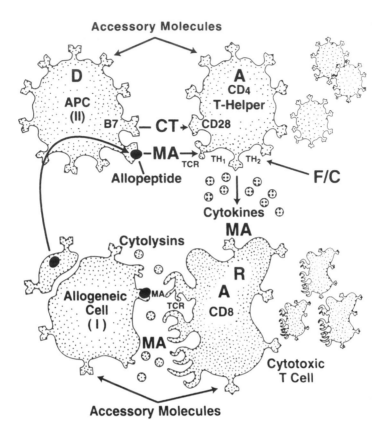

Figure 1.3. A schematic representation of the antiallograft immune response showing the cell surface proteins that participate in antigen recognition and signal transduction, the contribution of cytokines and the sites of action of the diverse agents that prolong graft survival. Antigen (allopeptide) recognition via the T cell receptor (TCR) and the role of accessory molecules can be blocked by monoclonal antibodies (MA), as can cytokine receptor expression. Deoxyspergualin (D) is believed to inhibit the function of antigen-presenting cells (APC). FK506 (F, now tacrolimus) and cyclosporine (C) inhibit cytokine gene expression within T helper (TH) cells, whereas rapamycin (R) blocks the responses of T cells to interleukin (IL)-2. By inhibiting DNA synthesis, the antimetabolite drugs (A) act later than F, C or R to block lymphocyte proliferation. CTLA4-Ig (CT) is a new agent that blocks transmission of second signal (the B7-CD28 pathway) essential for T cell activation. F/C, FK506/CsA (cyclosporin A). (I) and (II) indicate major histocompatibility complex (MHC) antigens classes I and II, respectively.

lymphocyte-oriented cell culture (in vitro) systems. These labors were rewarded by a Nobel Prize (to Baruj Benacerraf, 1980) and the Lasker Prize in Basic Science of 1995, which was shared by four Americans and one Swiss (Doherty 1995; Unanue 1995; Zinkernagel 1995). The conceptual model that emerged provided an explanation of cell-mediated immunity (Figure 1.3). In the context of the one-way paradigm, the details of the putative allogeneic reaction (rejection) included its dependence on antigen-presenting cells, the necessity for a co-stimulatory molecule(s) (the two-signal concept of self/non self discrimination), an important role of accessory molecules, and cytokine control of clonal expansion of T helper lymphocytes as well as of the cytotoxic T cells that are the agents of allograft destruction. The bewildering mass of details to which thousands of investigators had contributed over three decades (Janeway and Travers 1994) had long since overwhelmed most clinicians interested in applying the new information.

Mechanisms of drug action

However, the foregoing information allowed precise documentation of the surprising diversity of drugs with which long-term or permanent graft survival could be induced, no matter what the level of intervention in the immune reaction (Thomson and Starzl 1994). This is summarized in Figure 1.3. Deoxyspergualin was said to alter the function of antigen-presenting cells, of which dendritic cells have been conceded to be the most important. The anti metabolite drugs (including azathioprine) prevented clonal expansion of lymphocytes by inhibition of DNA synthesis. Cyclosporine and tacrolimus (FK506) disrupt signals from T cell receptor sites to the nucleus. Monoclonal antibodies (MAs) interrupt the immune reaction at the various specific targets (Figure 1.3), and rapamycin interdicts the effector events even after the secretion of the cytokine interleukin 2 (formerly called the "T cell growth factor"). The new immunosuppressive fusion protein CTLA4-Ig blocks the transmission of a "second signal" (the B7-CD28 pathway). All appear to be permissive of a natural event that became specific only by virtue of the presence of donor antigens.

The immunologic barrier: the two-way paradigm

Whole-organ transplantation

Insight into what had happened to the pioneer organ recipients was obtained in retrospect by studies, at the University of Pittsburgh nearly 30 years later, of a group of kidney and liver recipients from the earliest clinical trials at the University of Colorado, who still had good function of their original grafts. Donor leukocytes of bone marrow origin that are part of the structure of all complex grafts ("passenger leukocytes" (Snell 1957; Steinmuller 1967)) were found in 1992 to have migrated from the organs and survived ubiquitously in the patients for up to three decades (Starzl et al. 1992, 1993). Thus, organ allograft acceptance was associated with the cryptic persistence of a small fragment of extramedullary donor marrow, including stem cells (depicted as a bone silhouette in Figure 1.1(c)). These cells had been assimilated into the overwhelmingly larger immunologic network of the host. The leukocyte movement was in both directions, with small numbers of residual donor leukocytes (microchimerism) in both the graft and host.

The discovery was instinctively understood by most patients to whom it was explained, and it had a surprisingly great emotional impact. The point was not lost that the physical intimacy of the donor to the recipient was greater than anyone had ever imagined. It was closer and more lasting than that of a gestational fetus with its mother. The woman applying lipstick in the morning was touching that unknown cadaveric male donor of 30 years ago whose live cells were everywhere in her own tissue. She was not the recipient of an organ only. The realization was usually moving, and it was invariably sobering.

Scientifically, a revision of transplantation immunology was mandated in which the immunologic confrontation following whole-organ transplantation could be seen as a bidirectional and mutually cancelling (graft-versus-host (GVH) as well as host-versus-graft (HVG)) interaction (Figure 1.4), provided the two participants in the David (donor)/Goliath (recipient) mismatch could survive the initial confrontation. Clinically, but not in several animal models, this outcome requires an umbrella of immunosuppression that protects both cell populations equally (Figure 1.1(c)).

Understanding the amplification device by which the small number of donor cells can so profoundly affect the immunologic vision of, and eventually be assimilated by, the vast recipient army against which it is arrayed is of intense scientific interest. The chimeric leukocytes are multilineage (Starzl et al. 1992, 1993; Demetris et al. 1993; Qian et al. 1994). However, the antigen-presenting dendritic cells (DCs) of Steinman and Cohn (1973; Steinman 1991) are thought to be the key to the reciprocal tolerogenic process because they can modify in both cell populations the expression of cell interaction, MHC, and adhesion molecules. All of these interactions determine how antigen signals are responded to by T cells (Steinman 1991). Evidence confirming the original observations, allowing a more complete understanding of the tolerogenic mechanisms, has been summarized recently (Starzl and Zinkernagel 1998).

Historical enigmas

With the two-way paradigm, the reason for virtually every previously unexplained experimental or clinical observation after whole-organ transplantation became either transparent, or at least susceptible to experimental inquiry (Starzl et al. 1992, 1993). It could be understood why organ grafts are inherently tolerogenic and therefore "accepted" by the recipient. With the

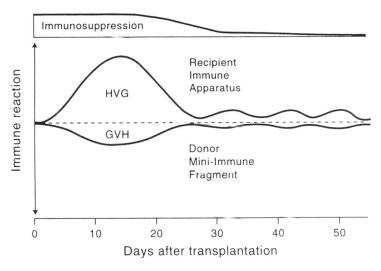

Figure 1.4. The pattern of convalescence after either organ or bone marrow transplantation in the framework of the two-way paradigm. HVG, host-versus-graft; GHV, graft-versus-host.

two-way mutual cancellation implicit in this concept, the loss or blunting of an HLA-matching effect was comprehensible. With each further level of histoincompatibility, the reciprocal effect apparently escalates both ways under the umbrella of an effective immunosuppressant (Figure 1.5). The consequent dwindling of the matching effect as donor-specific and recipient-specific nonreactivity evolves accounts for "blindfolding" of the expected HLA influence.

In addition to explaining why the HLA-matching effect is mitigated, the mutual functional cancellation of the two cell populations explains why GVHD does not develop after liver, intestinal, multivisceral, and heart–lung transplantation, despite the heavy lymphoid content of those organs. The safety of these procedures depended on leaving the recipient immunologic system intact until the time of transplantation.

Augmentation of spontaneous chimerism
Because the acquisition of immunologic tolerance in the originally Billingham–Brent–Medawar and derivative models depended on donor leukocyte (splenocyte or bone marrow) infusion (Billingham et al. 1953, 1956; Main and Prehn 1955), sporadic attempts had been made to improve organ allograft outcome by infusing adjuvant donor bone marrow (Monaco, Clark, and Brown 1976; Barber et al. 1991) or blood (Salvatierra et al. 1980; Anderson, Sicard, and Etheredge 1982; Sollinger et al. 1984). These were

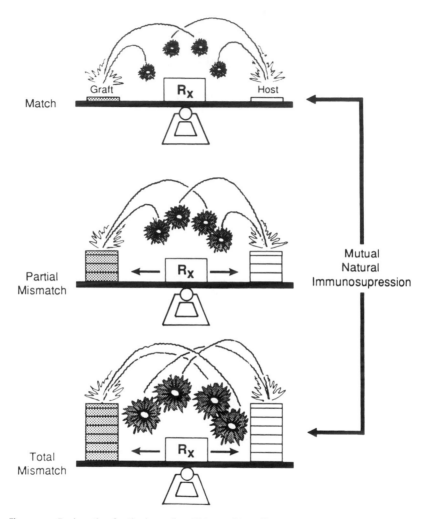

Figure 1.5. Explanation for the loss of an HLA-matching effect with whole-organ transplantation. R_x: immunosuppression.

hampered by the assumption that the infused cells would be destroyed unless there was recipient preconditioning with irradiation or myelotoxic drugs. In turn, the prospect of recipient cytoablation engendered anxiety about causing GVHD. Most importantly, the appropriate timing of the cell infusions was controversial. Consequently, the strategy of donor leukocyte augmentation never gained a clinical foothold.

The discoveries of leukocyte chimerism in 1992 (Starzl et al. 1992, 1993) exposed a perioperative window of opportunity during which unaltered

Two-Way Paradigm (Heart)

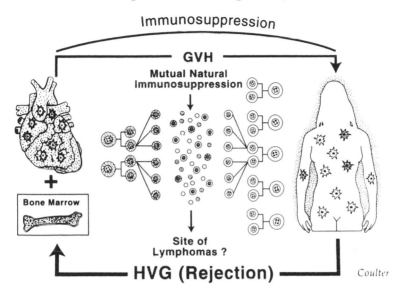

Figure 1.6. Iatrogenic augmentation of the graft-versus-host (GVH) component of the two-way paradigm by infusing 3 10⁸ to 6 10⁸/kg unaltered donor bone marrow cells at the same time as heart or other whole-organ transplantation. When the recipient is not cytoablated, there is essentially no risk of GVHD.

HLA-incompatible bone marrow or donor-specific blood transfusion was predicted to be safe without recipient preparation or any other deviation from the generic noncytoablative practices of immunosuppression for whole-organ transplantation that had evolved over the years from the original azathioprine–prednisone formula (Starzl et al. 1963). The validity of this expectation was verified recently in nonpreconditioned recipients of cadaveric kidneys, livers, hearts, and lungs who were given adjuvant bone marrow cells at 3×10^8 to 5×10^8/kg at the same time as organ transplantation under standard tacrolimus–prednisone treatment (Figure 1.6) (Fontes et al. 1994).

Chimerism estimated to be > 1000 times that occurring in conventional whole-organ recipients was reliably and safely produced and sustained. The persistent blood chimerism (usually $>1\%$), trend toward donor specific nonreactivity, and high rate of patient and graft survival, have marked these bone marrow augmented recipients as an advantaged cohort. They are the first patients to undergo HLA-mismatched cadaveric organ transplantation with the hope of eventually becoming drug free. The process of tolerance induction and drug weaning is expected to take 5 to 10 years, but in some the drug-free state may never be attainable.

The drug-free state

The concept that organ transplantation is equivalent to a small bone marrow transplantation (and that this explains allograft acceptance) has been confirmed and greatly extended in animal models, principally by Qian et al. (1994) and by Demetris et al. (1993) and Murase et al. (1995). The cardinal principle is that the long and continuing survival of an organ allograft means, by definition, that donor leukocyte chimerism is present. Failure to demonstrate chimerism in such recipients connotes an inadequate search (Murase et al. 1995).

However, donor leukocyte chimerism is merely a prerequisite for graft acceptance (Starzl et al. 1992). Is the demonstration of chimerism an indication to stop immunosuppression? Emphatically no! However, knowledge of the chimerism mechanism makes it clear why drugs can in fact be stopped permanently after organ transplantation in some cases. In late 1995, 12 (28%) of the 43 longest surviving liver recipients in the world (14 to 26 years) have been off drugs for 1 to almost 19 years. Complementing these observations, Ramos et al. (1995) have reported a prospective weaning trial for liver recipients, limited for the most part to patients who were 5 to 10 years post-transplantation. Freedom from rejection for at least 5 years was a prerequisite for admission to the trial, which has expanded to 80 patients. Forty-four (55%) of these liver recipients have come off drugs completely or have moved uninterruptedly in that direction; in 22 whose weaning is complete, the drug-free time averages $2\frac{1}{2}$ years. Weaning is being carried out more slowly now than at the beginning of the trial because of a 30% incidence of rejection. It was evident that the vast majority of the 80 liver recipients had been at a level of immunosuppression higher than they needed. It is more dangerous to attempt weaning after kidney transplantation, and we rarely recommend this. However, five of our longest-surviving living related kidney recipients have been off all immunosuppression for 2 to 30 years. A recent report has documented these results (Mazariegos et al. 1997).

Rejection after drug discontinuance

The benefits of weaning for organ recipients are obvious. However, it is equally important to recognize that there was a 30% overall risk of rejection in the prospective liver trial. Successful weaning was achieved consistently only in the patients being weaned from an azathioprine–prednisone regimen or from monotherapy with tacrolimus (Ramos et al. 1995). When weaning failed, biopsy-proved rejection was diagnosed 1 to 29 months after drug withdrawal was started and usually was classed histopathologically as minimal to mild. Restoration of the previous baseline immunosuppression was the only adjustment required in most cases, but four patients with moderate or severe rejection required rescue treatment with tacrolimus; this included

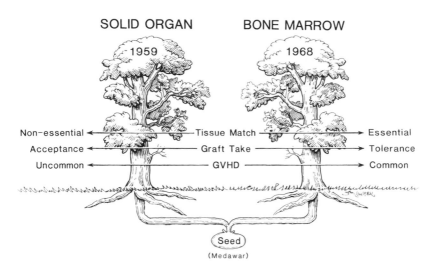

SOLID ORGAN   BONE MARROW
1959   1968

Non-essential	Tissue Match	Essential
Acceptance	Graft Take	Tolerance
Uncommon	GVHD	Common

Seed
(Medawar)

Figure 1.7. The growth, as separate disciplines, of bone marrow (right) and whole-organ transplantation (left) from the seed planted by Peter Medawar during World War II. It was recognized in 1992 that these seemingly disparate disciplines were mirror images caused by different treatment strategies as explained in the text. GVHD, graft-versus-host disease.

one who became jaundiced, with a peak bilirubin of 12 mg%. Although no patients or grafts were lost in our trial, Sandborn et al. (1994) encountered rejection in 6 of 12 patients at the Mayo Clinic whose rapid weaning from cyclosporine-based triple drug therapy was attempted after only three post-transplant years; two of the six died. It would be foolhardy to ignore such a warning.

Bone marrow transplantation

When it was discovered that successful whole-organ transplantation was associated with spontaneous chimerism, it was realized that the seemingly vast gap between the bone marrow and whole-organ transplantation fields reflected entrenched differences in treatment strategy (Figure 1.7). The mutually censoring immunologic limbs were being left intact with organ transplantation, whereas the recipient limb was deliberately removed (cytoablation) in preparation for bone marrow grafting procedures. Although it was long assumed that the entire recipient immune system had been eliminated with successful bone marrow transplantation (Figure 1.1(b)), a trace population of recipient leukocytes has been detected with sensitive techniques in the blood of almost all such patients (Przepiorka et al. 1991; Wessman et al. 1993).

These bone marrow recipients were in fact mirror images of those successfully bearing whole-organ allografts, the difference being that their own residual leukocytes rather than those of the donor constituted the trace population. Under both circumstances, other findings such as the appearance of veto and suppressor cells, enhancing antibodies, and changes in cytokine profile could be construed as by-products, of and accessory to, the seminal event of the mutual cell engagement (Figure 1.1(c) and (d)).

Conclusions

In this chapter, a generic explanation has been provided for what has been one of the most remarkable and in some respects conceptually enigmatic developments in the history of medicine. Successful engraftment of the kidney (Merrill et al. 1960), pancreas (Lillehei et al. 1970), liver (Starzl et al. 1968), heart (Barnard 1968), lung (Derom et al. 1971), and multiple abdominal viscera (Starzl et al. 1989) intestine (Goulet et al. 1992) were empirical achievements, accomplished largely by dogged trial and error. Each organ-defined specialty has had its historians who track their story back to one of the foregoing milestones where the trail goes cold. The reason is that such accounts have been preoccupied with a succession of events rather than the biologic principles that are applicable to all organ allografts. Escape from this intellectual cul de sac became possible with the discovery in 1992 that donor leukocyte chimerism occurs spontaneously after organ transplantation, and the development of evidence that this is the basis of graft acceptance.

Beacons of understanding shine forward as well as back. Comprehension of the history of transplantation in terms of the two-way paradigm (Starzl and Demetris 1995) provides the conceptual means to devise better treatment strategies, including the achievement of drug-free tolerance. If the goal of xenotransplantation is attained (and it may be soon), the same ubiquitous mix of two genetically different leukocyte populations as that following allotransplantation will be a necessary condition. Although the diffuse distribution of donor leukocytes in organ recipients is not thought to affect central nervous system changes, the emotional and psychiatric implications of creating animal/human genetic composites via xenotransplantation cannot be taken lightly.

Acknowledgments

From the Thomas E. Starzl Transplantation Institute, University of Pittsburgh Medical Center, Pittsburgh, PA. This work was supported in part by research grants from the Veterans Administration and Project Grant no. DK-29961 from the National Institutes of Health, Bethesda, MD.

References

Anderson, C. B., Sicard, G. A., and Etheredge, E. E. (1982). Pretreatment of renal allograft recipients with azathioprine and donor-specific blood products. *Surgery*, **92**, 315–41.

Bach, F. H. (1968). Bone-marrow transplantation in a patient with the Wiskott–Aldrich syndrome. *Lancet*, **2**, 1364–6.

Bach, F. and Hirschhorn, K. (1964). Lymphocyte interaction: a potential histocompatibility test in vitro. *Science*, **143**, 813–14.

Bain, B., Vas, M. R., and Lowenstein, L. (1964). The development of large immature mononuclear cells in mixed leukocyte cultures. *Blood*, **23**, 108–16.

Barber, W. H., Mankin, J. A., Laskow, D. A. et al. (1991). Long-term results of a controlled prospective study with transfusion of donor specific bone marrow in 57 cadaveric renal allograft recipients. *Transplantation*, **51**, 70–5.

Barnard, C. N. (1968). What we have learned about heart transplants? *J Thorac Cardiovasc Surg*, **56**, 457–68.

Billingham, R. and Brent, L. (1957). A simple method for inducing tolerance of skin homografts in mice. *Transplant Bull*, **4**, 67–71.

Billingham, R. E., Brent, L., and Medawar, P. B. (1953). "Actively acquired tolerance" of foreign cells. *Nature*, **172**, 603–6.

Billingham, R., Brent, L., and Medawar, P. (1956). Quantitative studies on tissue transplantation immunity. III. Actively acquired tolerance. *Phil Trans R Soc Lond B Biol Sci*, **239**, 357–412.

Brown, J. B. (1937). Homografting of skin: with report of success in identical twins. *Surgery*, **1**, 558–63.

Burnet, F. M. (1961). The new approach to immunology. *N Engl J Med*, **264**, 24–34.

Calne, R. Y. (1960). The rejection of renal homografts: inhibition in dogs by 6-mercaptopurine. *Lancet*, **1**, 417–18.

Calne, R. Y. (1961). Inhibition of the rejection of renal homografts in dogs with purine analogues. *Transplant Bull*, **28**, 445.

Calne, R. Y., Rolles, K., White, D. J. G. et al. (1979). Cyclosporin A initially as the only immunosuppressant in 34 recipients of cadaveric organs: 32 kidneys, 2 pancreases, and 2 livers. *Lancet*, **2**, 1033–6.

Dausset, J. (1990). The HLA adventure. In *History of HLA: Ten Recollections*, ed. P. I. Terasaki, pp. 1–20. UCLA Tissue Typing Laboratory: Los Angeles.

Demetris, A. J., Murase, N., Fujisaki, S., Fung, J. J., Rao, A. S., and Starzl, T. E. (1993). Hematolymphoid cell trafficking, microchimerism, and GVHD reactions after liver, bone marrow, and heart transplantation. *Transplant Proc*, **25**, 3337–44.

Derom, F., Barbier, F., Ringoir, S. et al. (1971). Ten-month survival after lung homotransplantation in man. *J Thorac Cardiovasc Surg*, **61**, 835–46.

Doherty, P. C. (1995). The keys to cell-mediated immunity. *JAMA*, **274**, 1067–8.

Elion, G. B., Bieber, S., and Hitchings, G. H. (1955). The fate of 6-mercaptopurine in mice. *Ann NY Acad Sci*, **60**, 297–303.

Fontes, P., Rao, A., Demetris, A. J. et al. (1994). Augmentation with bone marrow of donor leukocyte migration for kidney, heart, and pancreas islet transplantation. *Lancet*, **344**, 151–5.

Gatti, R. A., Meuwissen, H. J., Allen, H. D., Hong, R., and Good, R. A. (1968).

Immunological reconstitution of sex-linked lymphopenic immunological deficiency. *Lancet*, **2**, 1366–9.

Goulet, O., Revillon, Y., Brousse, N. et al. (1992). Successful small bowel transplantation in an infant. *Transplantation*, **53**, 940–3.

Hamburger, J., Vaysse, J., Crosnier, J., Auvert, J., LaLanne, A. M., and Hopper, J., Jr. (1962). Renal homotransplantation in man after radiation of the recipient. *Am J Med*, **32**, 854–71.

Hume, D. M., Jackson, B. T., Zukoski, C. F. et al. (1960) The homotransplantation of kidneys and of fetal liver and spleen after total body irradiation. *Annals of Surgery*, **152**, 354–78.

Janeway, C. A., Jr. and Travers, P. (1994). *Immunobiology*. Garland Publishing Inc.: New York.

Kuss, R., Legrain, M., Mathe, G., Nedey, R., and Camey, M. (1962). Homologous human kidney transplantation. Experience with six patients. *Postgrad Med J*, **38**, 528–31.

Lillehei, R. C., Simmons, R. L., Najarian, J. S., Weil, R., Uchida, H., Ruiz, J. D., Kjellstrand, C. M., and Goetz, F. C. (1970). Pancreaticoduodenal allotransplantation: experimental and clinical observations. *Ann Surg*, **172**, 405–36.

Main, J. M. and Prehn, R. T. (1955). Successful skin homografts after the administration of high dosage X radiation and homologous bone marrow. *J Natl Cancer Inst*, **15**, 1023–9.

Mannick, J. A., Lochte, H. L. Ashley, C. A., Thomas, E. D., and Ferrebee, J. W. (1959). A functioning kidney homotransplant in the dog. *Surgery*, **46**, 821–8.

Mathe, G., Amiel, J. L., Schwarzenberg, L., Cattan, A., and Schneider, M. (1963). Haematopoietic chimera in man after allogenic (homologous) bone marrow transplantation. *Br Med J*, 1633–5.

Mazariegos, G. V., Reyes, J., Marino, I. et al. (1997). Long-term follow-up of weaning of immunosuppression in liver transplant recipients. *Transplantation*, **63**, 243–9.

Medawar, P. B. (1944). The behavior and fate of skin autografts and skin homografts in rabbits. *J Anat*, **78**, 176–99.

Meeker, W., Condie, R., Weiner, D., Varco, R. L., and Good. R.A. (1959). Prolongation of skin homograft survival in rabbits by 6-mercaptopurine. *Proc Soc Exp Biol Med*, **102**, 459–61.

Merrill, J. P., Murray, J. E., Harrison, J. H., Friedman, E. A., Dealy, J. B., Jr., and Dammin, G. J. (1960). Successful homotransplantation of the kidney between non-identical twins. *New Engl J Med*, **262**, 1251–60.

Merrill, J. P., Murray, J. E., Harrison, J. H., and Guild, W. R. (1956). Successful homotransplantation of the human kidney between identical twins. *JAMA*, **160**, 277–82.

Monaco, A. P., Clark, A. W., and Brown, R. W. (1976). Active enhancement of a human cadaver renal allograft with ALS and donor bone marrow: case report of an initial attempt. *Surgery*, **79**, 384–92.

Murase, N., Starzl, T. E., Tanabe, M. et al. (1995). Variable chimerism, graft versus host disease, and tolerance after different kinds of cell and whole organ transplantation from Lewis to Brown-Norway rats. *Transplantation*, **60**, 158–71.

Murray, J. E., Merrill, J. P., Dammin, G. J., Dealy, J. B., Jr., Alexandre, G.W., and Harrison, J. H. (1962). Kidney transplantation in modified recipients. *Ann Surg*,

156, 337–55.

Murray, J. E., Merrill, J. P., Harrison, J. H., Wilson, R. E., and Dammin, G. J. (1963). Prolonged survival of human-kidney homografts by immunosuppressive drug therapy. *New Engl J Med*, **268**, 1315–23.

Padgett, E. D. (1932). Is iso-skin grafting practicable? *South Med J*, **25**, 895–900.

Przepiorka, D., Thomas, E. D., Durham, D. M., and Fisher, L. (1991). Use of a probe to repeat sequence of the Y chromosome for detection of host cells in peripheral blood of bone marrow transplant recipients. *Hematopathology*, **95**, 201–6.

Qian, S., Demetris, A. J., Murase, N., Rao, A. S., Fung, J. J., and Starzl, T. E. (1994). Murine liver allograft transplantation: tolerance and donor cell chimerism. *Hepatology*, **19**, 916–24.

Ramos, H. C., Reyes, J., Abu-Elmagd, K. et al. (1995). Weaning of immunosuppression in long term liver transplant recipients. *Transplantation*, **59**, 212–17.

Rapaport, F. T., Bachvaroff, R. J., Mollen, N., Hirasawa, H., Asano, T., and Ferrebee, J. W. (1979). Induction of unresponsiveness to major transplantable organs in adult mammals. *Ann Surg*, **190**, 461–73.

Salvatierra, O., Jr., Vincenti, F., Amend, W. J. et al. (1980). Deliberate donor-specific blood transfusions prior to living related renal transplantation: a new approach. *Ann Surg*, **192**, 543–52.

Sandborn, W. J., Hay, J. E., Porayko, M. K. et al. (1994). Cyclosporine withdrawal for nephrotoxicity in liver transplant recipients does not result in sustained improvement in kidney function and causes cellular and ductopenic rejection. *Hepatology*, **19**, 925–32.

Schwartz, R. and Dameshek, W. (1959). Drug-induced immunological tolerance. *Nature*, **183**, 1682–3.

Schwartz, R. and Dameshek, W. (1960). The effects of 6-mercaptopurine on homograft reactions. *J Clin Invest*, **39**, 952–958.

Simonsen, M. (1957). The impact on the developing embryo and newborn animal of adult homologous cells. *Acta Path Microbiol Scand*, **40**, 480–500.

Snell, G. D. (1957). The homograft reaction. *Annu Rev Microbiol*, **11**, 439–58.

Sollinger, H. W., Burlingham, W. J., Sparks, E. M., Glass, N. R., and Belzer, F. O. (1984). Donor-specific transfusions in unrelated and related HLA-mismatched donor-recipient combinations. *Transplantation*, **38**, 612–15.

Starzl, T. E. (1992). *The Puzzle People*. University of Pittsburgh Press: Pittsburgh.

Starzl T. E. and Demetris, A. J. (1995). Transplantation milestones: viewed with one- and two-way paradigms of tolerance. *JAMA*, **273**, 876–9.

Starzl, T. E., Demetris, A. J., Murase, N., Ildstad, S., Ricordi, C., and Trucco, M. (1992). Cell migration, chimerism, and graft acceptance. *Lancet*, **339**, 1579–82.

Starzl, T. E., Demetris, A .J., Trucco, M. et al. (1993). Cell migration and chimerism after whole organ transplantation: the basis of graft acceptance. *Hepatology*, **17**, 1127–52.

Starzl, T. E., Groth, C. G., Brettschneider, L. et al. (1968). Orthotopic homotransplantation of the human liver. *Ann Surg*, **168**, 392–415.

Starzl, T. E., Marchioro, T. L., Porter, K. A., Iwasaki, Y., and Cerilli, G. J. (1967). The use of heterologous antilymphoid agents in canine renal and liver homotransplantation and in human renal homotransplantation. *Surg Gynecol Obstet*, **124**, 301–18.

Starzl, T. E., Marchioro, T. L., and Waddell, W. R. (1963). The reversal of rejection in human renal homografts with subsequent development of homograft tolerance. *Surg Gynecol Obstet*, **117**, 385–95.

Starzl, T. E., Rowe, M., Todo, S. et al. (1989). Transplantation of multiple abdominal viscera. *JAMA*, **261**, 1449–57.

Starzl, T. E., Todo, S., Fung, J., Demetris, A. J., Venkataramanan, R., and Jain, A. (1989). FK 506 for human liver, kidney and pancreas transplantation. *Lancet*, **2**, 1000–4.

Starzl, T. E. and Zinkernagel, R. (1998). Antigen localization and migration in immunity and tolerance. *N Engl J Med*, **339**, 1905–13.

Steinman, R. M. (1991). The dendritic cell system and its role in immunogenicity. *Annu Rev Immunol*, **9**, 271–96.

Steinman, R. M. and Cohn, Z. A. (1973). Identification of a novel cell type in peripheral lymphoid organs of mice. I. Morphology, quantitation, tissue distribution. *J Exp Med*, **137**, 1142–62.

Steinmuller, D. (1967). Immunization with skin isografts taken from tolerant mice. *Science*, **158**, 127–9.

Terasaki, P. I. (ed.) (1990). *History of HLA: Ten Recollections*. UCLA Tissue Typing Laboratory: Los Angeles.

Thomas, E. D. (1991). Allogeneic marrow grafting – a story of man and dog. In *History of Transplantation: Thirty-Five Recollections*, ed. P.I. Terasaki, pp. 379–394, UCLA Press: Los Angeles.

Thomson, A. W. and Starzl, T. E. (eds.) (1994). *Immunosuppressive Drugs: Developments in Anti-Rejection Therapy*. Edward Arnold: .

Trentin, J. J. (1957). Induced tolerance and "homologous disease" in X-irradiated mice protected with homologous bone marrow. *Proc Soc Exp Biol Med*, **96**, 139–44.

Unanue, E. R. (1995). The concept of antigen processing and presentation. *JAMA*, **274**, 1071–3.

Wessman, M., Popp, S., Ruutu, T. Volin, L., Cremer, T., and Knuutila, S. (1993). Detection of residual host cells after bone marrow transplantation using non-isotopic in situ hybridization and karyotype analysis. *Bone Marrow Transplant*, **11**, 279–84.

Zinkernagel, R. M. (1995). The MHC-restricted T-cell recognition. *JAMA*, **274**, 1069–71.

Zukoski, C. F., Lee, H. M., and Hume, D. M. (1960). The prolongation of functional survival of canine renal homografts by 6-mercaptopurine. *Surg Forum*, **11**, 470–2.

2

Psychosocial screening and selection of candidates for organ transplantation

James L. Levenson M.D. and Mary Ellen Olbrisch Ph.D.

Overview

Since the earliest days of organ transplantation, psychiatrists and other mental health professionals have been involved in the screening and selection of candidates to receive these surgeries. Postoperative psychiatric disorders were common among the first disorders noted in patients undergoing transplant surgery, and these outcomes, while less common and more manageable today, still influence selection of patients, since pretransplant psychopathology is a predictor for post-transplant psychopathology. As a result of the growing shortage of organ donors relative to the number of persons in need of transplant surgery, there is increased pressure to select the patients most likely to benefit from the surgery, from medical and psychosocial perspectives. Concerns include the patient's ability to cope with the stresses of surgery, postoperative complications and a rigorous medical regimen, capacity to comply with lifestyle changes necessary to minimize morbidity and mortality, and attainment of a satisfactory rehabilitation and quality of life following transplant. In this chapter on psychosocial screening of transplant candidates, we discuss in turn relevant medical issues, the rationale behind screening, characteristics of screening processes (evaluation process, criteria, outcome) instruments and psychological tests used, and clinical issues related to disability law in the USA.[1]

Patient selection – medical issues

Over the past decade, consensus within the transplant community has developed regarding some criteria for organ candidate selection and position on waiting lists. In general, the sickest patients with the least life expectancy and most limited functional capacity move to the top of the list, while patients with fewer lifestyle restrictions and with the ability to wait longer are given lower priority. Organs are allocated within geographic regions in recognition

[1] Much of our discussion is based on the organ allocation and distribution system in the USA; policy issues and the law may differ in other countries.

of the practical limitations of ischemia time and in deference to the belief that use of organs for near neighbors inspires a greater sense of community and commitment than exportation of organs to distant regions. It was once routine for patients to travel long distances to the limited number of transplant centers, but with more centers available, the necessity for long distance travel has decreased until recently. However, patients in the USA are now being asked to travel to the transplant center preferred by the insurer or government payer, making geographic convenience less relevant.

Time already on the waiting list is one factor influencing patient standing. This reflects the "first come, first served" principle, the stress associated with long waits, and the perceptions of unfairness that occur when recently evaluated patients are given priority over those who have been waiting for months.

These criteria for candidate prioritization are not without dissenters. Some believe that the sickest patient poses the worst risk and may skew outcome data negatively. Others defend this practice because of the relative gain, compared with early death as the likely outcome without transplantation. Despite the consensus built through the United Network for Organ Sharing (UNOS) on how to prioritize patients on the waiting list, there are deep divisions within the transplant community regarding the criteria that determine which patient should be placed on the list. (These divisions became more visible in the recent controversy over a proposed change that would give precedence to patients with acute liver disease over those with chronic liver disease.) Transplant centers that have longer lists are perceived as having an advantage over programs with shorter lists in getting donors, because it appears that the former have greater need. Thus, some physicians worry that patients who are inappropriate transplant recipients in some way (those who can benefit from alternative treatments, patients who are too old, etc.) are listed for the advantage of the transplantation program rather than for the welfare of the individual. Another controversy is racial inequality in organ allocation, deriving from biomedical criteria. For example, the renal transplant list gives priority to patients with a six-antigen match, though this guideline results in successful matching much more often in white than in black renal failure patients. Whether the marginal improvement over the success of transplants matched only for blood type justifies the consequent reduced access for minority recipients is a topic of current debate.

Each transplant program determines its own criteria for choosing patients to list, though not without influences from external forces. Medicare legislation in the USA delineates medical conditions for which specific transplant surgeries may be offered and restrict what programs can do, at least for individual patients. Private insurers increasingly play a role in program decisions about listing patients, based on their understanding of the indications and contraindications for the surgery as established in the medical literature. Programs vary in the degree to which they are willing to accept higher risk patients or to push past the boundaries of established indications and contraindications.

Rationale for psychosocial screening

Psychosocial as well as physiological and medical factors are included in program selection criteria and also reflect the effects of external forces. Though there is significant variation among transplantation programs in their psychosocial assessment criteria and procedures, there are eight clinical reasons why psychosocial evaluations are conducted (a given assessment, however, may not include all eight):

1. To predict how the patient will cope with the stresses of surgery and screen out or intervene when a patient appears to be unable to cope effectively.
2. To identify co-morbid mental illness and plan interventions for these conditions.
3. To determine whether the patient can be sufficiently educated for the transplant patient role and ensure that the patient has an adequate understanding of the transplantation procedure in order to give informed consent.
4. To learn whether the patient will be able to form a collaborative relationship with physicians and comply with the medical regimen.
5. To assess substance abuse history and recovery, and predict the patient's ability to maintain long-term abstinence.
6. To help the transplant team know the patient better as a person in order to provide more effective clinical care.
7. To learn about the psychosocial needs of the patient and family, and plan for services during the waiting, recovery, and rehabilitation phases of the transplantation process.
8. To establish baseline measures of mental functioning in order to be able to monitor postoperative changes.

Though psychosocial evaluations are not conducted to determine the "social worth" of the transplant candidate, the belief persists that this is the purpose of psychosocial evaluations. This inaccurate perception is expressed openly by some patients and families, and less overtly by health professionals. Perhaps this is because many of the topics explored during a typical interview by a mental health professional do have some relation to concepts of social worth. Social support, educational attainment, occupational history, legal problems, and financial status all have implications for patient care during

Table 2.1. Psychosocial factors associated with poor transplant outcome

Poor social support

Psychiatric disorders likely to compromise adequate postoperative compliance (affective disorders, psychosis, anxiety disorders, etc.)

Self-destructive behaviors including nicotine, alcohol and drug abuse

Poor compliance with medical treatment (combined with a continued failure to appreciate the necessity of change)

Intractable maladaptive personality traits (such as oppositionality or counter-dependence)

the transplantation process, but raising such issues risks creating misconceptions that they are used to rank order or rule out socially undesirable individuals.

The notion that patients are rank ordered according to psychosocial criteria is inaccurate (except perhaps in some cases where persons of prominent social standing or celebrity appear to have jumped to the top of the list). Psychosocial screening is performed, then, not to rank-order patients, but as a gatekeeping function. However, psychosocial screening does contribute to the selection process by identifying risk factors that might exclude candidates from further consideration or identify a need for more psychiatric or psychosocial interventions so that transplantation and aftercare can be more successful. A patient might not be put on the list because of individual psychosocial, medical, or financial factors or a combination thereof that indicate the likelihood of poor outcome. Psychosocial factors that increase the risk of poor outcome are listed in Table 2.1.

Initial screening for such psychosocial factors may be performed by a transplant nurse coordinator, transplant physician, social worker, psychologist, or psychiatrist. Once a patient "passes" whatever psychosocial screening process the transplantation program uses, placement on the list is determined by specific parameters agreed upon by the transplant community (via UNOS) that serves patients with a need for the particular organ. These parameters include expected survival without transplant (sometimes determined by the patient's physical location – intensive care unit, hospital, at home, or still working) and length of time on the waiting list. There are no provisions to move a physician ahead of a plumber, a married person who is a parent over a childless single person, or a well-adjusted individual ahead of a person with a history of major depression or with a personality disorder. If social worth does play a role in who gets a transplant, it is not through manipulation of the list but rather through exclusion from evaluation or acceptance of the patient as a candidate (much of which may be done by referring physicians rather than transplantation programs themselves) or through disregarding usual criteria used to exclude patients, e.g., a decision to list an alcoholic physician for transplantation, even though he/she does not meet the criterion of six months' abstinence expected of all other patients within that program.

Characteristics of psychosocial screening

In this section, we summarize the findings from surveys that we conducted of all cardiac, liver, and kidney transplant programs within the USA (Levenson and Olbrisch 1993), and of cardiac transplantation programs internationally (Olbrisch and Levenson 1991) Survey methods are detailed elsewhere (Olbrisch and Levenson 1991; Levenson and Olbrisch 1993); response rates were 64% to 71% for US programs and 45% for non-US programs.

Evaluation process

Nearly all US transplantation programs (over 95%) utilize some form of pretransplant psychosocial evaluation process, while just over half of non-US cardiac programs do. In the majority of programs, each potential transplant candidate is interviewed by a mental health professional to determine suitability on psychosocial grounds. About one-quarter of US cardiac transplantation programs also require formal psychological testing as part of the screening process, but this occurs much less often among liver and kidney transplantation programs. A substantial minority of the liver and kidney programs require only that a mental health professional conduct the evaluation if the nonpsychiatric physician becomes aware of psychosocial concerns during the evaluation. US kidney transplant programs use psychiatrists and psychologists less often than do cardiac and hepatic programs; all rely heavily on social workers. In 1990, 23% of cardiac transplantation programs, 14% of liver transplantation programs, and 7% of renal transplantation programs indicated that they used formal psychosocial criteria for candidate selection. Thus, most programs utilize informal, unwritten psychosocial criteria for selection.

How often transplantation programs seek a second opinion in cases where the patient would be rejected as a candidate for transplantation (based on the first opinion) is highly variable, as is how often an explanation is provided to patients rejected on psychosocial grounds. Both are detailed in Table 2.2.

Selection criteria

Tables 2.3, 2.4, and 2.5 show what percentage of US transplantation programs regard each psychosocial criterion as an absolute or relative contraindication to transplantation, or irrelevant. Table 2.3 presents social variables,

Table 2.2. Frequency (%) of second opinions and provisions of explanations in cases where patient is rejected for transplant

	Cardiac		Liver		Renal	
	n	%	n	%	n	%
Second opinion frequency						
Always	21	28.8	14	35.0	43	31.2
Most of the time	16	21.9	9	22.5	36	26.1
Sometimes	21	28.8	14	35.0	48	34.8
Never	15	20.5	3	7.5	11	8.0
Frequency of explanation provided						
Always	25	34.2	27	65.9	81	58.7
Most of the time	22	30.1	11	26.8	38	27.5
Sometimes	17	23.3	3	7.3	15	10.9
Never	9	12.3	0	0.0	4	2.9

n, number of patients.
From Levenson and Olbrisch 1993. Reprinted with permission from the Academy of Psychosomatic Medicine and the American Psychiatric Press.

Table 2.3. Social contraindications to organ transplantation in the USA (given in % number of centers)

	Cardiac	Liver	Renal		Cardiac	Liver	Renal
Not a US citizen				*Recent death or loss*			
Absolute	10.3	4.3	3.9	Absolute	0.0	0.0	0.0
Relative	32.1	30.4	20.0	Relative	29.5	32.6	21.9
Irrelevant	57.7	65.2	76.1	Irrelevant	70.5	67.4	78.1
Not resident of your state				*Current felony prisoner*			
Absolute	00.0	2.2	0.6	Absolute	46.2	39.1	20.6
Relative	16.7	13.0	5.8	Relative	29.5	30.4	37.4
Irrelevant	83.3	84.8	93.5	Irrelevant	24.4	30.4	41.9
No support system				*Hx sig. criminal behavior*			
Absolute	9.0	6.5	2.6	Absolute	29.5	17.4	5.2
Relative	66.7	67.4	33.5	Relative	47.4	45.7	52.9
Irrelevant	24.4	26.1	63.9	Irrelevant	23.1	37.0	41.9

Hx sig., history significant.

including citizenship, social support, and criminal deviance. Table 2.4 presents the findings for variables related to psychopathology. Table 2.5 includes other variables related to the patient's ability to cooperate with care and engage in preventive behaviors, including compliance, lifestyle adjustments,

Table 2.4. Psychopathology contraindication to organ transplantation in the USA (given in % number of centers)

	Cardiac	Liver	Renal		Cardiac	Liver	Renal
Family Hx mental illness				*Hx multiple suicide attempts*			
Absolute	1.3	0.0	0.0	Absolute	71.8	41.3	38.7
Relative	47.4	41.3	26.6	Relative	24.4	45.7	47.1
Irrelevant	51.3	58.7	73.4	Irrelevant	3.8	13.0	14.2
Active schizophrenia				*Current suicidal ideation*			
Absolute	92.3	67.4	72.9	Absolute	75.6	50.0	56.8
Relative	5.1	23.9	19.4	Relative	17.9	39.1	27.7
Irrelevant	2.6	8.7	7.7	Irrelevant	6.4	10.9	15.5
Controlled schizophrenia				*Dementia*			
Absolute	33.3	15.2	6.5	Absolute	71.8	54.3	43.2
Relative	51.3	65.2	61.9	Relative	23.1	26.1	40.0
Irrelevant	15.4	19.6	31.6	Irrelevant	5.1	19.6	16.8
Current affective disorder				*Personality disorder*			
Absolute	44.9	17.4	31.0	Absolute	14.1	8.7	5.2
Relative	47.4	71.7	47.1	Relative	62.8	65.2	56.1
Irrelevant	7.7	10.9	21.9	Irrelevant	23.1	26.1	38.7
Hx affective disorder				*Mental retardation, IQ < 70*			
Absolute	5.1	0.0	1.3	Absolute	25.6	10.9	2.6
Relative	62.8	63.0	45.8	Relative	59.0	69.6	51.3
Irrelevant	32.1	37.0	52.9	Irrelevant	15.4	19.6	46.1
Recent suicide attempt				*Severe retardation, IQ < 50*			
Absolute	51.3	17.4	27.7	Absolute	74.4	45.7	24.0
Relative	41.0	63.0	56.1	Relative	19.2	41.3	51.9
Irrelevant	7.7	19.6	16.1	Irrelevant	6.4	13.0	24.0
Distant suicide attempt							
Absolute	12.8	0.0	1.3				
Relative	64.1	60.9	54.8				
Irrelevant	23.1	39.1	43.9				

Hx, history.

substance use, and appreciation of one's illness and the transplantation process.

Overall, cardiac programs were more likely to consider items as contraindications than were liver programs, which in turn were more stringent in general than kidney programs. The major recognized psychiatric contraindications to cardiac transplantation (regarded as an absolute contraindication by more than 70% of programs) have been schizophrenia with active psychotic symptoms, current suicidal ideation, history of multiple suicide attempts, dementia, severe mental retardation (IQ less than 50), current heavy drinking,

Table 2.5. Lifestyle and behavioral contraindications to organ transplantation in the USA (given in % number of centers)

	Cardiac	Liver	Renal		Cardiac	Liver	Renal
Significant obesity				*Other current tobacco use*			
Absolute	25.6	2.2	13.0	Absolute	15.4	0.0	0.0
Relative	59.0	60.9	56.5	Relative	43.6	30.4	15.6
Irrelevant	15.4	37.0	30.5	Irrelevant	41.0	69.6	84.4
Dietary noncompliance				*Current heavy EtOH use*			
Absolute	11.5	8.7	5.2	Absolute	80.8	80.4	41.6
Relative	71.8	56.5	53.2	Relative	17.9	13.0	42.9
Irrelevant	16.7	34.8	41.6	Irrelevant	1.3	6.5	15.6
Medication noncompliance				*EtOH abuse in 6 months*			
Absolute	51.3	32.6	35.7	Absolute	21.8	23.9	14.9
Relative	47.4	60.9	51.9	Relative	69.2	58.7	47.4
Irrelevant	1.3	6.5	12.3	Irrelevant	9.0	17.4	37.7
AMA hospital discharge Hx				*Current addictive drug use*			
Absolute	26.9	8.7	5.8	Absolute	92.3	84.8	69.5
Relative	61.5	73.9	58.4	Relative	7.7	8.7	24.0
Irrelevant	11.5	17.4	35.7	Irrelevant	0.0	6.5	6.5
Excessive caffeine use				*Addictive drugs in 6 months*			
Absolute	0.0	0.0	0.0	Absolute	35.9	32.6	17.5
Relative	29.5	21.7	9.1	Relative	56.4	54.3	60.4
Irrelevant	70.5	78.3	90.9	Irrelevant	7.7	13.0	22.1
Current cigarette smoking				*Transplant not understood*			
Absolute	2.6	0.0	0.0	Absolute	21.8	15.2	16.9
Relative	48.7	28.3	14.9	Relative	60.3	71.7	48.7
Irrelevant	48.7	71.7	85.1	Irrelevant	17.9	13.0	34.4

Hx, history; EtOH, ethyl alcohol.
From Levenson and Olbrisch 1993. Reprinted with permission from the Academy of Psychosomatic Medicine and the American Psychiatic Press.

and current use of addictive drugs. Liver programs regard only current heavy alcohol or addictive drug use as major contraindications. For renal programs only active schizophrenia is regarded as an absolute contraindication by more than 70% of programs, though current addictive drug use comes close.

Disagreements about patients who are current felony prisoners occur in all three types of transplantation programs in the USA. Cardiac programs are also very divided about patients with significant past criminal behavior. Kidney programs are very divided about current affective disorder and severe mental retardation. Liver programs are almost as divided over dementia.

Comparing US and non-US cardiac transplantation programs, one finds similar attitudes for the majority of criteria (Olbrisch and Levenson 1991).

Non-US programs tend to be more lenient about current smoking, substance abuse, criminality, and lack of social support. They are also more likely than US programs to refuse a transplant to patients with personality disorders, medical noncompliance, mental retardation, and controlled schizophrenia, perhaps because legal and fairness concerns with regard to access to services by the handicapped may be more recognized in the USA (Robertson 1987; Orentlicher 1996).

Kidney transplantation programs are the most lenient regarding specific criteria. Individual transplantation programs tend to become more lenient regarding psychosocial selection criteria over time (Mai 1987), and kidney programs have existed longer than other types of transplantation. Kidney transplantation programs may also place less weight on psychosocial criteria in the USA because, with nearly universal Medicare coverage, renal transplant recipients are likely to have better and more sustained aftercare. When kidneys are obtained from living related donors, the recipient is not competing with others on a list, perhaps reducing the ethical pressure to optimize outcome.

In degree of leniency of criteria, liver programs more closely resemble renal than cardiac programs, with the notable exception of alcohol abuse. Perhaps the particular philosophy and approach to candidate selection of the initial leading transplant centers leave their stamp on the field, e.g., Stanford and the Medical College of Virginia in heart transplantation, and the University of Pittsburgh in liver transplantation.

Just and fair access in transplantation is not served by widely differing psychosocial criteria. Although there are scant empirical data from which to judge the reliability and validity of any of the psychosocial selection criteria (Olbrisch and Levenson 1995), the face value of some widely used criteria seems at least questionable. In 1990, three-quarters of cardiac and liver transplantation programs still considered "no support person available" as a relative or absolute contraindication for transplantation. Many programs absolutely reject current felony prisoners as potential candidates. In the absence of data demonstrating a relationship between these variables and poor compliance or poor medical outcome, it seems likely that social values and prejudices are strongly influencing some currently used criteria, an observation that is consistent with other reports (Annas 1985; Kilner 1988).

Refusal rates

US transplantation programs decline to evaluate very few patients on psychosocial grounds (2.7% for US cardiac, 1.2% for liver, and 1% for kidney programs), tending to turn them down after completing the pretransplant psychosocial evaluation process (5.6% for cardiac, 2.8% for liver, 3.0% for renal programs). However, refusal rates range widely, from 0 to nearly 40%. It is difficult to assess why there is so much variability in the number of patients rejected for transplant on psychosocial grounds across centers. Differences in acceptance and rejection rates might be due to variation in how the criteria are actually applied (including informal prescreening), differences in the psychosocial resources available within the transplant center, and/or differences in the prevalence of psychosocial difficulties in the referral pools of different centers. The use of standardized evaluation formats across centers might be helpful in achieving consistency and equity (see next section).

US cardiac programs are more likely than non-US programs (5.6% vs. 2.4%) to refuse a patient for transplantation on psychosocial grounds. For US cardiac and liver transplant candidates, refusal rates on financial grounds are comparable to psychosocial refusal rates, with refusals for medical reasons much more common. While the total refusal rates for all reasons are lower for renal than for cardiac and liver transplant candidates, psychosocial refusals by kidney transplantation programs constitute a larger percentage of their total because renal patients are much less likely to be turned down for medical or financial reasons because of Medicare coverage. Interestingly, a program's psychosocial refusal rate does not seem to correlate with the program's psychosocial contraindications list or its size.

Instruments for psychosocial screening

We developed a new rating scale for the Psychosocial Assessment of Candidates for Transplant (PACT). The PACT was developed on the basis of clinical experience and published literature. It was designed as a brief yet comprehensive scale that could be completed in a minute or two following the evaluation interview (shown in Table 2.6). Details regarding the design and use of this instrument are described elsewhere (Olbrisch, Levenson, and Hamer 1989). For clinical, ethical, legal, and financial reasons, reliability and validity of decision-making about treatments in medicine have become a focus of close attention and empirical analysis. Psychiatric screening and selection of candidates for organ transplant is no exception in the recognition of how crucial it is to assess for reliability and validity.

PACT interrater reliability has been studied at the Medical College of Virginia in heart, liver, and bone marrow potential transplant candidates. In heart and liver patients, interrater reliability was high, with overall 96% agreement between raters on whether to give a transplant to a particular patient (Olbrisch et al. 1989). Interrater reliability for the eight subscales of the PACT ranged from about 0.6 to 0.8. Very similar results were found in bone marrow patients (Presberg et al. 1995). This does *not* mean that using the PACT will guarantee the same "rating" results regardless of who the examiner is, since different examiners may be using different criteria based on their own individual value judgments. If instead, examiners share the same selection criteria (based on policy consensus of the transplant team), one can expect reliably similar ratings using the PACT that are independent of the particular examiner.

Psychosocial transplant selection criteria should also have demonstrated validity. We compared the PACT with another rating scale for screening transplant candidates, the Transplant Evaluation Rating Scale (TERS) (Twillman et al. 1993). The TERS consists of ten items covering domains similar to, but not identical with, the PACT, and generates a weighted summary score. Both the PACT and the TERS have reasonable internal consistency, i.e., the individual items correlate with the final rating (though the contribution of a particular item varies with the population assessed). Conceptually similar items on the PACT and TERS correlate fairly highly with each other, and the two scales have comparable interrater reliability. We also compared the relevant subscales of the PACT to well-established psychometric instruments validated in medically ill populations. PACT subscales for current psychopathology and risk for psychopathology as well as PACT final ratings correlate well with clinically relevant Minnesota Mutiphasic Personality Investory (MMPI) subscales. Similarly, PACT subscales for social support correlate well with other measures of social support, e.g. Norbeck Social Support Questionnaire (Olbrisch et al. 1994; Olbrisch 1996).

While all of these forms of reliability and validity are potentially important, in the final analysis we should be most interested in predictive validity. Preliminary pilot data suggest that the PACT final rating may predict mortality in bone marrow transplant recipients independent of age, gender, diagnosis, or type of transplant, and may predict hospital length of stay following liver transplantation (Levenson et al. 1994). The PACT subscale "Risk for Psychopathology" predicts psychopathology requiring referral and treatment after liver, heart, and bone marrow transplantation (Levenson et al. 1994).

Standardized psychological tests in transplant patient evaluation

Clinical interviews are the most common approach to the psychosocial assessment of transplant candidates. Standardized psychological tests have been studied as predictors of transplant outcome on a very limited basis. Psychopathology is not an uncommon finding on pretransplant psychological tests (Stilley et al. 1998), but may reflect the stress of the illness and need for transplant, with unknown prognostic significance. Maricle et al. (1991) found that pretransplant psychological distress as measured on the Symptom Check list-90 (SCL-90) was not related to rejection, infection, or mortality,

Table 2.6. Scale for the Psychosocial Assessment of Candidates for Transplant (PACT) to be completed after the evaluation interview

Patient Name:———————————————— Date:————————

Rater:————————

Psychosocial Assessment of Candidates for Transplantation (PACT)

Initial Rating of Candidate Quality

(Use categories 1–4 only for those patients you think should be accepted for surgery)

0	1	2	3	4	
poor, surgery contraindicated	borderline, acceptable under some conditions	accepable with some reservations	good candidate	excellent candidate	unable to rate

I. SOCIAL SUPPORT

1. Family or Support System Stability

1————2————3————4————5 ———————

| | | | | | unable to rate |

No strong interpersonal ties or highly unstable relationships

some stable relationships: some problems evident

stable, committed relationships; strong family commitment; good mental health in supporters

2. Family or Support System Availability

1————2————3————4————5 ———————

unable to rate

Support unavailable

support availability limited emotional or geographical factors

in town with patient thru process; emotionally supportive

unstable relationships

good mental health in supporters

II. PSYCHOLOGICAL HEALTH
3. Psychopathology, Stable Personality Factors

1————2————3————4————5

1	3	5	
severe ongoing psychopathology (e.g., schizophrenia, recurrent depression, personality disorder)	moderate personality or adjustment/coping problems (e.g., significant reactive anxiety, situational depression)	well-adjusted	unable to rate

4. Risk For Psychopathology.

1————2————3————4————5

1	3	5	
strong family history of major psychopathology; previous significant psychiatric history in patient	periods of poor coping; some psychological sensitivity to medications: some family history of major psychopathology	no history of major psychopathology in family, self, no periods of poor coping	unable to rate

II. LIFESTYLE FACTORS
5. Healthy Lifestyle, Ability to Sustain Change in Lifestyle

1————2————3————4————5

1	3	5	
sedentary lifestyle; major dietary problems; ongoing smoking; reluctant to change	some lifestyle change may require further education to reduce controling risk	major, sustained changes in lifestyle, no major risk factors, willing to change	unable to rate

Table 2.6. (cont.)

6. Drug and Alcohol Use

1	2	3	4	5	
dependence, reluctant to change		moderate, non-daily use willing to discontinue		abstinence or rare use	unable to rate

7. Compliance with Medications and Medical Advice

1	2	3	4	5	
unreliable compliance; unconcerned; does not consult physician		knowledgeable re meds; near adequate compliance; not vigilant, usually consults physician		knowledgeable re meds; vigilant; keeps records; consults physician	unable to rate

IV. UNDERSTANDING OF TRANSPLANT AND FOLLOW-UP
   8. Relevant Knowledge and Receptiveness to Education

1	2	3	4	5	
no idea of what is involved; views transplant as cure, no long range picture		some knowledge gaps or denial, generally good understanding		able to state risks and benefits; realistic	unable to rate

Final Rating of Candidate Quality (Do not average above responses)

(Use categories 1–4 only for those patients you think should be accepted for surgery)

0	1	2	3	4
poor, surgery contraindicated	borderline, acceptable under some conditions	accepable with some reservations	good candidate	excellent candidate

Which of the above items contributed most heavily to your final rating 7 (Circle) 1 2 3 4 5 6 7 8
List any factors that went into your final rating other than those included above: _____

_____

_____

_____

_____

but their sample was small ($n = 58$). While the SCL-90 is frequently used in research, it is not commonly used as a primary method of detecting psychopathology in clinical populations. The correlation between psychological distress and substance abuse history (Stilley, Miller, and Tarter 1997), however, suggests that certain patient populations should be chosen for closer scrutiny and more aggressive psychological interventions. Chacko et al. (1996a) evaluated 91 heart transplant candidates using clinical interviews, the Mini-Mental State examination, the Beck Depression Inventory (BDI), the Millon Behavioral Health Inventory, and the Psychosocial Adjustment to Illness Scale (PAS). Stress proneness and health behavior maladjustment (as measured by a factor on the Millon BHI) and psychiatric distress (as measured by the PAS) as well as compliance and social support as assessed by interview were associated with post-transplant survival. In addition, Axis I disorders were associated with longer hospitalizations after transplantation. In another study of 311 heart, kidney, lung and liver transplant candidates, Chacko et al. (1996b) found that patients with DSM-III-R Axis I disorders tended to have poorer psychosocial adjustment and health status, while patients with Axis II disorders had more medical compliance problems. Patients with both Axis I and Axis II disorders had the poorest coping and more marital disharmony. However, these psychiatric diagnoses and other factors were assessed concurrently, and should not be interpreted as prospective and predictive of actual transplant outcome. More recently, however, Harper et al. (1998) demonstrated that the coping scales of the Millon BHI significantly discriminated good and poor pretransplant compliance, and that the Millon BHI was superior to interview judgments in predicting post-transplant survival and medical care utilization.

Shapiro and colleagues (1995) prospectively rated 125 heart transplant patients on an array of pretransplantation psychosocial variables and then measured medical and compliance outcomes. Noncompliance was associated with substance abuse history, personality disorder, living arrangements, and global psychosocial risk. Global psychosocial risk also was associated with the number of rejection episodes. Dew et al. (1996a) studied 101 heart transplant recipients and found that persistent noncompliance was frequent over the year following transplantation, and worsened over time. Preoperative psychosocial characteristics were strong and significant predictors of noncompliance. In another study, Dew et al. (1996b) found that preoperative history of psychiatric disorders increased recipient risk for psychiatric disorders after transplantation. Poor social support and avoidance coping strategies also predicted poor psychological outcome. The strong association between development of post-traumatic stress disorder related to the transplant experience and survival found by Dew et al. indicates a need for continued vigilance regarding the mental health of transplant recipients. Other literature using standardized personality tests documents an improvement in psychological status following transplantation, but investigators for these studies have not really attempted to look at the relationship between pretransplantation psychological functioning and transplant outcome. Other literature using standardized personality tests documents an improvement in psychological status following transplantation (e.g. Cohen et al. 1998), but investigators for these studies are only beginning to look at the relationship between pretransplant psychological functioning and transplantation outcome (e.g. Deshields et al. 1996; Gregurek et al. 1996; Mongeau et al. 1997; Cohen et al. 1998).

Neuropsychological or cognitive evaluation approaches have been studied more frequently than have standardized personality tests. Cognitive dysfunction is common among patients with end-stage organ failure, related to factors such as poor perfusion, toxicity, and co-morbidities (e.g., alcoholic dementia among cirrhotic patients). Cognitive deficits may have an important impact on the patient's ability to comply with a complex medical regimen, as well as overall quality of life and probability of survival. Neuropsychological testing in pretransplant patients is more likely to reveal organic brain dysfunction than will routine clinical examinations. Cognitive tests have been used to document both the potential for organ transplantation to result in improved cognitive functioning as well as the enduring nature of some deficits. The relationship between pretransplant cognitive functioning and transplant outcomes such as morbidity and mortality is less well studied, but an important area for further research. Deshields et al. (1996) found that cardiac transplant patients improved on both cognitive measures and measures of psychological distress in the first year after surgery, but anxiety, depression, and impaired cognition were associated with rejection episodes. These findings may suggest a predictive role for psychological measures, but may also reflect the effects of rejection episodes and the treatments for them, such as high dose steroids. Longitudinal studies would be useful to help sort out causal explanations. Farmer's (1994) comprehensive review of neuropsychological findings in patients with end-stage heart, kidney, and liver failure supports the need for development of comprehensive normative data bases for various categories of organ failure and stages of disease.

Screening and the Americans with Disabilities Act

Recently attention has been drawn to potential legal problems with psychosocial screening, specifically with regard to the Americans with Disabilities Act (ADA) (see Orentlicher 1996). The ADA considers any physical or psychological illness a disability if it "substantially limits" major life activities. Even if an illness is treatable, it may qualify as a disability. The law also includes as a potential disability the history of a disabling illness or perception by others that one is substantially limited in major life activities. As described earlier in this chapter, transplantation programs routinely screen candidates for depression, psychosis, cognitive dysfunction, and substance abuse, all of which fall under the ADA's definition of disability.

Orentlicher (1996) concluded that the ADA would seem to prohibit the use of criteria for transplant candidacy that screen out all individuals with a particular diagnosis, e.g., mental retardation or schizophrenia. The ADA also prohibits seemingly neutral criteria that systematically screen out persons with disabilities. On the other hand, ADA permits selection criteria that are based on risk assessment, i.e., giving preference to candidates who are at lower risk for transplant-related morbidity and mortality. ADA also allows the use of eligibility criteria considered necessary to operate a transplantation program (e.g., excluding a patient who has threatened or assaulted caregivers).

Thus, it appears that transplantation programs can use psychosocial selection criteria as long as the criteria distinguish potential candidates in terms of their likelihood of benefiting from transplant. This corresponds closely to how most transplantation programs proceeded before the passage of ADA, but there remains the potential for much legal dispute and confusion. On what basis can a transplantation program reasonably conclude that a patient's psychiatric or behavioral problem creates too much risk for successful transplantation? In a formal legal challenge to such a decision, citing the program's "clinical experience" may well be considered insufficient. In the absence of studies showing validity and reliability for the criteria, the court will be more likely to find discrimination on the basis of disability. This is especially likely when some investigators have reported equivalent transplant outcomes in selected patients with and without the disability (e.g., alcohol dependence and liver transplantation).

Another potential legal complexity is the principle of reasonable accommodation, which requires that even if a disability renders patients less suitable as candidates, the transplant team has a responsibility to provide support and treatment that can improve their chances (e.g., Nelson et al. (1995) described behavioral contracting interventions). Finally, while outcome research examines groups, ADA requires an individualized assessment for the particular patient. Even if it were well-established that continued abuse of alcohol was associated with a high rate of transplant failure, programs would still be expected to consider whether the individual alcoholic had extenuating circumstances rather than apply an exclusionary rule by rote (no active drinkers). Transplantation programs' candidacy decisions may be legally challenged as discriminatory either for failing to consider individual factors or for individualizing too much, not treating the patient equivalently with others with that diagnosis or trait. There has been little actual litigation to date, but it is expected.

Summary

Psychological screening of organ transplant candidates is routine at most transplant centers, but the methods of evaluation and the criteria employed appear to vary greatly among centers. Psychosocial evaluations are conducted in order to screen out patients who demonstrate enduring behavioral problems in areas such as compliance and substance abuse or who exhibit serious psychopathology likely to affect survival. In addition, these evaluations allow transplantation programs to identify problems that will respond to appropriate intervention. Evidence for the reliability and validity of clinical interviews, the most commonly used evaluation approach, is provided by studies employing two frequently used rating scales, the PACT and the TERS. Standardized psychological tests measuring personality, psychopathology, and some social variables show promise in predicting outcome. Cognitive tests document significant correlates of end-stage organ failure that may not be apparent on routine clinical examination and are also promising as predictors of compliance, quality of life, and survival. Ethical and legal concerns related to psychosocial evaluations of transplant candidates must be considered by clinicians conducting them, as the potential for judging patients on the basis of perceived social worth and discrimination against patients with disabilities is always present and must be guarded against. The Americans with Disabilities Act creates new demands for transplantation programs in the USA to offer mental and behavioral health treatment and rehabilitation to patients who might reasonably benefit, as patients who are excluded from surgery without adequate accommodation present risk for litigation. In addition, these concerns point to a need for more research documenting the relationship between psychosocial variables and transplant outcomes.

Acknowledgments

We are grateful to the Academy of Psychosomatic Medicine and the American Psychiatric Press for permission to use material published earlier in *Psychosomatics*.

References

Annas, G. J. (1985). The prostitute, the playboy, and the poet: rationing schemes for organ transplantation. *Am J Public Health*, **75**, 187–9.
Chacko, R. C., Harper, R. G., Gotto, J., and Young, J. (1996a). Psychiatric interview

and psychometric predictors of cardiac transplant survival. *Am J Psychiatry*, **153**, 1607–12.

Chacko, R. C., Harper, R. G., Kunik, M., and Young, J. (1996b). Relationship of psychiatric morbidity and psychosocial factors in organ transplant candidates. *Psychosomatics*, **37**, 100–7.

Cohen, L., Littlefield, C., Kelly, P., Maurer, J., and Abbey, S. (1998). Predictors of quality of life and adjustment after lung transplantation. *Chest*, **113**, 633–44.

Deshields, T. L., McDonough, E. M., Mannen, R. K., and Miller, L. W. (1996). Psychological and cognitive status before and after heart transplantation. *Gen Hosp Psychiatry*, **18**(6 Supplement), 62S–69S.

Dew, M. A., Roth, L. H., Schulberg, H. C. et al. (1996b). Prevalence and predictors of depression and anxiety-related disorders during the year after heart transplantation. *Gen Hosp Psychiatry*, **18** (6 Supplement), 48A–61S.

Dew, M. A., Roth, L. H., Thompson, M. E. et al. (1996a). Medical compliance and its predictors in the first year after heart transplantation. *J Heart Lung Transplant*, **15**, 631–45.

Farmer, M. E. (1994). Cognitive deficits related to major organ failure: the potential role of neurological testing. *Neuropsychol Rev*, **4**, 117–60.

Gregurek, R., Labar, R., Mrsic, M. et al. (1996(Anxiety as a possible predictor of GVHD. *Bone Marrow Transplant*, **18**(3), 585–9.

Harper, R. G., Chacko, R. C., Kotik-Harper, D., Young, J., and Gotto, J. (1998). Self-report evaluation of health behavior, stress vulnerability,a nd medical outcome in heart transplant recipients. *Psychosom Med*, **60**, 563–9.

Kilner, J. F. (1988). Selecting patients when resources are limited: a study of U.S. medical directors of kidney dialysis and transplantation facilities. *Am J Public Health*, **78**, 144–7.

Levenson, J. L., Best, A., Presberg, B. et al. (1994). Psychosocial assessment of candidates for transplantation (PACT) as a predictor of transplant outcome. In *Proceedings of the 41st Annual Meeting of the Academy of Psychosomatic Medicine*, p. 39.

Levenson, J. L. and Olbrisch, M. E. (1993). Psychosocial evaluation of organ transplant candidates: a comparative survey of process, criteria and outcomes in heart, liver and kidney transplant programs. *Psychosomatics*, **34**, 314–23.

Mai, F. M. (1987). Liaison psychiatry in the heart transplant unit. *Psychosomatics*, **28**, 44–6.

Maricle, R. A., Hosenpud, J. D., Norman, D. J. et al. (1991). The lack of predictive value of preoperative psychological distress for postoperative medical outcome in heart transplant recipients. *J Heart Lung Transplant*, **10**, 942–7.

Mongeau, J. G., Clermont, M. J., Robitaille, P. et al. (1997) Study of psychosocial parameters related to the surival rate of renal transplantation in children. *Pediatric Nephrol*, **11**, 542–6.

Nelson, M. K., Presberg, B. A, Olbrisch, M. E. et al. (1995). Behavioral contingency contracting for substance abuse and high risk health behaviors in patients being considered for transplant surgery. *J Transplant Coordination*, **5**, 35–40.

Olbrisch, M. E. (1996). Picking winners and grooming the dark horse: psychologists evaluate and treat organ transplant patients. *Health Psychologist*, **18**, 10–11.

Olbrisch, M. E. and Levenson, J. L. (1991). Psychosocial evaluation of heart transplant candidates: an international survey of process, criteria, and outcomes. *J Heart Lung Transplant*, **10**, 948–55.

Olbrisch, M. E. and Levenson, J. L. (1995). Psychosocial assessment of organ transplant candidates: current status of methodological and philosophical issues. *Psychosomatics*, **36**, 236–43.

Olbrisch, M. E., Levenson, J. L., and Hamer, R. (1989). The PACT: a rating scale for the study of clinical decision making in psychosocial screening of organ transplant candidates. *Clin Transplant*, **3**, 164–9.

Olbrisch, M. E., Levenson, J. L., Sherwin, E. D. et al. (1994). Validation of psychosocial assessments of cardiac transplant candidates. *J Heart Lung Transplant*, **13**, S70.

Orentlicher, D. (1996). Psychosocial assessment of organ transplant candidates and the Americans with Disabilities Act. *Gen Hosp Psychiatry*, **18**, 3S–12S.

Presberg, B. A., Levenson, J. L., Olbrisch, M. E. et al. (1995). Rating scales for the psychosocial evaluation of organ transplant candidates: comparison of the PACT and TERS with bone marrow transplant patients. *Psychosomatics*, **36**, 458–61.

Robertson, J. A. (1987). Supply and distribution of hearts for transplantation: legal, ethical, and policy issues. *Circulation*, **75**, 77–87.

Shapiro, P. A., Williams, D. L., Foray, A. T. et al. (1995). Psychosocial evaluation and prediction of compliance problems and morbidity after heart transplantation. *Transplantation*, **60**, 1462–6.

Stilley, C. S., Miller, D. J., Gayowski, T., and Marino, I. R. (1998). Psychological characteristics of candidates for liver transplantation. *Clin Transplant*, **12**, 416–24.

Stilley, C. S., Miller, D. J., and Tarter, R. E. (1997). Measuring psychological distress in candidates for liver transplantation: a pilot study. *J Clin Psychol*, **53**, 459–64.

Twillman, R. K., Manetto, C., Wellisch, D. K. et al. (1993). The Transplant Evaluation Rating Scale: a revision of the psychosocial levels system for evaluating organ transplant candidates. *Psychosomatics*, **34**, 144–53.

3

Psychosocial issues in living organ donation

Galen E. Switzer Ph.D., Mary Amanda Dew, Ph.D.,
Robert K. Twillman Ph.D.

Introduction

The theme of the gift, of freedom and obligation in the gift, of generosity and
self-interest in giving, reappear in our own society like the resurrection of a
dominant motif long forgotten. (Marcel Mauss, *The Gift*, 1954.)

The living donation of organs or bone marrow entails significant sacrifice on
the part of the donor and can be legitimately classified as a unique and
important form of gift giving. There are, however, features of organ donation
that distinguish it from other types of gift giving, including its impersonal
context, few if any penalties for refusing to donate (particularly for unrelated
donors), no expectation of reciprocal gift giving, and consequences of the gift
to prolong life (Titmuss 1972). Volunteer donors undergo significant discomfort, inconvenience, and physical risk to provide such gifts, suggesting
uniqueness to the psychological issues surrounding the decision to donate,
and factors that impact on donors' postdonation physical and psychological
experiences.

Composing a coherent summary of current research and issues involved in
living organ donation is a daunting task. First, unlike the case of the organ
recipient, whose condition is dire regardless of what type of organ he or she is
receiving, the physical risk of organ donation varies greatly across organ
types. Bone marrow donation is minimally invasive and involves a regenerating body part, while kidney, liver lobe, and lung lobe donations require major
surgery to remove organ or organ portions that do not regenerate (except
some liver tissue). Second, donor–recipient pairs represent all possible types
of relationship, including unrelated strangers, acquaintances, emotional
partners/spouses or close friends, and genetic relations. Receiving the necessary life-saving organ may be the paramount issue for the recipient at the time
of transplantation, though the type of donor–recipient relationship may have
important and enduring effects on the donation experience for the donor and
may ultimately affect the recipient as well. Further, the type of donor–

recipient relationship is likely to be associated with organ type. Bone marrow donors, for example, are less likely to be genetically related to the recipient than are other types of donor.

There are surprisingly few studies of psychosocial issues in organ donation, kidney donation being most often studied. Standardized measures across investigations are used infrequently, and there is a lack of consensus – at even the most basic level – about which domains should be routinely assessed. This is in striking contrast to the number and sophistication of studies concerned with transplant recipients (Borgida, Conner, and Manteufel 1992; Andrykowski 1994a,b). In Chapter 4, Dew et al. review 144 separate studies of organ recipients' quality of life. This emphasis on organ recipients may be related to the greater numbers of recipients compared to living donors, resulting partly from the large number of organs that are harvested from cadavers. Moreover, the fact that the transplantation process literally rescues the recipients from certain death lends a certain drama to their medical and psychosocial issues (Hirvas et al. 1980; Steinberg, Levy, and Radvila 1981; House and Thompson 1988). The organ donor literature is therefore still in early stages.

Our approach to organizing existing information about donation issues has been first to divide the issues into two groups according to their pertinence to pre- or postdonation. Predonation issues include donor motives, donor decision-making, and donor ambivalence. Because none of these areas has been well investigated, the few studies that have been conducted are discussed under a single heading regardless of the type of organ that is being donated. Postdonation issues – including both the physical and psychosocial outcomes addressed in a number of investigations – are divided into three sections corresponding to the three organs (kidney, bone marrow, liver lobe) that are most commonly donated by living donors. Unless otherwise specified, these data apply to the USA only.

Predonation psychosocial issues

Individuals who become organ or bone marrow donors come from a wide range of social backgrounds, religious perspectives, and family contexts. Thus, it is likely that donors approach the donation process guided by a variety of underlying motives and relying on diverse sets of decision-making strategies that may lead them to be more or less highly committed to the donation process.

Donor motives

Despite the importance of investigating donor motivation, systematic attempts to assess it are rare (Andrykowski 1994a,b). This is surprising given the demonstrated relationship between donor motivation and outcomes in other volunteer settings. For example, volunteers' motivations predict longer-term participation in the volunteer activity, volunteer/donor effectiveness, and volunteer/donor satisfaction in studies of blood donors and acquired immune deficiency syndrome (AIDS) hospice workers (Callero and Piliavin 1983; Piliavin and Callero 1991; Snyder and Omoto 1992). Though some outcomes, such as long-term participation, may not be a central concern for certain types of organ donation, it is still important to understand how donors' evaluations of themselves and the donation process may affect their reasons for donating.

Organ donors are probably motivated by a variety of intrinsic factors (e.g., acting in accordance with religious convictions) and extrinsic factors (e.g., social pressures) that may operate simultaneously to inspire and/or dissuade the donor. Furthermore, the particular combination of motivational forces differs depending on whether or not the donor is related to the recipient. The majority of all living organ donations (kidney, liver, lung, etc.) occur between genetically or emotionally related individuals. In this context, physicians and transplantation researchers have assumed that family members or emotional partners are naturally motivated by the prospect of saving the life of a loved one (Fellner and Schwartz 1971).

In the largest study of psychosocial issues among living related donors to date, Simmons, Klein and Simmons (1977) gathered predonation information on kidney donors' motives. As expected, 83% of donors cited "helping to save the recipient's life" as the primary reason for donating. In addition, 78% of donors felt that the donation would make their *own* lives more worth while. The authors anticipated, however, that related donors' motives might be more complex than had been originally assumed. They conducted a series of studies focused on assessing the potential for overt and subtle social pressures on the donor (Simmons, Klein, and Thornton 1973; for a comprehensive discussion of this topic, see Simmons, Klein Marine, and Simmons 1987). Based on in-depth interviews, Simmons and colleagues found that 11% of donors experienced significant direct family pressure to donate, and that an additional 43% experienced subtle family pressure. A substantial number of donors may donate due to guilt for past actions (25%) or fear of future disapproval if they did not donate (14%). Although the majority of donors do not report less socially desirable motives, such as atonement for past wrongs and anticipated guilt, these motives may be substantially underreported by donors (Simmons et al. 1977).

In contrast to widespread acceptance of the idea that one would be willing to donate an organ to a relative, willingness to donate to a stranger has been viewed as unusual or even pathological (Fellner and Schwartz 1971). In the early years of kidney transplantation, individuals who contacted transplant centers volunteering to donate a kidney to a stranger were regarded with distrust and suspicion by members of the medical profession (Hamburger and Crosnier 1968). However, in a community study of public attitudes toward kidney donation, Fellner and Schwartz (1971) found that 54% of metropolitan residents expressed willingness to donate a kidney to an unrelated stranger. They concluded that attitudes toward unrelated organ donation were much more favorable than the medical community had previously anticipated.

Unrelated donors provide the majority of bone marrow for transplantation in the USA (Silberman et al. 1994). In contrast, the availability of cadaveric and living related organs has restricted the number of unrelated solid organ transplants performed in part because of concerns that any system of unrelated living organ donation could be abused. Bone marrow donation bears similarities (a) to blood donation because it involves a less invasive medical procedure to share regenerative tissue, and (b) to solid organ donation because it involves surgery under general anesthesia to assist a specific patient. Motivations of blood donors are relevant to living organ donation because they provide information about motivations for medical donation in general, and because bone marrow donors often are recruited from blood donor lists.

The first studies on the motivation of blood donors were conducted in the same decade as the first studies on the motivation of organ donors, and reached similar conclusions. Altruistic/humanitarian motives for donating were most common (Oswalt 1977; Simmons et al. 1977). A more recent study showed that first-time donors often were motivated by less altruistic forces, such as external social pressures (e.g., obligations to a group), but that, if donation continued, these donors developed an internal "donor self-image" (Callero and Piliavin 1983; Callero 1985; Callero, Howard, and Piliavin 1987; Charng, Piliavin, and Callero 1988; Piliavin and Callero 1991; Gardner and Cacioppo 1995; Royse and Doochin 1995) and began to see themselves as "the kind of person who donates". A similar process may occur with bone marrow donors, under conditions that may involve high levels of social pressure, who subsequently make a series of small incremental decisions leading up to the donation (Stroncek et al. 1989). Medical donor self-images may generalize across donation types. Frequent blood donors are 3 to 12 times more likely to join the bone marrow registry than less frequent blood donors (Briggs, Piliavin, and Becker 1986; Beatty et al. 1989; Cacioppo and Gardner 1993; Sarason et al. 1993).

Bone marrow donor motives and the relationship between such motives and donation outcomes was studied in a cohort of 343 original National Marrow Donor Program (NMDP) marrow donors (Switzer et al. 1997). The most common type of motive was "exchange-related" (45%), in which donors emphasized the low costs to themselves and/or the high potential benefits to the recipient (e.g., "I got something freely, and if I can give it back, let's do it.") Other commonly reported motive types included "idealized helping" (37%), in which donors indicated helpful attitudes without specific reasons (e.g., "I guess I was just glad to be able to help."); "normative motives" (26%), in which donors expressed moral correctness (e.g., "I think it's kind of a social responsibility."); "positive feeling" (25%), in which donors discussed the psychic gains they might receive (e.g., "The bottom line here is I can do something that's going to make me feel pretty good about myself."); and "empathy-related" motives (18%), in which donors had mentally and emotionally placed themselves in the recipient's position (e.g., "It struck me this week how happy the recipient must be to be getting so close, because I am."). Less frequently, donors reported being motivated by past life experiences (e.g., blood donation experiences, or having had an ill relative) or, without giving specific reasons, expressed incredulity at *not* volunteering (e.g., "Why would anyone not donate?"). In general, these motive types are similar to motives described in other studies of medical volunteerism (e.g., Oswalt 1977; Simmons et al. 1977; Callero and Piliavin 1983; Piliavin and Callero 1991; Snyder and Omoto 1992; Omoto and Snyder 1995).

The relationship between demographic characteristics and motive types was examined (Switzer et al. 1997). Females were more likely to report empathy and positive feeling motives, and younger donors more often reported exchange-related motives. Overall, donors who expected to experience psychic gains from donating (positive feeling motives) were more likely to have positive donation experiences; they reported less predonation ambivalence about going ahead with the donation, and greater feelings of postdonation self-worth. Donors whose motives were focused more externally on the recipient (e.g., exchange and idealized helping) seemed to experience the donation process more negatively in terms of higher predonation ambivalence.

In summary, donors agree to donate for a variety of psychological and social reasons. Though the exact nature of the relationship between donor characteristics, such as demographic factors and family context, and donor motives have not been fully investigated, there is promising evidence that such a relationship exists. There is also evidence that these motivations, in turn, may be related to donors' donation experiences.

Donor decision-making

Factors influencing the donor decision-making process are likely to vary dramatically depending on the donor–recipient relationship and the physical component to be donated. For example, the decision-making process that characterizes the donation of a kidney to a sibling or an emotional partner may differ significantly from the process of deciding to donate marrow to an unrelated stranger. A better understanding of the decision-making process should lead to the development of more effective recruitment procedures, better donor educational techniques, and ultimately more positive donation outcomes.

Most studies of donor decision-making have focused on the rapidity with which individuals made the decision to become potential donors. Decision making swiftness may be an indicator of the type of decision being made. Simmons et al. (1977) described two competing social psychological donor decision-making models: the moral model, and the rational or deliberative model. Moral decision-making involves (a) awareness that one's actions can affect another, (b) self-ascription of responsibility, (c) acceptance of the norm governing the behavior, and (d) conformity to that governing norm (Schwartz 1970). Simmons and others (e.g., Fellner 1976/77) have argued that moral decision-making – because it does not involve weighing the costs and benefits of a given behavior but, instead, is based on norms governing that behavior – is likely to lead to nondeliberative, instantaneous decisions.

In contrast, the rational decision-making model includes several steps specifically focused on gathering information and evaluating alternatives: (a) identification of the problem, (b) collection of relevant information, (c) constructing alternatives, (d) evaluation of alternatives, (e) selection of one alternative, (f) implementation of the decision, and (g) evaluation of the outcome (Simon 1957; Brim et al. 1962; Hill 1970). According to this model, the decision-making process involves deliberation, and therefore will not be swift.

Until recently, virtually all the evidence concerning donor decision making indicated that the decision to donate – regardless of the donor-recipient relationship and donation type – was most often instantaneous and non-deliberative. In a series of psychosocial studies of related kidney donors, Fellner and colleagues found that practically all donors reported having made voluntary and immediate decisions characteristic of the "moral" decision-making process (Fellner and Marshall 1968, 1970; Fellner 1976/77). Based on their investigations, these authors observed that the immediacy of the dona-tion decision differs markedly from the typical deliberative and reasoned analysis by which individuals make important decisions (Fellner and Mar-shall 1981; Sherman and Fazio 1983). In the first systematic study of the decision-making process among related kidney donors, Simmons et al. (1977) also found support for a moral rather than a rational decision-making process; 68% of donors surveyed reported volunteering without deliberating, immediately upon hearing of the need. In light of these findings, the authors argued that the term "decision-making" may be inappropriate for describing the instantaneous process by which related individuals become donors.

An investigation of decision processes of unrelated bone marrow donors also lends support to the idea that donation decisions are made spontaneous-ly (Switzer, Simmons, and Dew 1996). The first 849 individuals to donate marrow through the NMDP were surveyed one to two weeks predonation, one to two weeks postdonation, and one year postdonation. Predonation survey results indicated that 80% of donors found it "not at all hard" to decide to donate, 71% said that they decided "right away that they would definitely be a donor when they first heard about the program," and 77% said that they did not postpone at all the decision to donate. These findings bolster the argument that donors perceive themselves as making instantaneous, nondeliberative decisions. Other studies of related and unrelated kidney donors (e.g., Sadler et al. 1971; Steinberg et al. 1981; Higgerson and Bulechek 1982; Smith et al. 1986; Horton and Horton 1991), bone marrow donors (Stroncek et al. 1989), and individuals who simply agree to sign organ donor cards (Simmons et al. 1974) all suggest that the large majority of volunteers reported making spontaneous decisions.

Though the evidence supporting spontaneous decision-making processes is substantial, there are some problems with these studies. First, most data gathered from donors are either retrospective or were collected shortly before donation, after donors were already thoroughly committed to the process. Thus, donors' retrospective reports (or memory) of the decision process may have been influenced by the fact that they had publicly committed themselves to donating. Any former doubts and worries, or periods of weighing costs and benefits, may have been overlooked or minimized, and factors indicating the donors' commitment may have been magnified in a process known as "bolstering" (Janis and Mann 1977). A second problem is that almost none of these studies included nondonors in their analyses of the decision-making process (Simmons et al. (1977) is an exception).

To address the shortcomings of previous investigations, Borgida et al. (1992) conducted a prospective study of individuals who contacted one US transplant center to seek information about donating a kidney to a relative or friend. All individuals who requested information received and completed a questionnaire, and subsequently decided either to donate ($n = 52$) or not to donate ($n = 102$). These authors argued that donors often do deliberate about the donation decision, and predicted that their findings would support a planned behavior model rather than an instantaneous or moral model. The planned behavior model, based on Ajzen's (1985) theory of reasoned action, suggests that intentions to donate are predicted by attitudes toward donation, normative pressure perceived from others, and control perceived over donation. Intentions to donate, in turn, best predict actual donation. The authors argue that the strong link found between intentions to donate and actual donation is evidence of planned decision-making, contrary to previous claims based on retrospective data (Borgida et al. 1992).

However, there may be several limitations to the findings. First, it is not clear whether the study sample included all possible family members available for kidney donation during this period, or some subsample who sought further information about the donation process. The latter would tend to bias the sample against individuals making spontaneous decisions to donate and toward those seeking additional information about the donation process.

Second, the study did not operationalize normative pressure or intentions to donate in a way that could have shown support for the moral model. Subjective normative pressures were measured with items asking whether the prospective donor's parents, brothers and sisters, and other relatives, thought he or she should donate. However, adherence to overarching societal level norms governing altruistic behavior (e.g., norms about general helpfulness and family responsibility) that are central to moral decision-making, were not assessed. In addition, though intentions to donate were measured with straightforward items (e.g., "I intend to donate a kidney to X"), there was no measure of how rapidly donors developed such intentions to donate. Therefore, the possibility that powerful normative forces are associated with instantaneous decisions to donate, as is suggested by the moral decision-making model, cannot be discounted.

Finally, and perhaps most importantly, the investigation treats donors and nondonors as a homogeneous group, when, in fact, the decision-making processes may differ substantially for these two groups. Even Simmons et al. (1977), who provided the strongest empirical support for moral decision-making, found that while 68% of donors followed a moral decision-making pattern, only 21% of nondonors fit this model. In fact, 31% of nondonors seemed to follow a rational decision-making pattern. Perhaps individuals who decide not to donate are those who weigh the costs and benefits of donating. Societal-level norms concerning altruism that lead donors to make immediate decisions to donate, probably do not produce similarly spontaneous decisions among donors not to donate. In the Borgida et al. study, the fact that nondonors (who might be expected to deliberate more about donation) comprised two-thirds of the total sample may have led to the false conclusion that most potential donors also made deliberative decisions.

Further research about how potential donors reach the decision of whether or not to donate should focus on prospectively examining the decision-making processes both of volunteer donors and of nondonors. A better understanding of the forces operating during the critical decision-making period will allow medical teams and recruitment coordinators to adjust their informational and educational efforts to enhance donation outcomes.

Donor ambivalence

Regardless of whether donors make moral, spontaneous or rational, deliberative decisions to donate, there are potential costs to themselves during donation. For solid organ donors, these costs include the loss of a body part, the medical risks of the surgical procedure, and the potential for longer-term physical consequences (Simmons et al. 1987). Because bone marrow regenerates, its donation involves fewer long-term risks than solid organ donation, though it still entails risks associated with a surgical procedure under general anesthesia (Bortin and Buckner 1983; Buckner et al. 1984). In addition, potential psychological costs to donors include concern and worry about their own health and the health of the recipient. Donors' awareness of these potential costs produce "mixed feelings" or ambivalence about donating. Such donor ambivalence has proved, in turn, to be a central predictor of postdonation outcomes (Simmons et al. 1977; Switzer et al. 1996).

Simmons et al. (1977), who were the first investigators to systematically assess ambivalence in organ donation, developed a seven-item ambivalence measure for use with related kidney donors. Items assessed difficulty in making the decision to donate, doubts and worries about donating, and whether donors would still want to donate, even if someone else could do it. The authors concluded that though the majority of donors were very positive about their impending donation, as many as 50% of donors reported at least some predonation ambivalence, and a substantial minority reported experiencing very high levels of ambivalence. In addition, donors were willing to express concerns about donation during the research that they had not related to their physicians. Given the social desirability of appearing positive about donation, true levels of ambivalence may be underestimated even during research.

Married donors who were siblings or children of the recipient were more ambivalent than unmarried donors, while female donors and parents donating to their children were less ambivalent than their counterparts (Simmons 1981). Perhaps married donors, on the one hand, feel a dual sense of obligation to their immediate families and their families of origin, a conflict heightened because these donors are often actively discouraged from donating by their spouses and in-laws. On the other hand, females and parents may experience less ambivalence because of their socially constructed roles as caregivers for their families.

A more recent study (Switzer et al. 1996) assessed predonation ambivalence among 343 unrelated bone marrow donors with items similar to those employed by Simmons and colleagues in 1977. Table 3.1 compares kidney and bone marrow donors' responses to these seven ambivalence items. Despite the differences in donation organ type and relationship to the recipient, the pattern of responses for both groups is quite similar, suggesting that there are fairly constant and unavoidable levels of ambivalence about medical donation within any population. It is also possible that the higher potential gains of related kidney donation (saving the life of a loved one versus that of a stranger) counterbalance its higher costs (i.e., loss of a nonregenerating versus a regenerating body part) to produce comparable levels of donor ambivalence between these two types of donation.

Ambivalence items were combined to form an ambivalence scale ranging from $0 = $ no ambivalence to $7 = $ very high ambivalence. Over a third of the bone marrow donors (38%) had scores of 0 on the ambivalence scale, indicating no ambivalence about their impending donation (Switzer et al.

Table 3.1. Ambivalence among related kidney donors and unrelated bone marrow donors [a]

Ambivalence item	Agree a lot	Agree a little	Disagree a little	Disagree a lot
I sometimes feel unsure about donating.	5%	21%	5%	70%
	1%[a]	*20%*	*18%*	*61%*
I sometimes wish the patient were getting the transplant from someone else (a cadaver) instead of from me.	2%	11%	7%	79%
	1%	*9%*	*20%*	*70%*
I would really want to donate myself even if someone else could do it.	60%	26%	8%	6%
	62%	*27%*	*9%*	*2%*

	Very disappointed	A little disappointed	A little relieved	Very relieved
How would you have felt if you found out that you could not donate for some reason?	65%	23%	11%	1%
	49%	*46%*	*5%*	*0%*

	Very hard	Somewhat hard	A little hard	Not hard
How hard a decision was it for you to decide to donate?	4%	10%	3%	72%
	1%	*5%*	*15%*	*79%*

	Knew right away	Thought it over
Did you know right away you would donate or did you think it over?	78%	22%
	71%	*29%*

	Yes	No
Did you ever have any doubts or worries about donating?	36%	64%
	41%	*59%*

[a] Bone marrow donor percentages are italicized.

1996). However, the remainder (62%) experienced at least some uncertainty about donating, with a notable percentage (12%) reporting high levels of predonation ambivalence (scores of 5–7 on the scale).

Using hierarchical regression, Switzer et al. (1996) also assessed the relationship of predonation ambivalence with a set of demographic characteristics (gender, education, age, and marital status) and psychosocial characteristics (frequency of blood donation, level of happiness, optimism about the recipient's chances of survival, and having been discouraged from donating by someone). Among demographic factors, only higher education was directly related to higher levels of ambivalence. Among psychosocial variables, having been discouraged from donating was related to greater ambivalence, while frequent blood donation, happiness, and optimism about the recipient's chances were all associated with lower levels of ambivalence. Unlike the Simmons et al. (1977) study, this survey did not find strong evidence that donors' gender was directly associated with ambivalence, though women were both less likely to have been frequent blood donors and more likely to have been discouraged from donating marrow.

In summary, there is strong evidence that predonation ambivalence is an important predictor of postdonation outcomes across different types of organ donation. As has been suggested elsewhere, these findings indicate that transplant teams should be especially aware of statements made by donors that seem to indicate reluctance to donate and treat these as a signal to more carefully discuss the risks and benefits of the donation (Simmons 1977; Switzer et al. 1996).

Postdonation physical and psychosocial issues

Table 3.2 summarizes studies of donation outcomes for kidney, bone marrow, and liver donation. Each entry in the table represents either a single study, or a series of studies by a single research group examining similar donation outcomes. Different postdonation outcomes for one sample of donors are often published in multiple reports. Table entries for clusters of studies from such cohorts are indicated by matching numerical superscripts. Unlike investigations of recipient quality of life (QOL) outcomes (see Dew et al. Chapter 4, this volume), donation investigations often have not utilized standardized instruments or have not measured outcomes within an established set of domains.

Two types of postdonation outcome were most common among the studies we reviewed: donor perceptions concerning the physical aspects of donation, and donor psychosocial reactions (e.g., self-esteem, anxiety, happiness). Across all 31 studies listed in Table 3.2, approximately 642 kidney donors, 2092 bone marrow donors (30 related, 2,062 unrelated), and 48 liver donors were studied. A single large archival study of bone marrow donors (Buckner et al. 1984; $n = 1549$) accounted for nearly 75% of the total bone marrow donors studied. In fact, sample size varied greatly across studies, ranging from 7 kidney donors (Kemph 1966, 1967) to 1549 bone marrow donors (Buckner et al. 1984), as did study design, ranging from cross-sectional postdonation to prospective pre- and postdonation. Investigations have focused more on psychosocial outcomes (90%) than on subjective physical outcomes of donation (48%). Postdonation physical condition of most donors is clinically determined to be good (Fellner 1976/77; Simmons 1977), so that donors' perceptions of their physical status might be presumed by some researchers to be positive.

Kidney donation outcomes

Early psychosocial studies of kidney donors were conducted in an atmosphere of medical and public skepticism about the efficacy and advisability of living organ donation (Fellner and Marshall 1968). Little was known at that time about the potential long-term physical consequences of donation, and even less was known about psychological reactions postdonation. Many researchers imagined the worst, suggesting that related kidney donors would experience feelings of having given up some part of themselves for nothing in return – a feeling potentially compounded by grief or guilt if the transplant failed (Kemph 1966, 1967). Thus, initial psychosocial investigations highlighted the unanticipated beneficial effects on donors as a result of donating (Fellner and Marshall 1968, 1970, 1981; Fellner 1976/77; Simmons et al. 1977).

Perhaps most striking is that only one investigation of those cited above that assessed both costs and benefits of kidney donation failed to report any donation benefits, and instead found almost universal feelings of depression and injustice among donors (Kemph 1966, 1967). However, this study had a very small sample size ($n = 7$), and was conducted prior to widespread use of the types of immunosuppressive drugs that greatly improve the recipients' chances of survival. Thus, donors' depression and feelings of having given something for nothing in return may have been related to their ill relatives' poor prognosis. Several other studies that only assessed postdonation psychiatric difficulties found a substantial proportion of donors who experienced mild to severe postdonation trauma (Hirvas et al. 1976, 1980) or other psychiatric symptoms, including anxiety or depression (Ewald et al. 1976). Other studies have found that many donors experienced at least some negative feelings one to two weeks postdonation, including depression (31%), and concerns about their own health (14%), sexuality (16%), or appearance (26%) (Simmons et al. 1987). Predonation ambivalence, unhappiness, and being male or married, were among the most prominent predictors of negative feelings postdonation (Simmons et al. 1987).

Most investigations of kidney donation, however, have found considerable donor benefits. Many prospective studies report pre- to postdonation improvements and controlled studies show gains in self-esteem, happiness, feelings of self-worth, and quality of the relationship with the recipient (e.g., Fellner and Marshall 1968, 1970; Simmons et al. 1977; Simmons 1981; see Table 3.2 for a complete list). Donor benefits occur not only in the weeks shortly after donation, but also can persist for many years (Marshall and Fellner 1977; Simmons and Anderson 1985).

Table 3.2. Postdonation physical and psychosocial outcomes in living donors

Author	Design and sample characteristics	Analyses	Postdonation outcomes	
			Perceived Physical	Psychosocial
Kidney donation				
Kemph (1966, 1967)	Cross-sectional postdonation evaluation of 7 related kidney donors	Post descriptive	—	Most experienced moderate to severe post depression which required psychotherapy; donors felt that they had given up something for nothing in return
Fellner (1976/77); Fellner and Marshall (1968, 1970)[a]	Cross-sectional/longitudinal postdonation survey/interview of 182 related kidney donors (total across studies)	Post descriptive	—	Most reported donation made life more meaningful, virtually all said they were proud of their donation and would donate again if asked
Ewald et al. (1976)	Longitudinal pre, 3 days postdonation psychiatric interview, long-term psychiatric follow-up 88 related kidney donors	Descriptive	—	17% predonation mental symptoms (e.g., anxiety, depression, alcoholism); 5% had postdonation symptoms (e.g., anxiety) related to donation; 24% had longer-term psychiatric symptoms (57% of these had had predonation symptoms)
Hirvas et al. (1976)	Cross-sectional 6 mth to 6 yr postdonation psychiatric assessment 64 related kidney donors, 10 patients with kidney removal for their own illnesses	Post descriptive, donor vs. control	—	37% mild post trauma, 19% moderate to severe post trauma; no difference in donor vs. control trauma levels; donor trauma not associated with donor–recipient relationship or transplant outcome

Marshall and Felner (1977)[a]	Cross-sectional 8–10 yr postdonation interview follow-up of 10 Fellner and Marshall (1968) related kidney donors	Post descriptive	All in good general health, several had minor physical complaints	Self-image gains in most donors
Simmons (1977); Simmons et al. (1977); Simmons et al. (1987)[b]	Longitudinal pre, 1 wk post, 1 yr post donation survey/interview, 111 related kidney donors, 174 family nondonors, 150 regional controls, 5430 national controls	Longitudinal comparison, donor vs. control	28% indicated substantial soreness shortly post, 34% did not feel completely normal 1 yr post	*Positive outcomes*: donors had pre–1 yr post self-esteem (53%) and happiness (44%) gains; no pre donor–nondonor–control differences in self-esteem or happiness – donor post scores were higher; 60% shortly post and 70% 1 yr post felt donation was high point of their life, 32% felt like better persons 1 yr post *Negative outcomes*: 31% somewhat depressed shortly post, some worried about own health (14%), sexuality (16%), or scar (26%), 26% have some negative feelings shortly post; donors who are male, married, not close to patient, family black sheep, receive less gratitude, less happy, and ambivalent, have more negative reactions

Table 3.2. (cont.)

Author	Design and sample characteristics	Analyses	Postdonation outcomes Perceived Physical	Psychosocial
Simmons (1981, 1983); Simmons and Anderson (1982, 1985)[b]	Longitudinal pre, 1 wk post, 1 yr post, 5–9 yr postdonation survey, 135 related kidney donors, 65 family nondonors	Pre–post comparison, donor vs. nondonor, successful vs. unsuccessful	—	Pre-1 wk post donor self-esteem increase; 1 wk and 5–9 yr post donor self-esteem higher than nondonor; 5–9 yr post unsuccessful donors had more regret and poorer sibling relationships than successful donors
Hirvas et al. (1980)	Longitudinal pre, 1 yr postdonation psychiatric assessment of 16 related kidney donors	Pre–post predictive	—	31% experienced moderate or severe psychiatric trauma; method developed for predicting which donors would experience trauma was unsuccessful
Weinstein et al. (1980)	Cross-sectional postdonation psychiatric assessment of 100 related kidney donors	Post descriptive	—	No donors experienced psychiatric or psychologic difficulties
Smith et al. (1986)	Cross-sectional 1–12 yr postdonation survey of 536 related kidney donors	Post descriptive	5% donation-related medical problem, 19% less physically active post, 8% donation had harmed health; donors who were white, female, felt underinformed, those who had financial problems perceived more physical problems	42% better post relationship with recipient, 2% post divorce related to donation; 23% donation was financial hardship (several spent ≥ $2,000 in donation-related costs)

Reference	Description	Comparison	Result	Result
Sharma and Enoch (1987)	Cross-sectional 5–10 yr postdonation survey of 14 related kidney donors and 9 family nondonors	Donors vs. nondonors, successful vs. unsuccessful		No difference in psychiatric morbidity between donors and nondonors or between successful and unsuccessful donors, all donors expressed positive feelings
Gouge et al. (1990)	Cross-sectional 5 yr postdonation survey of 36 related kidney donors and 30 family nondonors	Donors vs. nondonors	No difference in frequency of medical care hours/night slept, intercourse frequency, perceived health	No difference in life as a whole, general affect, well-being, positive/negative feelings, friendship satisfaction, marital satisfaction
Bone marrow donation				
Buckner et al. (1984)	Cross-sectional postdonation medical evaluation of 1549 unrelated marrow donors	Post descriptive	0.8% more painful than expected	—
Hill et al. (1989)	Longitudinal daily postdonation (1–13 days) donor verbal report of 30 related bone marrow donors	Post descriptive	Many patients experienced moderate to severe pain despite medication use, men reported more pain than women	—
Stroncek et al. (1989)	Cross-sectional postdonation survey of 20 unrelated marrow donors	Post descriptive	60% less painful than expected	95% happy they donated, 50% proud, 40% better person, 65% worried about recipient, 25% donation more negative than expected

Table 3.2. (cont.)

Author	Design and sample characteristics	Analyses	Postdonation outcomes	
			Perceived Physical	Psychosocial
Butterworth et al. (1993)[c]	Longitudinal pre, 2 wk post, 1 yr postdonation survey of 493 unrelated marrow donors	Post descriptive, longitudinal comparison	26% donation very/pretty stressful, 12% worried about own health, 20% more painful than expected; duration of anesthesia and duration of marrow collection predicted some perceived physical reactions	Generally positive about donation, 43% donation very/rather inconvenient, 23% could have been better prepared, 5% less emotionally positive than expected, 9% might not donate again; duration of anesthesia and marrow collection predicted some psychological reactions
Simmons et al. (1993)[b]	Longitudinal/cross-sectional pre, 2 wk post, 1 yr postdonation survey/interview, 966 unrelated bone marrow donors and 123 related kidney donors	Longitudinal comparison, marrow vs. kidney donors	—	Elevated pre-2 wk post self-esteem for *kidney donors only*; decline in pre-1 yr post self-esteem for marrow donors; marrow donors higher than kidney on self-esteem and better person measure at all timepoints; for marrow donors, recipient death was related to 1 yr post self-esteem and better person scores
Butterworth et al. (1992–93)[c]	Cross-sectional 1 yr postdonation survey/interview, of 330 unrelated marrow donors	Post descriptive, successful vs. unsuccessful	—	Universal feelings of grief among donors whose recipient died; both successful and unsuccessful donors would/did feel responsible for (33% vs. 19%)

Study	Design		
		or guilty about (23% vs. 22%) the donation outcome; successful donors felt more responsible than unsuccessful donors for donation outcomes	
Switzer et al. (1996)[c]	Longitudinal pre, 2 wk post, 1 yr postdonation survey of 343 unrelated marrow donors	Descriptive, path model for postdonation reactions	Majority of donors experienced at least moderate 2 wk post physical difficulty; females, younger donors, blood donors, and ambivalent donors had more physical difficulty	62% had some pre ambivalence; many had negative psychological reactions at 2 wk (38%) and 1 yr (33%) post; donor characteristics predict pre ambivalence; ambivalence is central predictor of post physical difficulty and negative psychological reactions

Related liver donation

Goldman (1993)	Longitudinal pre psychiatric interview and psychological tests post health and psychiatric status assessed informally by medical team and social worker for 22 related liver donors	Pre/post descriptive —	No postdonation depression or regression, higher post self-esteem and satisfaction
Sterneck et al. (1995)	Cross-sectional 6–31 mth postdonation survey of 26 related liver donors	Post descriptive	No serious medical complaints, 19% mild discomfort	27% financial difficulties, 19% professional difficulties, 35% family conflicts

a–c Table entries with identical notation numbers involve the same, or an overlapping group of, study participants.

Despite mostly positive psychosocial donation experiences, many kidney donors felt that the donation was relatively painful and many perceived long-term physical ill effects. Three of the four investigations that assessed donor physical health postdonation found self-reported medical problems among donors. Even several years postdonation (range 1 to 12 years), many donors (8% to 34%) felt that their health had not yet returned to normal or that the donation had permanently damaged their health (Smith et al. 1986; Simmons et al. 1987). Donors who were white or female felt underinformed about the process; those or who had financial problems related to donation were more prone to report medical problems (Smith et al. 1986). The contrast between negative physical and positive psychological consequences suggests that these domains are relatively unaffected by one another or that there is some bias in donor self-reporting. Though it has not been systematically investigated, some authors (e.g., Russell and Jacob 1993) argue that donor reports of psychosocial gains must be interpreted with caution because of donors' needs to maintain good feelings about having donated.

Bone marrow donation outcomes

Because the donation of bone marrow does not require general anesthesia and because it regenerates, it usually involves fewer medical risks to the donor and probably fewer long-term physical consequences. Though no studies have compared kidney and bone marrow donors' physical experiences, Simmons, Schimmel, and Butterworth (1993) compared these groups on two postdonation psychosocial outcomes: self-esteem and feelings of self-worth (e.g., feelings of being a "better person" postdonation). Both populations were assessed at one to two weeks predonation, one to two weeks postdonation, and one year postdonation. Overall, bone marrow donors' self-esteem and "better person" scores exceeded kidney donors' scores, except that kidney donors experienced self-esteem gains at the first postdonation assessment, while bone marrow donors did not. The relatively high levels of pre- and postdonation self-esteem among bone marrow donors as compared to kidney donors may have been partly due to demographic differences in that early bone marrow donors were highly educated and had above average occupational status. It is also possible that factors such as family pressure to donate that are inherent in the decision-making process for related, but not unrelated, donors might have preempted the self-image benefits that often result from making an uncoerced altruistic decision.

All but one of the studies concerning psychosocial issues in bone marrow donors come from Simmons' longitudinal investigation of the first 966 unrelated bone marrow donors to donate through the National Marrow Donor Program (the largest national bone marrow donor registry). Simmons' investigations (Butterworth, Simmons, and Schimmel 1992/1993;

Butterworth et al. 1993; Simmons et al. 1993; Switzer et al. 1996) and that of Stroncek et al. (1989) concur that the majority of bone marrow donors had positive experiences. Donors were happy that they donated (95%), proud of their donation (50%), felt like better people for having donated (40% to 71%), or felt that the donation had made their lives seem more worth while (75%). However, a significant percentage of donors *did* report at least some psychosocial difficulty with donation, including a feeling that they had been unprepared for the actual donation experience, concern about the marrow recipient, grief when the transplant failed, and more general negative feelings (e.g., having given up something for nothing in return). In terms of physical outcomes, many donors felt it was more painful and physically stressful than they had expected, and that they were concerned about their own long-term health. Although most studies did not examine predictors of physical difficulty with donation, one study did find that men reported more pain postdonation than did women (Hill et al. 1989).

One study examined the relationship of predonation demographic and psychosocial factors to postdonation physical and psychological difficulty (Switzer et al. 1996). Women, younger persons, frequent blood donors, and those with more predonation ambivalence all had more physical difficulty with donation than did their counterparts. These symptoms included fatigue, lower back pain, and more general feelings of "not being back to normal." Both short- and long-term negative postdonation psychological reactions were best predicted by predonation ambivalence. In addition, single persons, less frequent blood donors, less happy persons, and those having more physical difficulty with donation reported higher negative psychological reactions shortly postdonation than did their counterparts. The central finding of this study was the importance of predonation ambivalence in predicting postdonation physical and psychological reactions. Even when the effects of other variables were controlled, ambivalence exerted both direct and indirect effects on postdonation outcomes.

Liver donation outcomes

We could locate only two studies of perceived physical and psychosocial outcomes among living liver donors. One utilized a pre- to postdonation design in which the postdonation assessment was made informally by medical personnel in the course of routine medical examinations or by a social worker during incidental conversations with donors (Goldman 1993). This study found no psychiatric problems among donors and found elevated postdonation levels of self-esteem and life satisfaction, though outcomes data were not systematically gathered. The other study found that about one-fifth of donors continued to have minor physical discomfort several months after donation and that many experienced financial or professional difficulties, and family conflicts related to the donation (Sterneck et al. 1995).

In summary, living donors across several organ types experienced significant psychosocial benefits postdonation. Studies often report elevated self-esteem and happiness, and enhanced feelings of self-worth among donors. Donation "costs" include the small chance of developing psychiatric symptoms, negative feelings about having donated, pain and discomfort, and grief or feelings of responsibility if the recipient dies. Although few studies have examined the relationship of predonation factors to donation outcomes, the two large longitudinal studies concerned with this issue both found that predonation ambivalence was a central predictor of negative postdonation reactions (Simmons et al. 1977; Switzer et al. 1996). Finally, though direct comparisons of psychosocial issues across donation types have been rare, there is some evidence that more medically invasive donations and/or donations to a relative may produce less positive outcomes. It makes sense that kidney/liver donors would be more concerned about their long-term health status than would bone marrow donors and that related donors' experiences would be deeply affected by a personal relationship with the recipient and family anxiety about the donation outcome.

Conclusions and future research directions

Living organ donors make a unique contribution both to individual recipients and to broader society. Because their gift has such potentially high physical and psychological costs, it is incumbent upon us as a society to strive to fully understand the context in which decisions to donate are made. Such donation-related contexts include the full range of demographic and social factors that may affect donors' underlying motivations, their commitment to donation, and ultimately their physical and psychosocial donation experiences.

Most donors do not suffer from any lasting negative physical or psychosocial consequences of donation and, rather, experience significant psychic gains from helping another person. However, there is wide variability in the extent to which donors experience donation as positive. Less positive donation outcomes have been documented in large-scale longitudinal studies of both kidney and bone marrow donors and may well occur in other, newer forms of living donation such as liver and lung donation. Donors may feel that the donation has damaged their health or that their altruistic sacrifice has not been adequately appreciated – or they may feel partially responsible for the recipient's death, especially in cases of organ rejection or graft-versus-host disease. As advances in the medical technologies utilized in organ donation/transplantation become increasingly sophisticated, improved recipient prognosis may alleviate some postdonation guilt and feelings of responsibility among donors, as well as allay some of the donors' own health-related concerns. Conversely, routinization of the procedure may make members of the public and the medical community less sensitive to the magnitude of the donor's act, thereby enhancing his or her feelings of being unappreciated. In the current environment of rapidly advancing medical capabilities, it is crucial to continue to assess donation outcomes.

A second major conclusion that can be drawn from existing investigations is that less positive donation outcomes may be best predicted by predonation ambivalence or uncertainty about donation. That ambivalent feelings about donating can lead to less positive donation outcomes has not been appreciated until recently. This relationship – found in separate investigations of kidney and bone marrow donors – may be very useful in the practical settings of donor recruitment, education, and predonation counseling. Furthermore, investigations that explore the relationship of demographic, psychosocial, and social factors to ambivalence have the potential to inform applied and theoretical work in other healthy and ill populations.

Aside from these two fairly broad conclusions about donation experiences, many other important aspects about living donors are yet to be clarified. For example, donor motivations and decision-making processes remain only partially described and have not often been examined as predictors of donation outcomes. No comprehensive comparison of donation outcomes across organ types or across various combinations of donor–recipient relationships has been conducted. Psychiatric diagnostic evaluations are also lacking. Finally, broader issues of the social and political context within which organ donation occurs – including fears about AIDS or other diseases that could be transmitted during the donation, shifting norms about helpfulness to others, and religious barriers to donation – have rarely been investigated or even discussed.

References

Ajzen, I. (1985). From intentions to actions: A theory of planned behavior. In *Action-control: From Cognition to Behavior*, ed. J. Kuhl and J. Beckman, pp. 11–39. Heidelberg: Springer-Verlag.

Andrykowski, M. A. (1994a). Psychiatric and psychosocial aspects of bone marrow transplantation. *Psychosomatics*, **35**, 13–24.

Andrykowski, M. A. (1994b). Psychosocial factors in bone marrow transplantation: a review and recommendations for research. *Bone Marrow Transplant*, **13**, 357–75.

Beatty, P. G., Atcher, C., Hess, E., Meyer, D. M., and Slichter, S. J. (1989). Recruiting blood donors into a local bone marrow donor registry. *Transfusion*, **29**, 778–82.

Borgida, E., Conner, C., and Manteufel, L. (1992). Understanding living kidney donation: a behavioral decision-making perspective. In *Helping and Being Helped: Naturalistic Studies*, ed. S. Spacapan and S. Oskamp, pp. 183–211. Sage Publications: Newbury Park, CA.

Bortin, M. M. and Buckner, C. D. (1983). Major complications of marrow harvesting for transplantation. *Exp Hematol*, **11**, 916–21.

Briggs, N. C., Piliavin, J. A., and Becker, G.A. (1986). On willingness to be a bone marrow donor. *Transfusion*, **26**, 324–30.

Brim, O. G., Glass, D. C., Lavin, D. E., and Goodman, N. (1962). *Personality and Decision Processing*. Stanford University Press: Stanford, CA.

Buckner, C. D., Clift, R. A., Sanders, J. E. et al. (1984). Marrow harvesting from normal donors. *Blood*, 630–4.

Butterworth, V. A., Simmons, R. G., Bartsch, G., Randall, B., Schimmel, M., and Stroncek, D. F. (1993). Psychosocial effects of unrelated bone marrow donation: experiences of the national marrow donor program. *Blood*, **81**, 1947–59.

Butterworth, V. A., Simmons, R. G., and Schimmel, M. (1992–1993). When altruism fails: reactions of unrelated bone marrow donors when the recipient dies. *Omega*, **26**, 161–73.

Cacioppo, J. T. and Gardner, W. L. (1993). What underlies medical donor attitudes and behavior? *Health Psychol*, **12**, 269–71.

Callero, P.L. (1985). Role-identity salience. *Social Psychol Quart*, **48**, 203–15.

Callero, P. L., Howard, J. A., and Piliavin, J. A. (1987). Helping behavior as role behavior: disclosing social structure and history in the analysis of prosocial action. *Social Psychol Quart*, **50**, 247–56.

Callero, P. L. and Piliavin, J. A. (1983). Developing a commitment to blood donation: the impact of one's first experience. *J Appl Social Psychol*, **13**, 1–16.

Charng, H. W., Piliavin, J. A., and Callero, P. L. (1988). Role identity and reasoned action in the prediction of repeated behavior. *Social Psychol Quart*, **51**, 303–17.

Ewald, J., Aurell, M., Brynger, H. et al. (1976). The living donor in renal transplantation: a study of physical and mental morbidity and functional aspects. *Scand J Urol Nephrol*, **38**, 59–69.

Fellner, C. H. (1976/77). Renal transplantation and the living donor: decision and consequences. *Psychother Psychosomat*, **27**, 139–43.

Fellner, C. H. and Marshall, J. R. (1968). Twelve kidney donors. *JAMA* **206**, 2703–7.

Fellner, C. H. and Marshall, J. R. (1970). Kidney donors – the myth of informed consent. *Am J Psychiatry*, **126**, 79–85.

Fellner, C. H. and Marshall, J. R. (1981). Kidney donors revisited. In *Altruism and Helping Behavior: Social, Personality, and Developmental Perspectives*, ed. J. P. Rushton and R. M. Sorrentino, pp. 351–65. Lawrence Erlbaum: Hillsdale, NJ.

Fellner, C. H. and Schwartz, S. H. (1971). Altruism in disrepute: medical versus public attitudes toward the living organ donor. *New Engl J Med*, **284**, 582–5.

Gardner, W. E. and Cacioppo, J. T. (1995). Multi-gallon blood donors: why do they give? *Transfusion*, **35**, 795–8.

Goldman, L. S. (1993). Liver transplantation using living donors: preliminary donor psychiatric outcomes. *Psychosomatics*, **34**, 235–40.

Gouge, F., Moore, J., Bremer, B. A., McCauley, C. R., and Johnson, J. P. (1990). The quality of life of donors, potential donors, and recipients of living-related donor renal transplantation. *Transplant Proc*, **22**, 2409–13.

Hamburger, J. and Crosnier, J. (1968). Moral and ethical problems in transplantation. In *Human Transplantation*, ed. F. Rapaport and J. Dausset, pp. 37–44. Grune and Stratton: New York.

Higgerson, A. B. and Bulechek, G. M. (1982). A descriptive study concerning the psychosocial dimensions of living related kidney donation. *Am Assoc Nephrol Nurses Technicians*, **2**, 27–31.

Hill, R. (1970). *Family Development in Three Generations*. Schenkman: Cambridge, MA.

Hill, H. F., Chapman, C. R., Jackson, T. L., and Sullivan, K. M. (1989). Assessment and management of donor pain following marrow harvest for allogeneic bone marrow transplantation. *Bone Marrow Transplant*, **4**, 157–61.

Hirvas, J., Enckell, M., Kuhlback, B., and Pasternack, A. (1976). Psychological and social problems encountered in active treatment of chronic uraemia. *Acta Med Scand*, **200**, 17–20.

Hirvas, J., Enckell, M., Kuhlback, B., and Pasternack, A. (1980). Psychological and social problems encountered in active treatment of chronic uraemia. *Acta Med Scand*, **208**, 285–7.

Horton, R. L. and Horton, P. J. (1991). A model of willingness to become a potential organ donor. *Social Sci Med*, **33**, 1037–51.

House, R. M. and Thompson, T. L. (1988). Psychiatric aspects of organ transplantation. *JAMA*, **260**, 535–9.

Janis, I. L. and Mann, L. (1977). *Decision Making: A Psychological Analysis of Conflict, Choice, and Commitment*. Free Press: New York.

Kemph, J. P. (1966). Renal failure, artificial kidney and kidney transplant. *Am J Psychiatry*, **122**, 1270–4.

Kemph, J. P. (1967). Psychotherapy with patients receiving kidney transplant. *Am J Psychiatry*, **124**, 623–9.

Marshall, J. R. and Fellner, C. H. (1977). Kidney donors revisited. *Am J Psychiatry*, **134**, 575–6.

Omoto, A. M. and Snyder, M. (1995). Sustained helping without obligation: motivation, longevity of service, and perceived attitude change among AIDS volunteers. *J Personality Social Psychol*, **68**, 671–86.

Oswalt, R. M. (1977). A review of blood donor motivation and recruitment. *Transfusion*, **17**, 123–35.

Piliavin, J. A. and Callero, P. L. (1991). *Giving Blood: The Development of an Altruistic Identity*. Johns Hopkins University Press: Baltimore, MD.

Royse, D. and Doochin, K. E. (1995). Multi-gallon blood donors: who are they? *Transfusion*, **35**, 826–31.

Russell, S. and Jacob, R. G. (1993). Living-related organ donation: the donor's dilemma. *Patient Education Counsel*, **21**, 89–99.

Sadler, H. H., Davison, L., Carroll, C., and Kountz, S. L. (1971). The living, genetically unrelated, kidney donor. *Semin Psychiatry*, **3**, 86–101.

Sarason, I. G., Sarason, B. R., Slichter, S. J., Beatty, P. G., Meyer, D. M., and Bolgiano, D. C. (1993). Increasing participation of blood donors in a bone-marrow registry. *Health Psychol*, **12**, 272–6.

Schwartz, S. H. (1970). Elicitation of moral obligation and self-sacrificing behavior: an experimental study of volunteering to be a bone marrow donor. *J Personality Social Psychol*, **15**, 283–93.

Sharma, V. K. and Enoch, M. D. (1987) Psychological sequelae of kidney donation. A 5–10 year follow up study. *Acta Psychiatr Scand*, **75**, 264–7.

Sherman, S. J. and Fazio, R. H. (1983). Parallels between attitudes and traits as predictors of behavior. *J Personality*, **51**, 308–345.

Silberman, G., Crosse, M. G., Peterson, E. A. et al. (1994). Availability and appropriateness of allogeneic bone marrow transplantation for chronic myeloid leukemia in 10 countries. *New Engl J Med*, **331**, 1063–7.

Simmons, R. G. (1977). Related donors: costs and gains. *Transplant Proc*, 9, 143–5.

Simmons, R. G. (1981). Psychological reactions to giving a kidney. In *Psychonephrology*, vol. 1, ed. N. B. Levy, pp. 227–45. Plenum Press: New York.

Simmons, R. G. (1983). Long-term reactions of renal recipients and donors *Psychonephrology*, vol. 1, ed. N. B. Levy, pp. 275–87. Plenum Press: New York.

Simmons, R. G. and Anderson, C. R. (1982) Related donors and recipients: five to nine years post-transplant. *Transplant Proc*, **14**, 9–12.

Simmons, R. G. and Anderson, C. R. (1985). Social-psychological problems in living donor transplantation. *Transplant Clin Immunol*, **16**, 47–57.

Simmons, R. G., Bruce, J., Bienvenue, R., and Fulton, J. (1974). Who signs an organ donor-card: traditionalism versus transplantation. *J Chronic Dis*, **27**, 491–502.

Simmons, R. G., Klein, S. D., and Thornton, K. (1973). The family member's decision to be a kidney transplant donor. *J Comp Family Studies*, **4**, 88–115.

Simmons, R. G., Klein, S. D., and Simmons, R. L. (1977). *Gift of Life: The Social and Psychological Impact of Organ Transplantation*. A Wiley-Interscience: New York.

Simmons, R. G., Klein Marine, S., and Simmons, R. L. (1987). *Gift of Life: The Effect of Organ Transplantation on Individual, Family, and Societal Dynamics*. Transaction Books: New York.

Simmons, R. G., Schimmel, M., and Butterworth, V.A. (1993). The self-image of unrelated bone marrow donors. *J Health Social Behav*, **34**, 285–301.

Simon, H. A. 1957. *Administrative Behavior*, 2nd edn. Macmillan: New York.

Smith, M. D., Kappell, D. F., Province, M. A. et al. (1986). Living-related kidney donors: a multicenter study of donor education, socioeconomic adjustment, and rehabilitation. *Am J Kidney Dis*, **8**, 223–33.

Snyder, M. and Omoto, A.M. (1992). Volunteerism and society's response to the HIV epidemic. *Curr Directions Psychol Sc*, **1**, 113–16.

Steinberg, J., Levy, N. B., and Radvila, A. (1981). Psychological factors affecting acceptance or rejection of kidney transplants. In *Psychological Factors in Hemodialysis and Renal Transplantation*, ed. N. B. Levy, pp. 185–93. Plenum Press: New York.

Sterneck, M. R., Fischer, L., Nischwitz, U. et al. (1995). Selection of the living liver donor. *Transplantation*, **60**, 667–71.

Stroncek, D., Strand, R., Scott, E. et al. (1989). Attitudes and physical condition of unrelated bone marrow donors immediately after donation. *Transfusion*, **29**, 317–22.

Switzer, G. E., Dew, M. A., Butterworth, V. A., Simmons, R. G., and Schimmel, M. (1997). Understanding donors' motivations: a study of unrelated bone marrow donors. *Social Sci Med*, **45**, 137–47.

Switzer, G. E., Simmons, R. G., and Dew, M. A. (1996). Helping unrelated strangers: physical and psychological reactions to the bone marrow donation process among anonymous donors. *J Appl Social Psychol*, **26**, 469–90.

Titmuss, R. W. (1972). *The Gift Relationship: From Human Blood to Social Policy*. Vintage Books: New York.

Weinstein, S. H., Navarre, R. J., Loening, S. A., and Corry, R. J. (1980). Experience with live donor nephrectomy. *J Urol*, **124**, 321–3.

4

Quality of life in organ transplantation: effects on adult recipients and their families

Mary Amanda Dew Ph.D., Jean M. Goycoolea B.A.,
Galen E. Switzer Ph.D., Aishe S. Allen B.S.

Introduction

Over the past 25 to 30 years, the call to examine quality of life (QOL) as it is affected by transplantation has become stronger and more urgent. This has occurred because transplantation technology and immunosuppression have improved, leading transplants of many types to become more prevalent. The increasing prevalence of transplantation demands that we consider the full range of costs and benefits of these therapies to the individual recipient, his or her family, and society at large.

It is customary to begin articles focused on QOL in transplantation with the statement that QOL has seldom been investigated and/or that little is known about QOL in transplantation. In this review, we suggest that the first point is no longer true for the established types of transplantation in adults and, as regards the second, that more is known about QOL in transplantation than has been previously recognized. There are certainly gaps in what is known, and studies vary widely in their ability to contribute to this knowledge base depending on their design, the number of subjects and the types of comparison groups included. Nevertheless, as we have argued previously (Dew and Simmons 1990; Dew 1998), just as psychometric principles show that multi-item measures of any given domain increase the reliability of our overall assessment of the domain, so too do multiple studies of QOL – each with its own strengths and weaknesses – yield a more complete and accurate understanding of QOL in transplantation than that contained in any single investigation.

In the present chapter, we focus on QOL in the six types of transplantation in adults where surgical and other treatments are relatively well established and the probability of post-transplant survival is sufficiently high that the quality of that survival may be reasonably considered. These types are kidney, pancreas/combined kidney–pancreas, heart, lung/combined heart–lung, liver, and bone marrow transplantation. Across these transplant types, we will summarize evidence that addresses the following key questions:

Does QOL improve from pre- to post-transplantation?
Is QOL in transplant recipients better than QOL in other patient comparison groups?
Is QOL in transplant recipients similar to or better than QOL in healthy persons?
What effects does the transplantation experience have on QOL in recipients' families?

We begin with a brief overview of how QOL is typically defined and optimally measured in patients with chronic physical illness.

Quality of life and its measurement

The development of valid and reliable measures of QOL, plus growing evidence that QOL itself is sensitive and responsive to important biological and clinical changes, have led to its inclusion in clinical trials and quality-of-care evaluations across a spectrum of medical illnesses and conditions (Bombardier et al. 1986; Croog et al. 1986; Eschbach et al. 1989; McMillem et al. 1989; Canadian Erythropoietin Study Group 1990; Cleary et al. 1991; Tarlov 1992; Testa et al. 1993; Rogers et al. 1994; Hlatky et al. 1997; Pae et al. 1998; for reviews see Testa and Nackley 1994; Wilson and Cleary 1995; Bulpitt 1997; Revicki and Ehreth 1997; Fitzpatrick et al. 1998). For example, the National Heart, Lung and Blood Institute in the USA now routinely includes QOL assessments in clinical trials and efficacy studies of cardiovascular, lung, and blood therapies (Schron and Shumaker 1991; Schron, Gorkin, and Garg 1994; Avis et al. 1995; National Heart, Lung and Blood Institute 1995; Pae et al. 1998).

This emphasis is also growing in clinical practice settings and in health policy decision-making, where information about patients' QOL is increasingly being used by physicians and other health care providers for treatment decision-making and to plan allocation of resources (Edelson et al. 1990; Evans 1991; Freedberg et al. 1991; Their 1992; Patrick and Erickson 1993; Revicki and Ehreth 1997). For example, QOL was a key consideration in the Health Care Financing Administration's decision to extend Medicare coverage for recombinant human erythropoietin to dialysis-dependent end-stage renal disease patients (Edelson et al. 1990; Office of Technology Assessment 1990).

From a conceptual and medical ethics standpoint, the use of QOL as an indicator of treatment safety and efficacy is mandated by the World Health Organization's (WHO) definition of health as "a state of complete physical, mental, and social well-being and not merely absence of disease or infirmity"

(World Health Organization 1948). Indeed, the optimal assessments of QOL are multidimensional (as opposed to single, global indicators), incorporating the measurement of patients' functional status and well-being in each of the three dimensions in the WHO definition (Patrick and Deyo 1989; Dew and Simmons 1990). A multidimensional approach is essential in order to collect data adequate for the evaluation of the benefit/burden ratio associated with medical treatments (Testa and Nackley 1994; Revicki and Ehreth 1997). In reviewing studies of QOL in organ transplantation, we consider findings in each of the three domains of functioning and well-being defined above, in addition to patients' overall assessments of the quality of their lives. This latter component extends beyond how their health has affected any specific domain. Evans' work has shown that these global evaluations are often only modestly related to functioning in any specific domain and they provide additional insight into the QOL consequences of medical therapies (Evans 1990, 1991).

In terms of specific measurement approaches, two major categories of instrument have been designed to assess QOL in patient populations (Patrick and Deyo 1989; Patrick and Erickson 1993). Both rely primarily, although not exclusively, on patient self-report. First, a number of generic measures have been created that assess health status in broad terms. They provide overall evaluations of QOL domains that are relevant to every individual, regardless of specific illness. They are also useful because they allow comparisons across illness groups and across persons at different stages of the same illness. Second, disease- or illness-specific measures have been created to address symptoms and limitations unique to particular health conditions. Such measures are useful for understanding finer-grained differences between patients with similar conditions and are very important in clinical trials designed to improve certain symptoms or illness states that are related to specific diseases. Also in the category of specific measures are instruments designed to focus on particular areas of functioning, such as psychiatric status or cognitive status.

Currently, the QOL assessment approach that is considered to be optimal (Patrick and Deyo 1989; Stewart and Ware 1992; Testa and Nackley 1994; Fitzpatrick et al. 1998) and is becoming more commonplace in transplantation involves (a) selection of a generic measure to serve as the core instrument, and (b) supplementation of the core instrument with other measures to assess areas of particular concern to a given patient population. Such supplementation is important in transplantation studies because differences in procedures and treatments can lead to very different patient concerns. For example, QOL in the area of sexuality, though important for all transplant recipients, assumes particular significance for bone marrow recipients because infertility usually results from the irradiation prior to transplantation. Thus, although we focus below on broad differences in general physical functioning, mental health/cognitive status, social adjustment, and global QOL assessed across all transplant types, we also comment on QOL findings regarding issues of particular concern for specific areas of transplantation.

QOL studies included in the present review

Most studies of QOL in transplantation focus on the transplant recipient, and an examination of these studies' findings across approximately the first 20 years of research in this area constitutes the core of this review. Tables 4.1 to 4.6 summarize QOL studies of recipients in each of the six types of transplantation conducted through 1995. Although additional studies have appeared in the last four to five years, their findings are remarkably similar to those included in the tables (Dew, Switzer, and DiMartini 1998b; Dew et al. 1997; Joralemon and Fujinaga 1997). Individual qualitative reviews of specific QOL outcomes within each type of transplantation also continue to appear at a rapid rate (e.g., Gross and Raghu 1997: Dubernard et al. 1998; Goff, Glazner, and Bilir 1998; Gross, Limwattananon, and Matthews 1998; Neitzert et al. 1998; Wingard 1998), Their conclusions are very similar to those reached in the present review.

In the tables, each entry represents an independent investigation of a transplant sample, although any given investigation may have resulted in multiple publications that address different issues. The major publications available for each investigation are noted. The studies in the tables were retrieved via computerized literature searches using Medline, Current Contents, and Psychological Abstracts. The studies met several criteria. First, they were empirical studies of samples rather than case reports. Second, all respondents in the sample received systematic assessment (i.e., studies of only subsets of transplant recipients referred for special care were not included, nor were studies based upon medical records reviews alone). Information from special samples, for example, patients referred for psychiatric evaluation (Penn et al. 1971), are not generalizable to all transplant recipients. Finally, we were limited to reports published in English (with the exception of Bunzel et al. (1994a,b), which Dr. Bunzel discussed with us in English).

Tables 4.1 to 4.6 thus provide the "raw data" for our review of transplant recipient QOL outcomes. For each study, the country where the cohort was studied and the study design are noted (e.g., cross-sectional comparison of separate groups; longitudinal evaluation with more than one timepoint of data collection; prospective pre- and post-transplant evaluations). Sample size and timepoints for assessment relative to the transplant are noted. In studies with multiple samples, an asterisk indicates the key group for which we have summarized the findings (relative to the remaining comparison or

Table 4.1. Quality of life in samples of kidney transplant recipients

Author, country	Design and sample characteristics	Major instruments/ assessments[a]	Quality of Life Domains			
			Physical functional	Mental health/cognitive	Social	Overall QOL
Simmons et al. (1977, 1981, 1984) USA	Prospective *n ≥ 178; pre, 3 weeks, 1 year, 5–9 years post n = 130 family donors n = 186 family nondonors	Simmons health scales; Rosenberg Self-Esteem; Bradburn Happiness; Campbell QOL and Social Adjustment items	Sustained pre to post improvement in ability to do daily activities, ambulation, mobility; reduction of fatigue, pain	Pre to post improvement in depression, anxiety levels, with some decline by 5–9 years post; emotional well-being similar to that of nonpatient groups and norms	58% employed/ student by 1 year post; 62% by 5–9 years post; pre to post improvement in job, recreation, social, family roles and satisfaction; remained stable over time	Sustained pre to post improvement; levels became similar to nonpatient groups and norms
Procci et al. (1978); Procci (1980) USA	Cross-sectional/ retrospective *n ≥ 37; ≥ 6 mos. post[b] n = 16 dialysis patients	Social Disability Rating Scale; unnormed question	—	Slightly higher levels of depression than controls	19% employed in both groups; complaints of sexual dysfunction equal in both groups but txp patients reported that sexual activity improved	No differences between groups
Sophie and Powers (1979) USA	Cross-sectional n = 24, < 1 years to 9 years post	Cantril's Self-Anchoring Scale; unnormed questions	—	—	45.8% employed full-time, rate increased over pre-txp dialysis period; more satisfied with social life, no change in family life post-txp	QOL rated as better than pre-txp and expected to continue to improve

Table 4.1. (cont.)

Author, country	Design and sample characteristics	Major instruments/ assessments[a]	Quality of Life Domains			
			Physical functional	Mental health/cognitive	Social	Overall QOL
De-Nour and Shanan (1980) Israel	Prospective *n = 11; pre, 1 year n = 20 dialysis patients	Coping measure; sentence completion	—	Pre to post improvement in self-image; most had good psychological adjustment post-txp and better than controls	36% employed full-time, rate somewhat higher than controls; social adjustment/activities similar across groups	—
Frisk et al. (1980) Sweden	Cross-sectional n = 46; ≥ 10 years post	Unnormed questions	Majority reported excellent physical health, few disabilities	Majority reported excellent emotional well-being	80% employed	Overall QOL rated as similar to others of same age
Devins et al. (1981, 1982, 1983–1984, 1986–1987); Binik et al. (1982, 1986, 1989); Chowanec and Binik (1989) Canada	Cross-sectional *n = 45,[b] ≥ 1 year post n ≥ 53[b] dialysis patients (inc. txp failures)	Illness Intrusiveness; McGill Pain; SCL-90; BDI; HAM-D; POMS; ABS; Helplessness; Life Satisfaction; Locke–Wallace Marital Adjustment	Slightly less pain and less impact of illness on well-being than controls	Slightly less depression, helplessness than controls; slightly better self-esteem and overall mood/distress level than controls but poorer than norms	Approx. 55–59% employed, similar to controls; no differences in marital and sexual adjustment but lower than norms	Similar or lower life satisfaction and happiness than controls

Study	Design/Sample	Measures	Functioning	Psychological	Social/Employment	Quality of life
Johnson et al. (1982) USA	Cross-sectional *n=20; post n=20 txp candidates or failed txp n=19 dialysis only	Campbell QOL items; ABS; unnormed questions	Less fatigue than all controls	Mood and affect more positive than txp-related controls, but similar to dialysis controls and to norms	70% employed or housework, rate higher than controls; satisfaction with marriage and family similar to controls	QOL rated higher than txp-related controls, similar to dialysis controls and norms
Kalman et al. (1983) USA	Cross-sectional *n=57; ≥ 5 years post n=44 dialysis patients	GHQ; Beck Hopelessness Scale	—	No differences in psychiatric morbidity between groups; txp patients were slightly more distressed	No group differences in employment status	—
Keegan et al. (1983) Canada	Prospective n=27; pre, 1, 6, 12, 24 mos. post	MMPI; Perceived Effects of Illness	Pre to post decline in perceived impact of illness on activities	Depression higher than norms pre-txp, improved post-txp; anxiety low pre and post-txp	Less than 50% employed by 2 years post; pre to post improvement in social adjustment	—
Evans et al. (1985a,b); Hart and Evans (1987) USA	Cross-sectional *n=144, average 51 mos. post n=715 dialysis patients n=152 heart recipients	Karnofsky; SIP; Campbell QOL items	Low levels of impairment and better than other groups	Psychological affect better than dialysis and heart patients; similar to norms	54% employed; rate higher than in dialysis and heart patients; social adjustment better than other patients	Well-being and life satisfaction higher than other patients and similar to norms
Rodin et al. (1985–1986) Canada	Prospective *n=42; pre, 6 mos. post n=51 txp candidates or failed txp	SIP, BDI	Pre to post improvement in functional status and better than controls	Pre to post improvement in depression symptom levels and overall emotional well-being; better than controls	—	—

Table 4.1. (*cont.*)

Author, country	Design and sample characteristics	Major instruments/ assessments[a]	Quality of Life Domains			
			Physical functional	Mental health/cognitive	Social	Overall QOL
Kutner et al. (1986) USA	Longitudinal/ prospective, 3 assessments 18 mos. apart *n = 10; post only, median 35 mos. post *n = 10; pre, 18, 36 mos. post n = 50 dialysis patients	Zung Depression and Anxiety Scales; unnormed questions	Post-txp fatigue and overall health perceptions similar to controls; appetite better than controls	Post-txp depression, anxiety symptom levels tended to be higher than controls but declined from pre to post-txp	62% to 70% employed or student post-txp, higher than controls; satisfaction with leisure improved post-txp with some decline over time, but was stable in controls	—
Nadel & Clark (1986) USA	Cross-sectional *n = 15; post-txp n = 9 failed txp	Zung Depression Scale; unnormed questions	—	All but 2 had mild or major psychiatric disorder, rate higher than in failed txp group	47% employed, rate higher than failed txp group; less sexual dysfunction than failed txp group	Majority scored high, averaging above failed txp group

Study	Design	Measures				
Churchill et al. (1987); Russell et al. (1992) Canada	Cross-sect, prospective *n=79; ≥ 3 mos. post *n=27; pre, 1.5–52 mos. post n=115 dialysis patients (cross-sectional only)	Time Tradeoff Evaluation; MOS; Q-L Index	—	Similar post-txp levels of depression, anxiety as controls but higher levels of happiness	71% employed full-time, rate increased from pre-txp; more social activity, involvement post-txp than controls, similar to norms	Pre to post improvement; better perceived QOL post txp than controls
Hong et al. (1987) USA	Cross-sect, retrospective *n=15; ≥ 1 year post n=45 dialysis patients	SADS	—	Lower rate of major depression since ESRD onset than controls, but higher rate than controls since onset of current treatment	—	—
House (1987) UK	Longitudinal, 2 assessments 12 most. apart *n=20; post-txp n=40 dialysis patients	PSE; GHQ; SSAM	—	Lower rates of psychiatric disorder than controls at both assessments	Less work, social, family, marital, sexual disability than controls; all improved with time	—
Seedat et al. (1987) South Africa	Cross-sectional *n=46; 1–138 mos. post n=82 dialysis patients	Karnofsky; BDI; unnormed questions	Majority had no functional limitations; better than controls	Low average level of depressive symptoms; lower than controls	63% employed, rate higher than controls; more were satisfied with sexual activity than controls	Slightly higher life satisfaction than controls

Table 4.1. (*cont.*)

Author, country	Design and sample characteristics	Major instruments/ assessments[a]	Quality of Life Domains			
			Physical functional	Mental health/cognitive	Social	Overall QOL
Morris and Jones (1988, 1989) Australia	Cross-sectional *n=69; 5–174 mos. post n=69 dialysis patients	GHQ; unnormed questions	Higher level of satisfaction with health than controls	Distress levels were similar to controls and other patient populations	42% employed; more satisfaction with social functioning than controls; similar in sexual, family relationship satisfaction	Higher life satisfaction than controls
Parfrey et al. (1988a,b, 1989); Barrett et al. (1989) Canada	Longitud./ prospective, 2 assessments, 1 year apart *n=67; average > 3 years post *n=20 pre, post n=63 dialysis patients	Physical symptom scale; Karnofsky; Campbell QOL items; Q-L Index	Txp groups had fewer symptoms and activity limitations than controls; pre to post improvement in functional status unless txp failed; little change over time post-txp	All had similar mood, affect, overall emotional well-being at baseline; txp groups improved over time unless txp failed; dialysis group did not change	—	All had similar life satisfaction at base-line; txp groups improved with time unless txp failed
Simmons et al. (1988, 1990); Simmons and Abress (1990) USA	Cross-sectional *n=91; 1–4 years post, *n=82; 5–9 years post, *n=593 dialysis patients (from earlier 1977 study n=593 dialysis patients	Simmons health scales; Rosenberg Self-Esteem; Bradburn Happiness; Campbell QOL and Social Adjustment items	Both txp groups had higher levels of satisfaction, well-being, activity than controls	Txp groups had better mood and affect than controls, similar to norms	69% of txp groups employed/student full-time, rate higher than controls; satisfaction in job, social, recreation, sexual, family roles higher in txp groups than controls	Higher life satisfaction in txp groups than controls; levels similar to norms

Study	Design	Measures	Physical/functional	Emotional well-being	Employment/social	Life satisfaction/overall
Bremer et al. (1989) USA	Cross-sectional *n=187; ≥ 3 mos. post n=302 dialysis patients	Campbell QOL items; ABS; unnormed questions	Less fatigue, fewer activities avoided than controls; similar pain levels as controls; satisfaction with health higher than controls, equal to norms	Emotional well-being higher than controls and similar to norms; affect/happiness higher than controls and norms	48% employed full-time, higher than controls; satisfaction with friends, marriage, children similar across groups and slightly lower than norms	Higher life satisfaction than controls; similar to norms
Julius et al. (1989) USA	Cross-sectional *n=163; ≥ 6 mos. post n=296 dialysis patients	Katz and OARS ADL; SIP	Less ADL limitations than controls but more than norms; better physical functional status than controls but poorer than norms	—	—	—
Petrie (1989) New Zealand	Cross-sectional *n=30; post-txp n=75 dialysis patients n=126 primary care patients	GHQ; Mental Health Inventory	—	Distress levels lower than dialysis patients and similar to primary care patients	—	Better overall well-being than dialysis patients, similar to primary care patients
Sensky (1989) UK	Prospective n=51; pre, 1 year post	CIS; HADS	—	Pre to post decline in psychiatric disorder rate; decline in depression, anxiety symptom levels	—	—
Sutton and Murphy (1989) USA	Cross-sectional n=40; 0–48 mos. post	Baldree Stressor Scale	Physical activity limitations were among the most common problems endorsed	—	30% employed full-time; little stress reported in family, friend relationships	—

Table 4.1. (*cont.*)

Author, country	Design and sample characteristics	Major instruments/ assessments[a]	Quality of Life Domains			
			Physical functional	Mental health/cognitive	Social	Overall QOL
Andrykowski et al. (1990b) USA	Cross-sectional *n = 29; 17–97 mos. post n = 29 bone marrow recipients	SIP; FLIC; POMS; PAIS; PHQ	No group differences in perceived health or functional status; all rated health as poorer than other samples; no change with time post-txp	More depressed but otherwise similar to controls; all were more distressed than other samples; no change with time post-txp	31% employed, rate slightly lower than controls; similar in work, family, sexual, social adjustment; no change with time post-txp	—
Devins et al. (1990) Canada	Longitudinal, 2 assessments 6 weeks apart *n = 34, post-txp n = 65 dialysis patients	Illness Intrusiveness Scale; BDI; ABS; Beck Hopelessness Scale; Life Satisfaction	Lower impact of illness on physical well-being than controls; no differences in fatigue and daily activities	Similar levels of depression, hopelessness, general affect	Lower impact of illness on work and relationships than controls; no differences for social activity	Similar or lower life satisfaction than controls
Evans et al. (1990); Manninen et al. (1991); Evans (1992) USA	Longitudinal, retrospective *n = 396; 3–18 mos. post (204 reassessed 2.5–3.5 years post) n = 22 failed txp after 18 mos.	Limitations of Daily Activity; SIP	Limitations in vigorous activities, but fewer than controls; similar limitations in vision, carrying weights; better perceived health and satisfaction than controls	Good emotional well-being and better than controls	52% able to work; higher than controls; better social interaction and adjustment than controls	—

Study	Design & sample	Measures		Mood	Employment/social	Overall QOL
Gouge et al. (1990) USA	Cross-sectional *n=42; average of 57 mos. post; n=10 failed txp; n=36 kidney donors; n=30 potential donors	Campbell QOL items; ABS; unnormed questions	More activities avoided in patient than in donor groups; satisfaction with health lower in patient than in donor groups and lower than norms	Mood similar in txp and donor groups, and both similar to norms and better than dialysis patients; affect/happiness similar across all groups	43% employed full-time; higher than dialysis patients but lower than donor groups; all groups similar in adjustment to norms	Similar overall satisfaction to donors and to norms, better than dialysis patients
Koch and Muthny (1990) Germany	Cross-sectional retrospective *n=761; 2 mos.–12 years post; n=358 dialysis patients	Unnormed questions	Pre to post improvement in functioning and better than controls; fatigue noted as continuing problem	Pre to post decline in depression, fearfulness; levels somewhat better than controls	28% employed full-time, pre to post increase; pre to post improvement in family, social relationships, less change in work and sexual satisfaction, but all areas higher than controls	Reported pre to post QOL improvements; better than controls
Hauser et al. (1991) USA	Longitudinal n=39; early post (16–26 mos.); later post	Inpatient transplant interview	Most did not feel as well as expected and had continuing difficulties in resuming activities	—	36% employed full-time, increased with time; had more time for social activities, but relationships often worsened	—
Lai et al. (1992a,b) Taiwan	Cross-sectional *n=90; average 4 years post; n=198 dialysis patients	Parfrey health items; Campbell QOL items; Q-L Index	Most able to resume normal daily activities post-txp	—	—	Rated QOL higher than controls' ratings

Table 4.1. (cont.)

Author, country	Design and sample characteristics	Major instruments/assessments[a]	Quality of Life Domains			
			Physical functional	Mental health/cognitive	Social	Overall QOL
Park et al. (1992) Korea	Cross-sectional *n=96; average 40 mos. post n=114 dialysis patients	Unnormed questions	—	—	64% employed	Rated QOL above midpoint on scale; better than controls
Gorlen et al. (1993) Norway	Cross-sectional n=31; 10–22 years post	Unnormed questions	Majority rated physical health as medium to very good	Most reported no psychological or alcohol use problems post-txp	71% employed full-time; highly satisfied with family relationships; moderately satisfied with social activity	Majority rated QOL above midpoint on scale
Benedetti et al. (1994) USA	Cross-sectional n=151 aged 60+; 1–7 years post	SF-36	Lower than norms on physical functioning and limitations; similar to norms on general health, fatigue, pain	Similar to norms on emotional well-being	Similar or slightly lower than norms on role functioning	—
Yoshimura et al. (1994) Japan	Prospective n=109; pre, ≤ 2 years post	Unnormed questions	Pre to post improvement in activity, exercise, vision; worsening in bone/joint pain	Pre to post improvement in emotional well-being	Pre to post improvement in social relationships	—

Frazier et al. (1995) USA	Cross-sectional *n = 121; 3–46 mos. post n = 121 spouses	BDI: Dyadic Adjustment Scale	—	Recipients had higher depression levels than spouses, but both groups fell in nondepressed range of scale	Marital satisfaction levels similar to norms and to controls	—
Gudex (1995) UK	Cross-sectional *n = 367, post-txp n = 249 dialysis patients	Health Measurement Questionnaire	Less impairment than controls in mobility, self-care, sleep, energy, ability to daily activities, but worse than norms	Less depression, anxiety, overall distress than controls and similar to norms	Social, leisure, sexual activity less impaired than controls but worse then norms	—
Hilbrands et al. (1995) Netherlands	Longitudinal n = 120; 3, 6, 12 mos. post	SIP; CES-D; ABS; Campbell QOL items	Improvement in functional status; decline in weakness and fatigue over time post-txp	Low and stable levels of depression and negative mood over time post-txp	Social adjustment was high and increased over time post-txp	High levels of satisfaction with life, similar to norms
Ohkubo (1995) Japan	Cross-sectional retrospective n = 701; 3 mos.–21.25 years post	Unnormed questions	Pre to post improvement in perceived health status	—	87% employed full-time, increased from pre-txp; majority felt social adjustment and activity were similar to those of healthy persons	—

Asterisks denote study groups of key interest; QOL, quality of life; txp, transplant; mos., months; ESRD, end stage renal disease.

[a]Instrument abbreviations: ABS, Affect Balance Scale; BDI, Beck Depression Inventory; CES-D, Center for Epidemiologic Studies Depression Scale; CIS, Clinical Interview Schedule; FLIC, Functional Living Index – Cancer; GHQ, General Health Questionnaire; HADS, Hospital Anxiety and Depression Scale; HAM-D, Hamilton Rating Scale for Depression; MMPI, Minnesota Multiphasic Personality Inventory; MOS, Medical Outcomes Study Form; OARS ADL, Older Americans Resources and Services Activities of Daily Living; PAIS, Psychological Adjustment to Illness Scale; PHQ, Perceived Health Questionnaire; POMS, Profile of Mood States; PSE, Present State Examination; Q-L Index, Spitzer Quality of Life Index; SADS, Schedule for Affective Disorders and Schizophrenia; SCL-90, Symptom Checklist-90; SF-36, Medical Outcomes Study Short Form-36; SIP, Sickness Impact Profile; SSAIM, Structured and Scaled Interview to Assess Maladjustment.

[b] Multiple papers reported on partially overlapping samples; degree of sample overlap or total number of persons studied cannot be determined.

Table 4.2. Quality of life in samples of pancreas (P) or combined kidney–pancreas (K–P) transplant recipients.

Author country	Design and sample characteristics	Major instruments/ assessments[a]	Quality of life domains			
			Physical functional	Mental health/cognitive	Social	Overall QOL
Nakache et al. (1989, 1994) Sweden	Longitudinal *n = 14 K–P; ≥ 2 years post and 5 years later n = 16 kidney	Q-L Index; Reintegration Index; unnormed questions	Rated physical abilities, activity level and overall healthy similarly early post-txp; K–P group continued to improve subsequently, controls did not	—	90% employed full-time higher than controls; slightly higher reintegration into work, family, social roles; advantage over controls increased over time; pre to post decline in sexual satisfaction only in controls	Larger increase and somewhat better post-txp QOL ratings than controls
Voruganti and Sells (1989) UK	Cross-sectional *n = 10 K–P; 6–54 mos. post n = 6 kidney only	PAIS; Rosenberg Self-esteem; Bradburn Happiness; Campbell QOL items	—	No differences in mood, affect, psychological distress	50% employed, slightly higher than kidney group; rated work, home, sexual adjustment better, no differences in social activities/adjustment	Rated general well-being higher than controls
Corry and Zehr (1990); Zehr et al. (1991); Milde et al. (1992, 1995) USA	Cross-sectional *n = 41 K–P; 6 mos.–6 years post n = 13 K–P, failed P n = 28 kidney only	Karnofsky; Subjective Fatigue Scale; BDI; MAACL; Campbell QOL items	No group differences; fatigue, weakness were common in all groups; K–P group perceived overall health somewhat better than failed group and similar to kidney group	Low depression, anxiety, hostility levels; similar across groups	58% employed, somewhat higher than both control groups	Rated QOL slightly higher in K–P and kidney groups than failed group, but slightly lower than norms

Study	Design	Measures	Functional status/health	Mood/affect	Employment/satisfaction	QOL
Johnson et al. (1990) USA	Prospective n = 15 K–P; pre, 3, 6, 9, 12 mos. post	Karnofsky; unnormed questions	Pre to post improvement in functional status with minor activity limitations by 1 year post	—	40% employed	—
Nathan et al. (1991) USA	Prospective *n = 25 K–P; pre, ≥ 6 mos. post n = 14 kidney only	DCCT measure	Pre to post reduction in concern about diabetes only in K–P group	—	Pre to post reduction of worry about work only in K–P group	Pre to post rise in overall satisfaction only in K–P group
Piehlmeier et al. (1991) Germany	Cross-sectional *n = 31 K–P; 1–91 mos. post n = 29 K–P, failed P n = 15 K–P failed both n = 9 P alone, failed n = 73 P txp candidates	Scales utilized in Germany; SCL-90	Satisfaction with functional status best in K–P group, but majority felt impaired; only small differences from K–P group with failed P graft	Less depression, slightly less anxiety than other groups; K–P group most satisfied with subjective cognitive status but all groups reported high rates of such problems	26% employed, rate similar or lower than other groups; higher satisfaction with leisure, social, work, marriage, family than other groups; similar to other groups on sexual satisfaction	Rated QOL higher than other groups
Secchi et al. (1991) Italy	Cross-sectional *n = 17 K–P; 1–5 years post n = 13 K–P, failed P	Unnormed questions	Perceived health better than failed P group slightly more active	—	63% employed, rate slightly higher than failed P group; higher level of social activity	—
Zehrer and Gross (1991); Gross and Zehrer (1992) USA	Cross-sectional *n = 65 P or K–P only; 1–11 years post n = 66 failed P	Karnofsky; Simmons health items; Campbell QOL and Social Adjustment items; SF-20	Higher functional status, perceived health, ability to do daily activities; less pain than failed P groups, but all indices lower than norms	Better mood and affect than failed P group but lower than norms	37% employed full-time, rate similar to failed P group; low activity/role satisfaction; higher social functioning than failed P group but lower than norms	QOL rated higher than failed P group but lower than norms

Table 4.2. *(cont.)*

Author country	Design and sample characteristics	Major instruments/ assessments[a]	Quality of life domains			
			Physical functional	Mental health/cognitive	Social	Overall QOL
Gross and Zehrer (1993) USA	Cross-sectional *$n = 37$ K–P; 1–11 years post (subset of Zehrer and Gross, 1991) $n = 50$ kidney only	SF-36; DCCT Life Satisfaction and Lifestyle	Better perceived health and satisfaction with health than controls; slightly better functional status	No differences in emotional well-being	30% employed; better social functioning, somewhat better role function than controls; perceived less impact of health on family	Majority of both groups had moderate to high life satisfaction
Stratta et al. (1993) USA	Prospective *$n = 30$ K–P after dialysis; pre, 4–36 mos. post *$n = 31$ K–P, no past dialysis	Unnormed questions	—	—	50% employed full-time in group with past dialysis; rate slightly higher than other group but required longer rehabilitation; pre to post improvement in social activity similar across groups	—
Esmatjes et al. (1994) Spain	Cross-sectional *$n = 12$ K–P; ≥ 1 year post $n = 10$ kidney only (including failed P) $n = 10$ dialysis patients	Karnofsky; Q-L Index; unnormed questions	Functional status and perceived health higher in K–P group, but all groups did little exercise/sports activity	—	100% employed, slightly higher than other groups; slightly better reintegration into work, social, family roles	Rated QOL slightly higher than other groups

Study	Design/sample	Instruments				
Hathaway et al. (1994); Gaber et al. (1994) USA	Prospective *n=12 K–P; pre, 12 mos. post n=7 kidney only	SIP	Pre to post improvement in ambulation, body care, movement, overall functional status; slightly more improvement in K–P group	Pre to post improvement in emotional well-being; no group differences	Pre to post improvement in work, home, social functioning; slightly more improvement in K–P group	—
Kiebert et al. (1994) Netherlands	Cross-sectional, retrospective *n=17 K–P; 2–74 mos. post n=11 failed P and/or kidney n=23 kidney only	NHP; EuroQol: STAI	Successful K–P group had better mobility than kidney group; failed txp group had more fatigue than other groups and slightly less satisfaction with health	No differences in psychological well-being	More social isolation in failed txp group than other groups	Rated QOL similarly in K–P and kidney groups and better than failed txp group
Schareck et al. (1994) Germany	Cross-sectional, retrospective n=45 K–P; ≥ 1 year post	Unnormed questions	Majority had nausea; degree did not improve post-txp	—	38% employed	Pre to post improvement in QOL
Zehrer and Gross (1994) USA	Prospective *n=14 K–P; pre, 1 year post n=16 kidney only n=23 diabetes patients	SF-36; DCCT Life Satisfaction and Lifestyle	Pre to post improvement in perceived health, fatigue, pain in K–P and kidney groups but worse than norms; no differences in controls; functional status worse in kidney group	Slight improvement over time in all groups but poorer than norms	Pre to post improvement in social functioning but lower than norms; no change in controls; K–P group reported less impact of health on role function and family	—

Asterisks denote study groups of key interest; QOL, quality of life; txp, transplant; mos., months.

[a]Instrument abbreviations: BDI, Beck Depression Inventory; DCCT, Diabetes Control and Complications Trial; EuroQol, European Quality of Life Questionnaire; MAACL, Multiple Affect Adjective Checklist; NHP, Nottingham Health Profile; PAIS, Psychological Adjustment to Illness Scale; Q-L Index, Spitzer Quality of Life Index; SCL-90, Symptom Checklist-90; SF-20 and SF-36, Medical Outcomes Study Short Form-20 and -36; SIP, Sickness Impact Profile; STAI, Spielberger State-Trait Anxiety Inventory.

Table 4.3. Quality of life in samples of heart transplant recipients

Author, country	Design and sample characteristics	Major instruments/ assessments[a]	Quality of life domains				
			Physical functional	Mental health/cognitive	Social	Overall QOL	
Evans et al. (1984, 1985a,b); Evans (1987, 1992) USA	Cross-sectional *n = 152; post n = 540 kidney recipients n = 715 dialysis patients	Karnofsky; SIP; Campbell QOL items	Better functional status and perceived health than dialysis patients but worse than kidney recipients	Somewhat worse than other patient groups and norms on emotional well-being, but more happiness than other patients and norms	32% employed, rate lower than kidney recipients; social adjustment worse than kidney but better than dialysis patients	Rated QOL worse than other groups, lower than norms	
Samuelsson et al. (1984) USA	Cross-sectional n = 23; 1–6 years post	Unnormed questions	Majority rated status as good–excellent and similar or better than persons of same age; majority had few restrictions in daily activity, exercise, self-care	—	30% employed full-time; majority were satisfied with marital relationships; slightly less satisfied with sexual activity	Majority were satisfied with life since txp	
Buxton et al. (1985); Wallwork and Caine (1985); O'Brien et al. (1987); Caine and O'Brien (1989); Caine et al. (1990, 1992) UK	Cross-sectional/ prospective *n = 122; pre, every 3 mos. post *n = 45; once 6 mos.–2 years post n = 30 CABG patients	NHP; unnormed questions	Pre to post improvement in mobility, pain, sleep, energy, activity level in all groups; larger change in txp group who became similar to CABG group by 1 year post; all groups had continued sleep problems; little further change over time	Pre to post improvement in emotional well-being in all groups; txp patients were worse pre-txp but similar to CABG patients at 1 year post; all groups had better emotional well-being than norms; little further change over time	28% to 47% employed full-time by 1 year post; rate lower than CABG group; pre to post improvement in social involvement/ activities, sexual, family relations for all groups; no group differences and similar to norms; little further change over time	Pre to post improvement in QOL rating in txp patients; became similar to CABG patients	

Study	Design/Sample	Measures	Physical	Psychological	Social	Quality of life
Lough et al. (1985, 1987) USA	Cross-sectional, retrospective n = 75; 7 mos.–14 years post	Unnormed questions	Pre to post improvement in overall status, endurance; many still had pain, fatigue, sleep problems	Pre to post improvement in self-esteem; depression was common; many reported subjective cognitive complaints	Pre to post improvement in family, friend relationships; some sexual problems; more social activity post-txp	Rated QOL and satisfaction with QOL well above scale midpoint
McAleer et al. (1985); Meister et al. (1986) USA	Cross-sectional n = 40; 3 mos.–6 years post	Unnormed questions	Many reported chronic pain	Majority reported mood alterations; all showed psychological distress	32% employed by 1 year post; majority reported marital stress; sexual and family problems were common	—
Mai et al. (1986, 1990) Canada	Prospective n = 24; pre, 12 mos. post	PSE; SCL-90; GHQ; unnormed questions	Pre to post improvement in physical activity	Pre to post decline in rate of psychiatric disorder, decline in anxiety symptoms but not depression	71% employed, increased over pre-txp rate; majority had no sexual dysfunction	—
Brennan et al. (1987) USA	Cross-sectional retrospective n = 11; 9–15 mos. post	Unnormed questions	Majority perceived largest degree of pre to post improvement to be in physical health	—	45% employed; most perceived little pre to post change in social, vocational adjustment	Rated QOL very high post-txp
Freeman et al. (1988) USA	Prospective n = 40; ≤ 6 mos., 6–12 mos., annually thereafter	PAIS; STAI; Zung Depression Scale MMSE; unnormed questions	—	High rate of psychiatric problems post-txp, but depression, anxiety levels were better post-txp and continued to improve with time	Pre to post improvement in social adjustment, continued improvement over time	—

Table 4.3. (cont.)

Author, country	Design and sample characteristics	Major instruments/ assessments[a]	Quality of life domains			
			Physical functional	Mental health/cognitive	Social	Overall QOL
Harvison et al. (1988); Jones et al. (1990) Australia	Cross-sectional retrospective $n = 47 + 25$; 3 mos.–3 years post (overlapping samples)	Rosenberg Self-esteem, Happiness; Campbell QOL items; unnormed questions	High average ratings of physical well-being and activity level; better than pre-txp	Above midpoint of scales on self-esteem, happiness; moderate anxiety; high levels of overall affect	36% to 47% employed full-time; high levels of family, marital satisfaction; moderate sexual, social satisfaction	Level of overall satisfaction higher than norms
Jones et al. (1988, 1992a) Australia	Prospective $n = 38$; pre, discharge, 4, 8, 12 mos.; 3.5–5.2 years post	NHP; BDI; STAI; Campbell QOL and Social Adjustment items	At final assessment, mobility, pain, energy were similar or better than other patient groups	Pre to post improvement in depression, anxiety; low levels of depression, anxiety post-txp stable over time	50% employed full-time by 1 year post; majority satisfied with marriage, family	Pre to post improvement in QOL ratings
Kuhn et al. (1988, 1990) USA	Prospective $n = 40$; pre, ≥ 3 mos. post	Unnormed clinical interview	—	Pre to post decline in rate of psychiatric diagnoses	—	—
Niset et al. (1988) Belgium	Prospective $n = 62$; pre, ≤ 1 year post	SIP	Pre to post improvement in ambulation, mobility, body care, sleep; continued improvement over time post-txp	Pre to post decline in emotional well-being early post-txp; some improvement thereafter	71% returned to prior work by 4 mos. post; pre to post decline in social functioning early post-txp followed by improvement	—

Study	Design/Sample	Measures				
Aravot et al. (1989) UK	Prospective $n=21$; pre, 6 mos. post	NHP	Pre to post improvement in mobility, pain, sleep, energy; larger change than other QOL domains	Pre to post improvement in emotional well-being	Mild pre to post improvement in social involvement	—
Packa (1989) USA	Cross-sectional $n=22$; 6–39 mos. post	MHIQ; Cantril's Self-Anchoring Scale	Functional status rated satisfactory or better by all; better than emotional/social functioning	Emotional well-being rated satisfactory or better by all but worse than physical, social functioning	Social functioning rated satisfactory or better by all	Rated QOL as much improved from pre-txp
Schall et al. (1989) USA	Prospective $n=20$; pre, ≥ 3 mos. post	Standard cognitive tests	—	Pre to post improvement primarily in psychomotor speed; little or no change in memory, higher level information processing and poorer than norms	—	—
Shapiro and Kornfeld (1989) USA	Cross-sectional/longitudinal *$n=23$, pre, 1–12 mos. post *$n=41$, post only, 6 mos.–6 years	SCID; MMSE	—	Majority had mood, anxiety disorders post-txp; rates were same or worse than pre-txp	42% employed full-time; many had family, marital, sexual problems post-txp	—
Walden et al. (1989) USA	Cross-sectional *$n=24$; ≥ 6 mos. post, averaging 12 mos. post $n=20$ txp candidates	PAIS; MAACL; Functional Status Questionnaire	Better perceived functional status than controls; similar levels of fatigue	Both groups had elevated distress levels; no group differences in depression, anxiety, hostility	17% employed full-time, rate similar to controls; similar sexual, home, family functioning but social functioning was better in txp group	—

Table 4.3. (cont.)

Author, country	Design and sample characteristics	Major instruments/ assessments[a]	Quality of life domains			
			Physical functional	Mental health/cognitive	Social	Overall QOL
Bunzel et al. (1991, 1992, 1994a); Grundböck et al. (1992) Austria	Cross-sectional/ prospective *n = 38; 13–45 mos. post *n = 62; ≤ 7 years post (overlaps with 38) *n = 47; pre, 1 year post (overlaps with 62)	Dyadic Relationship Scale; unnormed questions	Status rated as improved from pre-txp, although some limitations remained; larger changes than in emotional, social functioning areas	Emotional, subjective cognitive status rated as improved from pre-txp; some cognitive limitations still reported	26% employed; improvement in work, leisure, family, marital, sexual relationships, although many continued to have sexual dysfunction; scores on family, marital relationships were similar to norms	QOL rated as better post-txp and considered satisfactory
Dew et al. (1991, 1993, 1994, 1996a,b); Dew 1994 USA	Longitudinal *n = 154; 2, 7, 12 mos. post n = 59 txp candidates	SIP; Karnofsky; SCL-90; SCID; Campbell QOL items; Dyadic Adjustment Scale; unnormed questions	Majority had few limitations in daily activity, perceived status as good–excellent; mobility, sleep, ambulation, body care/movement better than controls, improved with time but worse than norms	Lower depression, anxiety symptom levels than controls, improved over time, became similar to norms; rates of psychiatric disorders were similar to other chronically ill samples but worse than norms	22% employed, improved over time post; some perceived improvement in sexual activity, social interactions	Life satisfaction rated higher among recipients
Mulligan et al. (1991) USA	Cross-sectional retrospective n = 71; 3–80 mos. post	Fillenbaum ADL; HAM-D; unnormed questions	Perceived health as fair, on average	Low average level of depression	Majority reported adequate sexual interest but continuing sexual dysfunction post-txp	—

Baumann et al. (1992) USA	Longitudinal $n = 29$; 5–60 mos. post, reassessed 6 mos. later	SIP; Symptom Frequency and Distress Scale; POMS; Satisfaction with Life Scale	Improvement in mobility, ambulation, sleep, pain, fatigue over time post-txp	Mood improved over time post-txp; tension levels remained elevated; alertness worsened over time	28% ultimately employed; work, social interaction, leisure, home activities improved over time; majority were disturbed over sexual functioning with some improvement over time	—
Bohachick et al. (1992) USA	Prospective $n = 44$; pre, 6 mos. post	PAIS; POMS	—	Pre to post improvement in mood, distress levels, subjective cognitive impairment	14% employed full-time; pre to post improvement in work, home, sexual, social involvement/activity	—
Bornstein et al. (1992, 1995) USA	Prospective *$n = 7$; pre, average of 25 mos. post $n = 4$ txp candidates	Standard cognitive Tests; MMPI	—	Pre to post improvement in memory, psychomotor speed, overall cognitive status; controls did not change; both groups were lower than norms: depression worsened in both groups from: pre to post	—	—

Table 4.3. (cont.)

Author, country	Design and sample characteristics	Major instruments/ assessments[a]	Quality of life domains			
			Physical functional	Mental health/cognitive	Social	Overall QOL
Angermann et al. (1992); Bullinger et al. (1992) Germany	Cross-sectional/ prospective *n = 41; average 24 mos. post *n = 22; pre, 3 and 6 weeks, 6 and 12 mos. post n = 41 healthy controls (cross-sectional only)	POMS; ABS; PGWB Index	Pre to post lessening of fatigue, improvement in perceived health; more likely to feel bothered by symptoms than controls	Pre to post improvement in depression, overall mood, no change in anxiety; post scores similar to controls	29% employed (cross-sectional sample); work and sexual dysfunction were problematic	Pre to post improvement in QOL ratings; rated QOL high post-txp and similar to controls
Jones et al. (1992b) Australia	Prospective n = 43; pre, 4 mos. post	Standard cognitive tests	—	Pre to post improvement in short-term memory, psychomotor speed; no change in attention, concentration	—	—
Magni and Borgherini (1992) Italy	Prospective n = 26; pre, discharge, 3, 12 mos. post	SCL-90; Illness Behaviour Questionnaire	Pre to post improvement in sleep but high levels of impairment remained	Pre to post improvement in depression, anxiety, global distress; no further change over time	80% employed	—
Paris et al. (1992, 1993) USA	Cross-sectional n = 250; ≥ 3 mos. post	Unnormed questions	Majority felt physically able to be employed	—	45% employed	—

Study	Design	Measures				
Riether et al. (1992) USA	Prospective *n = 15; pre, 3, 6, 12 mos. post n = 19 liver recipients	SIP; BDI; STAI; cognitive tests	Pre to post improvement from worse than to better than liver recipients	Pre to post improvement in depression, cognitive status from similar or worse than liver patients to better than liver patients; anxiety levels stable in both groups	Pre to post improvement in social adjustment from worse than to similar to liver recipients	—
Strauss et al. (1992) Germany	Cross-sectional *n = 40; 1–43 mos. post n = 50 CABG patients	Standard cognitive tests; HAM-D; HAM-A; STAI; BDI	Slightly less satisfied with health status than controls	Lower levels of depression, anxiety than controls; more cognitive impairment than controls, particularly in memory	20% employed; no group differences in satisfaction with work, leisure, partner and family relationships, sexual activity	—
Erdman et al. (1993) Netherlands	Cross-sectional *n = 39; 7–47 mos. post n = 39 spouses	NHP; Zung Depression Scale	Sleep problems were similar to controls and to norms	Depression levels were higher than in controls and similar to other samples of ill patients	Social isolation levels were similar to controls and to norms	—
Mulcahy et al. (1993) UK	Cross-sectional n = 14; 10–33 mos. post	Standard exercise testing; unnormed questions	Majority showed good exercise capacity and reported no activity restrictions		71% employed full-time	—
Rector et al. (1993) USA	Cross-sectional *n = 143; post n = 42 txp candidates	SF-36	Better perceived health, fewer limitations in functional status, energy, daily activities than controls; slightly less pain; all scores worse than norms for persons with minor health problems	Somewhat better perceived emotional well-being than controls but worse than norms	Better social and role functioning than controls but worse than norms	—

Table 4.3. (cont.)

Author, country	Design and sample characteristics	Major instruments/assessments[a]	Quality of life domains			
			Physical functional	Mental health/cognitive	Social	Overall QOL
Rosenblum et al. (1993) USA	Cross-sectional n = 96; 6 mos.–9.7 years post	SIP; unnormed questions	Majority reported weakness; fatigue was common; limitations in sleep, ambulation, daily activities greater than norms and similar to or better than other patient groups	Emotional well-being and subjective cognitive status worse than norms and similar to or better than other patient groups	66% employed; sexual activity, social adjustment poorer than norms and similar to or better than other patient groups	—
Bunzel et al. (1994b) Austria	Prospective n = 50; pre, early post, 1 year post	Measures from German-speaking countries	Pre to post improvement in perceived physical health; majority rated health as good/excellent at 1 year	Pre to post improvement in affect, mood, except that irritability increased over time post-txp to pre-txp levels	—	Pre to post improvement but life satisfaction then declined slightly
Duitsman and Cychosz (1994) USA	Cross-sectional n = 132; average 3.2 years post	Rosenberg self-esteem; Bradburn Happiness; Anxiety; Campbell QOL items	—	Majority had depression, anxiety levels at lower end of scale; self-esteem was above midpoint of scale	34% employed	Overall QOL well above midpoint of scale
Paris et al. (1994) USA	Prospective n = 53; pre, 6–39 mos. post	Unnormed clinical interview	—	Some pre to post worsening in rate of psychiatric problems, mainly depression, anxiety	—	—

DeCampli et al. (1995) USA	Cross-sectional n = 26; 11–22 years post	NHP; General Well-Being Exam	Limitations in mobility, pain, sleep, energy similar to other heart txp samples but greater than norms	Psychological symptom levels similar to norms	52% employed; sexual dysfunction noted by many; levels of employment and sexual function similar to other heart txp samples	—
Fisher et al. (1995) USA	Longitudinal/ prospective *n = 62; 4, 8, 12, 24, 36, 48, 60 mos. post *n = 32; pre, 4, 8, 12 mos. post	SIP; BDI	Pre to post improvement in mobility, ambulation, sleep, body care, daily home activities; no further change post-txp	Pre to post improvement in depression and overall emotional well-being; no further change with time post-txp	53% employed at 60 mos. post; pre to post improvement in leisure activity with no further change; little change in social interaction or work limitations	—
Leedham et al. (1995) USA	Prospective n = 31; pre, discharge, 3, 6 mos. post	POMS; PAIS; unnormed questions	Pre to post improvement in functional status and ability to do daily activities; further improvement over time post-txp	Pre to post improvement to levels at or better than norms for emotional well-being	—	Pre to post improvement in global adjustment and overall QOL

Asterisks denote study groups of key interest; QOL, quality of life; txp, transplant; mos., months; CABG, coronary artery by-pass graft.
[a]Instrument abbreviations: ABS, Affect Balance Scale; ADL, Activities of Daily Living; BDI, Beck Depression Inventory; GHQ, General Health Questionnaire; HAM-D, HAM-A, Hamilton Rating Scale for Depression; Anxiety; MAACL, Multiple Affect Adjective Checklist; MHIQ, McMaster Health Index Questionnaire; MMPI, Minnesota Multiphasic Personality Inventory; MMSE, Mini Mental State Examination; NHP, Nottingham Health Profile; PAIS, Psychological Adjustment to Illness Scale; PGWB Index, Psychological General Well-Being Index; POMS, Profile of Mood States; PSE, Present State Examination; SCID, Structural Clinical Interview for DSM-III-R; SCL-90, Symptom Checklist-90; SF-36, Medical Outcomes Study Short Form-36; SIP, Sickness Impact Profile; STAI, Spielberger State-Trait Anxiety Inventory.

Table 4.4. Quality of life in samples of lung and heart–lung (H–L) transplant recipients

Author, country	Design and sample characteristics	Major instruments/assessments[a]	Quality of life domains			
			Physical functional	Mental health/cognitive	Social	Overall QOL
O'Brien et al. (1988) UK	Prospective *n* = 28 H–L; pre, 3, 6, 12 mos. post	NHP	Pre to post improvement in mobility, sleep, pain, energy, ability to do daily activities; smaller improvements over time post-txp; similar to norms at 1 year post	Pre to post improvement in emotional well-being; smaller improvements over time post-txp; better than norms at 1 year post	Pre to post improvement in work, leisure, social, sexual areas; smaller improvements over time post-txp; better than norms in all areas except work	—
Craven et al. (1990) Canada	Cross-sectional *n* = 22 lung; > 6 mos. post	Unnormed questions	Majority reported good–excellent satisfaction with status, but some limitations remained	Majority reported good–excellent satisfaction with emotional status	32% employed or volunteer full-time	Majority reported good–excellent satisfaction with life
Caine et al. (1991); Dennis et al. (1993); Scott et al. (1993) UK	Prospective *n* = 31 H–L; pre, 3–6 mos. post	NHP	Pre to post improvement in mobility, energy, ability to do daily activities; somewhat better sleep, less pain	Pre to post improvement in emotional well-being	Pre to post improvement in work, leisure, sexual activity; some improvement in family relationships	—

Study	Design/sample	Instruments[a]				Overall QOL
Busschbach et al. (1994) Netherlands	Cross-sectional, retrospective; *$n=3$ double lung; 12–16 mos. post; $n=3$ txp candidates	Karnofsky; EuroQol scale; Visual Analog Scale; Standard Gamble; Time Tradeoff	Better functional status than controls	—	—	Higher QOL ratings than controls
Al-Kattan et al. (1995) UK	Longitudinal *$n=17$ H–L; 1, 2, 3 years post; *$n=45$ single lung; 1, 2, 3 years post	NHP	H–L patients had more energy, mobility, slightly better sleep than lung patients; similar pain levels; both groups worse than norms; little change over time	H–L patients had slightly worse emotional well-being than lung patients and norms; little change over time	H–L patients had slightly better social adjustment than lung patients but worse than norms; little change over time	—
Ramsey et al. (1995a,b) USA	Cross-sectional *$n=23$ single or double lung; post $n=21$ txp candidates	SIP; Standard Gamble	Slightly better ambulation, sleep, ability to do daily activities than controls; poorer care/movement and similar mobility as controls	Slightly better emotional well-being than controls; worse subjective cognitive status than controls	Slightly more social, work, role activity and involvement than controls	Rated QOL better than controls

Asterisks denote study groups of key interest. QOL, quality of life; txp, transplant; mos., months.
[a]Instrument abbreviations: EuroQol, European Quality of Life Questionnaire; NHP, Nottingham Health Profile; SIP, Sickness Impact Profile.

Table 4.5. Quality of life in samples of liver transplant recipients

Author, country	Design and sample characteristics	Major instruments/ assessments[a]	Quality of Life Domains			
			Physical functional	Mental health/cognitive	Social	Overall QOL
House et al. (1983) USA	Cross-sectional $n = 20$; 6 mos.–12 years post	Unnormed clinical interview	—	All 20 had adverse psychiatric reactions post-txp	—	—
Tarter et al. (1984, 1988) USA	Cross-sectional *$n = 10$; averaging 3 years post *$n = 66$; 1 year post *$n = 10$ Crohn's disease	SIP; standard cognitive tests; SBAS; MMPI; Unnormed questions	$n = 10$: similar to controls but worse than norms on sleep, ambulation mobility, body care, overall health $n = 66$: majority reported little disability	$n = 10$: similar to controls but worse than norms on emotional status, perceptual motor performance $n = 66$: majority reported low depression, anxiety	$n = 10$: similar to controls but worse than norms in work, social activities $n = 66$: 38% employed full-time	$n = 66$: majority rated QOL as good to excellent
Williams et al. (1987) USA	Cross-sectional $n = 38$; 12–42 mos. post	Unnormed questions	Majority had few or no limitations in daily activities	—	34% employed full-time	—
Colonna et al. (1988) USA	Cross-sectional retrospective $n = 28$; 6 mos.–3 years post	Unnormed questions	Pre to post improvement in activity tolerance	—	Pre to post increase in employment; 75% employed post-txp	Pre to post improvement; majority rated QOL as good–excellent post
Eid et al. (1989) USA	Cross-sectional $n = 46$; 13–31 mos. post	Unnormed questions	—	—	85% employed	Majority reported good overall well-being

Foley et al. (1989) USA	Cross-sectional $n=45$; ≥ 6 mos. post	Unnormed questions	Most distressed about fatigue since txp	—	Majority rated QOL as good-excellent
Wolcott et al. (1989) USA	Cross-sectional $n=41$; 4–36 mos. post	Health ratings; POMS; Rosenberg Self-esteem; Campbell QOL and Social items; cognitive tests	Majority rated health good-excellent but also had restricted activity level; level improved with time post	Minimal mood disturbance, high self-esteem; on average, poorer than norms on cognitive learning tests but similar on other tests; worsened with time post-txp	25% employed full-time; low level of social interaction	Rated well-being lower than kidney recipients
Grant et al. (1990); Adams et al. (1995) Canada	Cross-sectional *$n=203$; ≥ 9 mos. post (only employment status reported) *$n=31$; 3–49 mos. post (subgroup of the 203)	Karnofsky; Campbell QOL and Social items; Evans QOL index	Majority had few limitations in functional status or daily activities	High level of perceived emotional adjustment; similar to norms	40% employed full-time; better perceived social adjustment, marital, family relationships than norms	Majority very satisfied with life
Kober et al. (1990); Küchler et al. (1991) USA & Germany	Cross-sectional/prospective *$n=38$; 1–47 mos. post *$n=29$; pre, 2, 6, 12, 24, 36 mos. post $n=12$ liver disease $n=15$ healthy persons (controls cross-sectional only)	EORTC QOL Questionnaire; STAI	Pre to post improvement in physical symptoms, but functional status, pain symptoms, pain worse than normals; longer-term survivors scored better than disease controls but worse than normals	Anxiety: no pre to post change, similar to disease controls, worse than normals; little change over time post-txp. Depression: pre to post improvement	Social integration ratings higher than disease controls, poorer than healthy controls	Pre to post improvement; better than disease controls, worse than healthy controls

Table 4.5. (*cont.*)

Author, country	Design and sample characteristics	Major instruments/ assessments[a]	Quality of Life Domains			
			Physical functional	Mental health/cognitive	Social	Overall QOL
Lowe et al. (1990) UK	Cross-sectional $n = 64$, at least 3 mos. post	NHP	Worse than norms in energy, pain, sleep; functioning worse with time post-txp	Better than norms in emotional well-being	Worse than norms on social isolation; better than norms on work difficulties	—
Robinson et al. (1990) USA	Cross-sectional $n = 31$, 3 years post	Unnormed questions	Majority had no activity limitations and moderate to normal endurance	—	39% employed full-time; majority had work-related adjustment difficulties	—
Felser et al. (1991) USA	Cross-sectional, retrospective $n = 126$, avg. 44 mos. post	Unnormed questions	Majority perceived health and sleep to have improved over time post-txp	Majority perceived depression, nervousness, mood swings to have lessened over time post-txp	Work, family, social activities perceived as stable or improved over time post-txp; sexual, family changes less common	—
Tarter et al. (1990a,b, 1991, 1992); Arria et al. (1991) USA	Prospective *$n = 62$; pre, > 6 mos. post $n = 22$ Crohn's disease $n = 38$ normal controls	SIP; SBAS; standard cognitive tests	Pre to post improvement in ambulation, mobility, body care and movement, but poorer than normal controls	Decline in disturbed behavior post-txp, became comparable to normal controls; pre to post improvement on emotional well-being and on some (not all) cognitive tests	84% employed, with pre to post improvement in rate; role performance improved and similar to normal controls; social interaction, recreation better but poorer than normal controls	—

Reference	Design	Measures				
Bonsel et al. (1990, 1992) Netherlands	Cross-sectional/ prospective *n = 46; 1 mo.–8 years post *n = 20; pre, 3 mos. post	NHP; STAI; Zung Depression; ADL; Campbell QOL items, Life Satisfaction	Pre to post improvement in mobility, pain, energy, sleep, but lower than norms	Pre to post improvement in anxiety, depression, but worse than norms	Pre to post decline in social isolation and similar to norms	Pre to post improvement; satisfaction similar to norms
Commander et al. (1992) UK	Cross-sectional n = 32; 6–31 mos. post	PAS; GHQ; SAS	—	Major depression, panic were most common; rates higher than norm; large subgroup with subjective cognitive complaints	19% employed full-time, no pre to post change; worse than norm in ratings of work, relations with family, partner; similar to norm on leisure, parent/household relationships	—
Hicks et al. (1992) USA	Cross-sectional n = 35; ≥ 3 mos. post	SIP, Perceived Health Status; POMS. QLI	Mobility, ambulation, body care/movement worsened with time post-txp; sleep was stable	Overall emotional well-being, depression, anxiety levels worsened with time post-txp	Satisfaction with social, work, leisure, family stable over time post-txp	Stable and high post-txp
Moore et al. (1992) Australia	Prospective *n = 22; pre, 1, 3, 9 mos. post n = 11 nonalcoholic cirrhotics	PAIS; Austin QOL Scale	Pre to post improvement in well-being, pain, nausea, appetite; no change over time among controls	Pre to post improvement in mood and distress level; no change over time among controls	Pre to post improvement in social interest and interaction; trend toward better relationships; no change in controls	Pre to post improvement; no change among controls

Table 4.5. (*cont.*)

Author, country	Design and sample characteristics	Major instruments/ assessments[a]	Quality of Life Domains			
			Physical functional	Mental health/cognitive	Social	Overall QOL
Riether et al. (1992) USA	Prospective *n = 19; pre, 3, 6, 12 mos. post n = 15 heart recipients	SIP; BDI; STAI; cognitive tests	No pre to post change; slightly more impaired than heart recipients by 12 mos. post	Depression and cognitive status improved pre to post but somewhat worse than heart recipients; similar anxiety levels in both groups over time	No pre to post change; similar to heart recipients at 12 mos. post	—
Leyendecker et al. (1993) Germany	Cross-sectional n = 47; 3–19 mos. post	Scales utilized in Germany	Higher levels of fatigue, rheumatism than norms; status improved with time post-txp	Depression, anxiety levels similar to hepatitis patients; overall mood, subjective cognitive status similar to healthy persons	Social activity level similar to healthy persons	Slightly more positive ratings of QOL than norms
Chen & Sun (1994) Taiwan	Cross-sectional n = 7; 2–8 years post	Karnofsky; unnormed questions	Pre to post improvement in overall status; health complaints mostly related to drug side effects	—	71% employed; most were satisfied with leisure and social activities	High levels of satisfaction post-txp
Belle and Porayko (1995) USA	Prospective n = 191; pre, 1 year post	SIP; Karnofsky; Bradburn Happiness item; SF-36; unnormed questions	Pre to post improvement in ambulation, mobility, body care/movement, sleep, perceived overall health	Pre to post improvement in mood and anxiety levels	Pre to post improvement in satisfaction with work, family, social life, sexual activity; no change in marital relation	Overall satisfaction high and similar to norms

Study / Country	Design	Instruments				
Boudet et al. (1995) France	Cross-sectional, retrospective $n=78$; 2–3 years post	SIP	—	—	53% returned to work post-txp	Somewhat lower than norms
Collis et al. (1995) UK	Cross-sectional/ prospective *$n=19$; 2–151 weeks post *$n=11$; pre, once 2–15 weeks post	NHP; CIS; GHQ; MMSE	Energy, sleep, mobility improved but limitations remained; pain did not improve	Psychiatric disorder rate higher than norms; no pre to post change and similar to other ill samples; no pre to post change in distress levels; little cognitive impairment	No improvement in home life ratings	—
Levy et al. (1995) USA	Prospective/cross-sect.[b] $n=150$; pre, 1, 2, 5 years post	SIP; Karnofsky; NHP; MOS; Campbell QOL items	Pre to post improvement in perceived health, functional status, ability to do activities; no change thereafter	Pre to post improvement in self-image and distress levels, no change thereafter	54% employed full-time by 5 years post; rate declined from pre to post-txp, then returned to original level	Pre to post improvement in positive feelings about life
Price et al. (1995) UK	Prospective *$n=27$; pre, 6, 12, 24, 30–42 mos. post $n=71$ candidates $n=11$ rejected candidates	NHP	Recipients improved by 6-mos. post with less improvement thereafter, largest change in energy; moderate change in mobility, sleep; controls did not improve	Recipients showed moderate improvement in emotional well-being by 6 mos. post, with little change thereafter; controls did not improve	Recipients had some improvement in social isolation by 6 mos. post, little change thereafter; controls did not improve	—

Asterisks denote study groups of key interest; QOL, quality of life; txp, transplant; mos., months.

[a]Instrument abbreviations: ADL, Activities of Daily Living; BDI, Beck Depression Inventory; CIS, Clinical Interview Schedule; EORTC QOL, European Organization for Research and Treatment of Cancer Quality of Life Questionnaire; GHQ, General Health Questionnaire; MMPI, Minnesota Multiphasic Personality Inventory; MMSE, Mini Mental State Examination; MOS, Medical Outcomes Study Form; NHP, Nottingham Health Profile; PAIS, Psychological Adjustment to Illness Scale; PAS, Psychiatric Assessment Schedule; POMS, Profile of Mood States; QLI, Ferrans Quality of Life Index; SAS, Social Adjustment Scale; SBAS, Social Behavior Assessment Schedule; SF-36, Medical Outcomes Study Short Form-36; SIP, Sickness Impact Profile; STAI, Spielberger State-Trait Anxiety Inventory.

[b]Different but overlapping subsets of the 150 persons were assessed at each timepoint.

Table 4.6. Quality of life in samples of bone marrow transplant recipients

Author country	Design and sample characteristics	Major instruments/assessments[a]	Quality of life domains			
			Physical functional	Mental health/cognitive	Social	Overall QOL
Wolcott et al. (1986) USA	Cross-sectional *n=26; 19–91 mos. post n=18 related donors	Health status items; POMS; Rosenberg Self-esteem; SAS	Majority rated functional status as good–excellent; ratings were better with time post-txp	Recipients show more depression, anxiety, anger, total mood disturbance than donors, but similar to norms; no change with time post-txp	35% employed full-time; social adjustment similar to norms but many reported low QOL in work, leisure, relationships with family, friends; no change with time post-txp	—
Hengeveld et al. (1988) Netherlands	Cross-sectional n=17; 12–60 mos. post	Karnofsky; BDI; SCL-90	Majority were able to carry on normal physical activities	Higher levels of depression and overall distress than norms	29% employed; sexual satisfaction levels were impaired	—
Andrykowski et al. (1989a,b) USA	Cross-sectional/longitudinal n=23; 3 annual assessments at average of 28, 37, 52 mos. post	SIP; FLIC; POMS	Functioning better than in other cancer samples; no change over time	More depression, anxiety, anger, overall distress than other cancer samples; no change over time; more subjective cognitive complaints, with worsening over time	50% ultimately employed; increased over time; more impaired social activity levels than other cancer samples; some gains with time	—

Reference	Design/sample	Measures	Physical	Psychological	Social/employment	Other
Andrykowski et al. (1990a,b) USA	Cross-sectional *n = 29; 12–96 mos. post n = 20 kidney recipients	SIP; FLIC; POMS; PAIS; PHQ	No group differences in perceived health or functional status; both groups rated health poorer than other samples; no change with time post-txp	Many reported cognitive complaints; less depressed but otherwise similar to controls; all were more distressed than other samples; no change with time	55% employed, rate slightly better than controls; similar levels of work, social, family, sexual adjustment; no change with time post-txp	—
Altmaier et al. (1991) USA	Cross-sectional *n = 12, 25–41 mos. post n = 10 cancer patients	Karnofsky; unnormed questions	Few or no limitations in physical activities or self-care; no differences from controls	Low levels of distress, no differences from controls	58% employed full-time; more relationship and sexual difficulties than controls	—
Baker et al. (1991, 1994); Wingard et al. (1991, 1992); Wingard (1994); Curbow et al. (1993) USA	Cross-sectional n = 135; 6–149 mos. post	Karnofsky; Health Perception Scale; MOS-short form; POMS; SLDS; Ladder of Life; ABS; Personal Change Scale	Majority were able to do normal physical activities; strength, health, body satisfaction rated above midpoint of scale; pain was a continuing problem; reported more negative than positive physical changes overall	Less depression, tension, confusion, more anger than other cancer samples and norms; greater positive and negative affect than community norms	51% employed full-time; reported high levels of social function but lower sexual satisfaction; little pre to post social role change except increased employment; reported more positive than negative social function change	Rated QOL well above scale midpoint
Baruch et al. (1991) UK	Cross-sectional n = 46; 6–154 mos. post	HADS; unnormed questions	Majority rated health as good-excellent	Anxiety and depressive symptoms were the most commonly reported, 13% extremely distressed	Global rating of sexual problems higher post-txp than before illness	—

Table 4.6. (*cont.*)

Author country	Design and sample characteristics	Major instruments/ assessments[a]	Quality of life domains			Overall QOL
			Physical functional	Mental health/cognitive	Social	
Jenkins et al. (1991) UK	Cross-sectional, retrospective $n = 33$; 3–67 mos. post	PAIS; HADS; CIDI	—	Anxiety levels similar to norm; depression rate higher than norm	Social and sexual adjustment similar to levels in other cancer samples	—
Vose et al. (1992) USA	Cross-sectional, retrospective $n = 50$, 12–62 mos. post	Unnormed questions	Activity level same or higher than pre-txp	Depression was only mental health problem reported post-txp	76% employed or students; sexual function rated poorer than pre-txp	—
Belec (1992) USA	Cross-sectional $n = 24$; 12–38 mos. post	QLI; unnormed questions	Majority reported good health and functioning; 50% reported lack of energy, fatigue; no change over time post-txp	Majority reported good emotional well-being; no change with time post-txp	Most reported good relationships with family; work and sexual difficulties were noted; no change with time	Majority rated QOL as acceptable or good
Chao et al. (1992) USA	Longitudinal $n = 58$; 3, 12 mos. post	Karnofsky; unnormed questions	Most described appetite and sleep to be good; Karnofsky showed little disability; all measures improved over time	—	64% employed full-time by 1 year, increased over time; lower satisfaction with sexual activity than pre-txp, no change over time	Rated QOL above scale midpoint, rating improved with time
Grant et al. (1992) USA	Cross-sectional $n = 179$; > 3 mos. post	Karnofsky; QOL-BMT Instrument	Majority had little impairment in daily activities	Emotional well-being rated as poorer than other areas of functioning	Social functioning and adjustment rated as very satisfactory	Rated QOL better than other cancer samples, worse than nonpatients

Study	Design/Sample	Measures	Functional	Psychological	Social/Vocational	QOL
Lesko et al. (1992); Mumma et al. (1992) USA	Cross-sectional *n=21; ≥1 year post n=49 cancer patients	Karnofsky; BSI; SAS; DFSI	Very little impairment on average, no group differences	More depression, anxiety, anger, overall distress than norms, no differences between groups	29% employed, lower than controls; more impaired in family, work than norms and worse than controls; no differences in satisfaction with sexual activity; for women, sexual activity lower than controls and poorer than healthy persons	—
Schmidt et al. (1993) USA	Cross-sectional n=162; ≥1 year post	Karnofsky; unnormed questions	Majority had little functional impairment; areas of most difficulty were appetite and sleep	—	87% employed full-time; sexual dissatisfaction frequently reported	Majority rated QOL as excellent
Syrjala et al. (1993) USA	Prospective n=67; pre, 3 mos., 1 year, 4.5–6 years post	Karnofsky; SIP; BDI; BSI	Pre to post decline in sleep, ambulation, mobility, body care/movement; some improvement with time	Higher levels of depression, anxiety than norms; no pre to post or later change over time	20% employed full-time at 1 year post; no pre to post change in social adjustment and was similar to norms	—
Jenkins et al. (1994) UK	Prospective n=36; pre, 1, 6 mos. post	PAIS; HADS; CIDI	—	33% had diagnosable anxiety or depression both pre and post; 14% to 18% had high distress levels post-txp, but improved over pre-txp	Mild pre to post improvement in family, social, sexual adjustment	—

Table 4.6. (cont.)

Author country	Design and sample characteristics	Major instruments/assessments[a]	Quality of life domains			
			Physical functional	Mental health/cognitive	Social	Overall QOL
Litwins and Rodrigue (1994) USA	Cross-sectional *n = 32; ≥ 1 year post n = 22 cancer patients	SIP	Physical functioning similar to controls and similar to norms	Emotional status similar to controls and similar to norms	56% unemployed; recreation and home life more impaired than other areas but no different from controls	—
Andrykowski et al. (1995a,b) USA	Cross-sectional n = 200; 12–127 mos. post	SIP; Recovery of Function; Health Perception Scale; Rosenberg Self-esteem; POMS; PAIS	43% impaired in physical activity; most difficulty with fatigue, stiff joints, sleep, headache; some improvement with time	13% subjective cognitive problems (mood measures not reported)	60% employed; high rate of sexual activity impairment; little social functioning impairment	QOL rated as lower than others of same age
Bush et al. (1995) USA	Cross-sectional n = 125; 6–18 years post	EORTC QOI; Ware Health Perceptions; POMS	Mild disability; highest in sleep, joint/muscle discomfort, pain, fatigue; better than cancer patients, no change with time	Less anxiety, confusion than cancer patient samples, but more anger and similar overall emotional well-being; similar levels of subjective cognitive impairment	74% employed; better role and social functioning than cancer samples; high rates of sexual impairment	Better global rating than cancer comparison samples

Asterisks denote study groups of key interest; QOL, quality of life; txp, transplant; mos., months.

[a]Instrument abbreviations: ABS, Affect Balance Scale; BDI, Beck Depression Inventory; CIDI, Composite International Diagnostic Interview: DFSI, Derogatis Sexual Functioning Inventory; EORTC QOL, European Organization for Research and Treatment of Cancer Quality of Life Questionnaire; FLIC, Functional Living Index – Cancer; HADS, Hospital Anxiety and Depression Scale; MOS, Medical Outcomes Study Form; PAIS, Psychological Adjustment to Illness Scale; PHQ, Perceived Health Questionnaire; POMS, Profile of Mood States; QLI, Ferrans Quality of Life Index; QOL-BMT, Quality of Life – Bone Marrow Transplant Instrument; SAS, Social Adjustment Scale; SCL-90, Symptom Checklist-90; SIP, Sickness Impact Profile; SLDS, Satisfaction with Life Domains Scale.

control groups). Major assessment instruments are listed, followed by study findings in any of the four central QOL domains. For example, the first entry in Table 4.1 concerns research from the Simmons group, which focused on a cohort of 178 kidney recipients who were studied prior to transplant, with follow-up assessments at 3 weeks, 1 year, and 5 to 9 years post-transplantation. Comparison groups followed during the study included 130 family members who were kidney donors to these recipients, and 186 nondonor relatives of the recipients. Multiple measures were used, and the study yielded findings in all four of the QOL domains under consideration.

A general summary of recipient QOL studies

We located 144 separate investigations, from a total of 19 countries, conducted during the period from 1977 through 1995. Table 4.7 shows the distribution of these studies across the six areas of transplantation. Studies of kidney recipients and heart recipients were equally prevalent, followed by liver, bone marrow, and pancreas/kidney–pancreas transplant studies. In general, the number of studies in a given area reflects how long the transplantation procedure has been utilized as a medical therapy. Thus, kidney transplantation was the earliest well-established area, while lung/heart–lung studies have appeared only relatively recently. It is interesting to note that, although studies of heart recipients and liver recipients were both first initiated in the early 1980s, the proportion of studies available about liver patients' QOL is considerably smaller. A similar distinction is evident for pancreas/kidney–pancreas studies and lung/heart–lung studies, which both began to appear in the late 1980s. Lung/heart–lung transplantation has not become as widely used a procedure as pancreas transplantation, with consequently fewer opportunities for QOL research.

Across the 144 studies, over 10 595 recipients were studied. (The exact number of recipients cannot be determined because some studies used partially overlapping samples, e.g., work by Binik and colleagues, Table 4.1). More kidney recipients were studied than any other type of transplant recipient. Compared with kidney, heart, liver and bone marrow recipients, very few pancreas/lidney–pancreas and lung/heart–lung patients were studied.

As can be seen in Tables 4.1 to 4.6, sample size varied widely across the individual investigations, from small samples of 15 or fewer recipients (e.g., Kutner, Brogan, and Kutner 1986; Brennan et al. 1987; Busschbach et al. 1994; Esmatjes et al. 1994) to moderately large samples of 150 or more persons (Simmons, Klein, and Simmons 1977; Evans et al. 1984; Bremer et al. 1989; Andrykowski et al. 1995a,b; Dew et al. 1996a) to very large samples of more than 700 recipients (Koch and Muthny 1990; Ohkubo 1995). Investiga-

Table 4.7. Summary information about 144 retrieved studies

Type of transplantation	No. of studies	% of Total studies	No. of respondents	% of total respondents
Kidney	40	27.7	4761	45.0
Pancreas/kidney–pancreas	15	10.4	380	3.6
Heart	39	27.1	2437	23.0
Lung/heart–lung	6	4.2	169	1.6
Liver	25	17.4	1573	14.8
Bone marrow	19	13.2	1275	12.0
Total	144	100.0	10 595	100.0

tions also differed regarding measures selected for QOL assessments, although not as widely as might be expected: some instruments have been used in many investigations across different types of transplantation. These include instruments that assess QOL across a broad range of areas: the Sickness Impact Profile (SIP; Bergner et al. 1981), Nottingham Health Profile (NHP; Hunt, McEwen, and McKenna 1985), Spitzer Q-L Index (Spitzer, Dobson, and Hall 1981), Karnofsky Index of Functional Impairment (Karnofsky and Burchenal 1949), and various forms of the Medical Outcomes Study (MOS) instrument, including the complete MOS form and the Short Form-36 (SF-36; Stewart and Ware 1992; Ware and Sherbourne 1992). Other commonly used instruments focus on mood and emotional status, including the Campbell QOL items (Campbell et al. 1976), Affect Balance Scale (ABS; Bradburn 1969), Profile of Mood States (POMS; McNair, Lorr, and Droppelman 1981); Psychosocial Adjustment to Illness Scale (PAIS; Derogatis 1976), Beck and Zung Depression Scales (Beck, Steer, and Garbvin 1988; Zung 1965), State-Trait Anxiety Inventory (STAI; Spielberger, Gorsuch, and Lushene 1970), and the Symptom Checklist-90 (SCL-90; Derogatis 1983).

The majority of studies utilized a cross-sectional design in which respondents were assessed once post-transplantation. Some included comparison or control groups within the study design; others referenced normative samples or other cohorts for comparison purposes. Over time a growing number of studies utilized the stronger prospective design, either with or without comparison groups, in which respondents were assessed both before and after transplantation. An additional sizable number of longitudinal studies enrolled respondents post-transplantation and then reassessed them periodically, usually for the first 1 to 2 years post-transplant, but occasionally for many more years (e.g., Andrykowski, Henslee, and Barnett 1989a; Nakache, Tyden, and Groth 1994; Al-Kattan et al. 1995).

We considered each study in Tables 4.1 to 4.6 according to the key questions about recipient QOL that we posed above. In the following discussion of our review questions, we first examine QOL effects in each of the four outcome domains. Then, we consider whether the pattern of QOL effects across the four outcome domains differs as a function of the type of transplant involved.

Does QOL improve from pre- to post-transplantation?

Although some cross-sectional investigations asked transplant recipients to retrospectively compare their post-transplantation QOL to memories of pretransplantation QOL, such retrospective accounts are subject to a variety of recall biases. Thus, in order to rigorously address the question of QOL improvement, only the 44 of the 144 studies that prospectively evaluated recipients both before and after transplantation were considered. Only 14 of these 44 studies included nontransplant comparison groups to control for temporal changes unrelated to the transplant, and the remaining studies followed only transplanted patients. The former design is more powerful than the latter in terms of causal inference, but it is more difficult to conduct. The 44 reports also varied in whether they assessed all or only some of the four QOL outcome domains. For all reports that considered a given domain (e.g., the 33 studies that examined physical functional status), we determined the proportion that reported either a large or statistically reliable improvement in QOL from pre- to post-transplantation (as opposed to a stable or declining QOL across time, or a mixed pattern of change within the QOL domain). The results are summarized in Figure 4.1, which plots the proportion of kidney recipient studies that reported improvement in each of the four QOL domains, the analogous proportion of heart recipient studies reporting improvement, and so on. For example, of kidney recipient studies, 66.7% found physical functional improvement, 100% found mental health improvement, 83% found social functioning improvement, and 100% found pretransplantation to post-transplantation improvements in perceptions of overall QOL. The bottom of Figure 4.1 provides the total number of studies available (across all types of transplantation) that addressed each QOL domain. Thus, while 33 studies examined pre- to post-transplantation improvement in physical functional QOL, 42 examined change in mental health QOL. For each QOL domain shown in Figure 4.1, Table 4.8 provides the number of relevant studies used in the calculation of the plotted proportions.

Figure 4.1 shows that 100% of investigations of pancreas, heart, lung/heart–lung, and bone marrow recipients found evidence of pre- to post improvement in patients' physical functional QOL, despite dramatic differences in length of post-transplantation follow-up across studies. (Because there was only one study of bone marrow recipients' physical functional QOL, the bone marrow point on the physical functional QOL dimension in Figure 4.1 should be viewed with caution.) In contrast to studies concerning these four types of transplantation, only 78% of liver recipient studies and only 66.7% of kidney recipient studies found physical functional improvements. Figure 4.1 shows that the median proportion of studies reporting QOL improvement in the physical functional domain (i.e., the median across the six separate types of transplantation) was 100% – quite an outstanding "success" rate.

Although physical functional QOL was defined and measured somewhat differently across studies, the vast majority considered such essential areas as ambulation, mobility, fatigue, pain, sleep, ability to perform daily activities, and/or general physical health perceptions. Ability to perform daily activities and perceptions of general physical health tended to show the most pre- to post-transplantation improvement. Results for other specific functional areas, such as sleep and pain were less pronounced across studies. In general, among the studies examining the physical functional domain, improvements were usually larger than the changes noted in any other QOL domain. The minority of studies reporting no improvement in physical functional QOL tended to report constant rather than declining physical functional status from pre- to post-transplantation.

Figure 4.1 similarly reports the proportion of studies for each transplant type that found pre- to post-transplantation improvements in mental health/ cognitive QOL. The results across studies were more variable than those for physical functional QOL. One hundred percent of kidney and lung/heart– lung transplant studies reported improvement, while only 50% of pancreas and bone marrow transplant studies found evidence of improvement. (It is important to note, however, that the latter two transplant types contained only two relevant studies each; see Table 4.8) The remaining types of transplantation lie between these two extremes. Studies reporting improvement in this domain of QOL generally found patients' cognitive status and self-reported emotional well-being to be better post-transplantation. But some of the studies noted actual declines in emotional well-being or psychiatric status (e.g., Niset, Coustry-Degré, and Degré 1988; Paris et al. 1994). Others reported a mixed pattern, with, for example, some improvement in cognitive status but a decline in emotional well-being (e.g., Bornstein et al. 1995), or improvements in some areas of psychiatric symptoms but not in others. Riether et al. (1992), for example, found that liver recipients' depression and cognitive status improved with the transplant, but anxiety levels showed no change. In contrast, Mai et al. (1990) found that heart recipients' anxiety levels improved whereas their depression levels did not. This variability across studies in mental health QOL findings may be related to the fact that the studies differed in whether they relied exclusively on recipients' self-reported status or whether self-reports were supplemented with standardized diagnostic assessments of these areas. The studies that incorporated clinician-administered diagnostic assessments were less likely to report pre- to post-

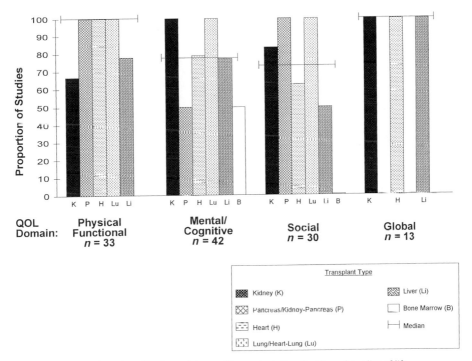

Figure 4.1. Proportion of studies in each type of transplantation that found quality of life (QOL) improvements from pre- to post-transplantation.

transplantation improvement in mental health and cognitive status than those that relied exclusively on self-report symptom severity data.

The third QOL domain, social functioning, appears to have produced even less consistent results across studies (see Figure 4.1). While employment status has historically been the most commonly considered variable in this domain, social functioning also encompasses satisfaction with and adjustment in relationships with family and others, leisure and social activity involvement, and intimacy and sexual activity. Of the studies evaluating any of these elements of social functioning, 100% of those focusing on pancreas and on lung/heart–lung recipients reported improved QOL, while fewer than 60% of studies of heart recipients and liver recipients reported improvement. Neither of the two studies of bone marrow recipients reported improvement, most likely due to the fact that reported sexual dysfunction generally increases with the infertility caused by the bone marrow transplantation process. Otherwise, studies that found no improvement in social QOL tended to find no change, rather than any decline, in social QOL with transplantation. Studies that found improved social functioning generally described better

Table 4.8. Number of available studies in each transplant area that addressed the central review questions in four QOL domains

QOL Domain	Pre to post QOL improvement?	Transplant patients have better QOL than ill controls?	Transplant patients have similar/better QOL than healthy norms?
Physical functional			
Kidney transplant	6	17	5
Pancreas	4	11	2
Heart	11	8	5
Lung/heart–lung	2	2	2
Liver	9	4	6
Bone marrow	1	6	1
Total	33	48	21
Mental health/cognitive status			
Kidney transplant	8	24	10
Pancreas	2	8	2
Heart	19	7	10
Lung/heart–lung	2	2	2
Liver	9	6	10
Bone marrow	2	7	7
Total	42	54	41
Social functioning			
Kidney transplant	6	20	8
Pancreas	4	12	2
Heart	8	5	3
Lung/heart–lung	2	2	2
Liver	8	4	9
Bone marrow	2	7	3
Total	30	50	27
Global QOL perceptions			
Kidney transplant	3	17	7
Pancreas	1	9	2
Heart	5	1	3
Lung/heart–lung	0	2	0
Liver	4	3	5
Bone marrow	0	2	1
Total	13	34	18

Types of transplantation in which only one study had been conducted concerning a specific review question (e.g., bone marrow studies of pre to post improvement in physical functional QOL) are not graphed in the corresponding Figures 4.1 to 4.3.

leisure and social activity, relationships with friends and extended family, and satisfaction with work and home roles.

In the fourth outcome domain, self-rated overall QOL, all reports for all transplantation types indicated improvement from pre- to post-transplantation. However, there were many fewer studies of global QOL change than studies of QOL improvement in the specific areas described above. Nevertheless, this uniform pattern of improvement in global QOL across all studies, in contrast to the more variable patterns of change within the specific functional areas, is consistent with Evans' argument that QOL evaluations must consider elements beyond those that are obviously influenced by health conditions. In other words, one's overall QOL is not determined solely by one's health, and assessing global QOL may provide a perspective on patients' lives that is different than inquiring only about specific health-related QOL domains.

Figure 4.1 can also be viewed in terms of domain-by-domain differences within a given type of transplantation. For example, studies of kidney recipients were less likely to find pre- to post-transplantation improvement in physical functional QOL than to find positive changes in mental health or social functioning. In contrast, heart transplant studies uniformly documented physical functional improvements, but were less likely to find mental health/cognitive status improvements, and were even less likely to find social QOL improvements. Bone marrow studies showed a pattern similar to heart studies, with little likelihood of finding improvement in mental health/cognitive or social domains. Studies of pancreas recipients were less likely to find mental health/cognitive improvements than to consistently find improvements in the other QOL domains, while studies of lung/heart–lung recipients showed improvement in all domains. Liver recipient studies were quite variable in their findings across the QOL domains. The fact that no single QOL area stood out as particularly improved by liver transplantation, relative to either other QOL areas or other types of transplantation, suggests that liver recipients have a difficult path to recovery and may take longer to realize the QOL benefits that other desperately ill patients (e.g., lung candidates) realize relatively quickly.

In summary, whether QOL improves with transplantation depends, first, on the QOL domain being considered. Figure 4.1 shows that physical functional QOL very often improves from pre- to post-transplantation, while improvement in mental health/cognitive status and social QOL is less certain. Superimposed on these differences are the QOL variations related to the specific type of transplant. Yet, these transplant-specific variations disappeared when recipients were asked about their global, overall perceptions of QOL. Every study examining global perceptions found improvements.

Is QOL in transplant recipients better than QOL in other similarly ill patient comparison samples?

From the pool of 144 studies retrieved, 61 primarily cross-sectional studies addressed this issue. The majority of these ($n = 52$) included comparison groups within the study design. The remainder compared their findings to patient samples described in other reports. Comparison groups most often consisted of persons who had illnesses similar in type and severity to those of the recipients. (In most reports, these were transplant candidates.) In a limited number of studies, however, comparison groups were recipients of other types of organs. For example, Riether et al. (1992) compared liver to heart recipients, and Andrykowski et al. (1990b) compared bone marrow to kidney recipients. Most of the pancreas transplant studies utilized kidney-only transplant comparison groups. (In addition to the 61 studies that are relevant here, several other investigations compared recipients to other types of patient who were considerably less ill than persons eligible for transplantation; these investigations will be summarized separately below.)

Figure 4.2 shows the proportion of studies for each transplant type that found recipients' QOL to be superior to QOL in similarly ill comparison groups. As was noted for pre- to post-transplantation comparisons (Figure 4.1), there was less variability in results across the different areas of transplantation in Figure 4.2 for physical functional QOL than for the other three QOL domains. The findings range from 75% of liver studies reporting physical functional advantages for recipients to only 37.5% of heart studies and 33.3% of bone marrow studies finding effects in this direction. Most studies reporting advantages for recipients focused on specific physical functional areas, such as ambulation or mobility. However, some reports also found better general perceptions of physical health status and better clinical ratings of functional status (e.g., on the Karnofsky Index), relative to comparison groups. It is noteworthy that studies which did not report recipient advantages in the physical functional domain generally found no differences between the groups; there was little evidence that recipients' QOL appeared any poorer than other similarly ill or transplanted groups.

Relative to the physical functional domain, studies were less likely to find recipient QOL advantages over comparison groups for mental health/cognitive status. In fact, except for heart transplant studies, studies of the five other transplant types were more likely to find that recipient mental health QOL was the same or poorer than that of comparison groups. Pancreas, lung/heart–lung and bone marrow recipients were particularly unlikely to have QOL advantages for mental health. However, while pancreas and lung/heart–lung recipients were usually found to be indistinguishable from comparison patients, bone marrow recipients were found in three of the seven relevant studies to actually have worse QOL than comparison groups in the mental

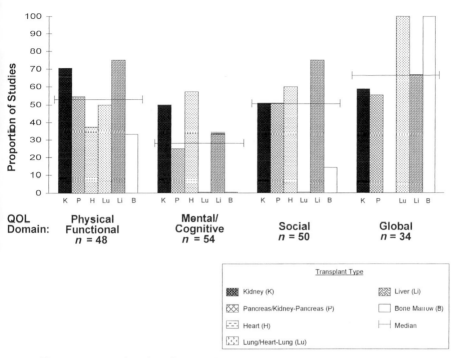

Figure 4.2. Proportion of studies in each type of transplantation that found recipients' quality of life (QOL) to be better than that of similarly ill comparison groups.

health/cognitive status domain. Andrykowski et al. (1989a; Andrykowski, Henslee, and Farrell 1989b), in particular, found that bone marrow recipients had poorer QOL in all emotional and cognitive areas assessed. In contrast, 57% of heart recipient studies found that recipients showed a QOL advantage in the mental health domain. Their heightened well-being appeared to be related to improvements in depression and anxiety levels, as well as improved cognitive status post-transplantation.

Results across the six transplant types were even more variable for social functioning QOL: while 50% or more of studies of liver, heart, and pancreas recipients found QOL advantages over comparison groups, studies of bone marrow recipients and lung/heart–lung recipients were unlikely to show advantages. Any social QOL advantages seemed to pertain to employment status and involvement and satisfaction with social/leisure activities. Among transplant types without consistent social QOL advantages, lung/heart–lung studies found that recipients appeared no worse in social functioning than did comparison groups. In contrast, several bone marrow studies found worse social QOL for recipients: Andrykowski et al. (1989a,b) reported more impairments in social activity, Altmaier, Gingrich, and Fyfe (1991) found higher levels of difficulty in interpersonal relationships and sexual function-ing, and Lesko and colleagues (Lesko et al. 1992; Mumma, Mashberg, and Lesko 1992) reported more difficulties in family, work and (for women) sexual activity areas than in comparison samples.

Finally, recipients' overall QOL in relation to other ill patients was ex-tremely variable. Although there were only two relevant studies each of bone marrow recipients and lung/heart–lung recipients, all four found recipients to report better overall QOL than that reported by controls. These recipients' global QOL advantages are especially interesting in light of their lack of advantage over comparison groups in the more specific domains of QOL already described. Liver, kidney, and pancreas recipient studies were mid-range in the proportion of each that found recipients to be advantaged over comparison groups; in each of these transplant types, more studies documented an advantage than a disadvantage (i.e., their "success" rate was over 50%). Only one study of heart recipients examined overall QOL. Although it did not find positive effects, it is difficult to place much emphasis on results from a single investigation.

Examination of domain-by-domain QOL differences for each specific type of transplantation suggests that only kidney studies consistently demonstrate, at above a 50% "success" level, that recipients' QOL was superior to QOL in comparison groups. For other transplantation types, recipients' advantages over comparison groups occurred only in certain QOL domains, but not in others. For example, the majority of liver transplant studies found recipient physical functional and social QOL advantages over comparison groups, but were considerably less likely to find mental health advantages. On the other hand, heart studies showed recipient mental health and social, but not physical functional, QOL advantages as compared to controls. Finally, even though bone marrow recipients rarely showed QOL advantages for any of the three specific QOL domains, they were consistently found to have higher perceptions of overall QOL than comparison groups. This discrepancy be-tween specific and general QOL evaluations among bone marrow studies again indicates that patients view health-related QOL areas very differently from how they view the overall quality of their lives.

In summary, as for the first central question addressed in this review, the answer to the second question, concerning whether transplant recipients have QOL advantages over similarly ill comparison groups, depends on the QOL domain under consideration. Among the three specific functional domains, the physical functional domain shows more consistently positive outcomes for transplant patients than do the mental health and social domains (i.e., the range of the bars in Figure 4.2 is more compressed for physical functional QOL than for other domains of QOL). There appears to be as yet little consensus about whether transplant recipients experience social functioning QOL advantages over patient comparison groups. It is again striking that, in general, global QOL, compared to other domains, is most likely to show transplant recipients to be advantaged relative to ill comparison groups.

Finally, there are a few studies that compared transplant recipients to other patient populations presumed to be less severely ill than transplant recipients had been pre-transplantation. Thus, the hypothesis implicit in these studies was not that transplant recipients would show any advantages over these other groups but, instead, that their QOL would appear similar to, and certainly no worse than, these other groups. Kidney recipients were compared to primary care patients (Petrie 1989), two sets of investigations compared heart recipients to coronary artery by-pass graft (CABG) patients (Wallwork and Caine 1985; Strauss et al. 1992), and liver recipients were compared to Crohn's disease patients (Tarter et al. 1984, 1988). Petrie found that kidney recipients had poorer mental health QOL but similar perceptions of global QOL as control patients. Wallwork and Caine and Tarter et al. found transplant recipients to be similar to comparison groups in all QOL domains. Strauss et al. obtained similar findings except that liver recipients had relatively poorer cognitive status. The limited number of studies precludes firm conclusions, but these four reports do suggest that transplant candidates can hope to achieve QOL comparable to that of much less severely ill persons.

Is QOL in transplant recipients similar to or better than QOL in healthy samples?

Forty-nine studies addressed this issue, generally with cross-sectionally collected data. The majority made comparisons solely to normative data or data from healthy cohorts published elsewhere. Five of the 49 studies included healthy comparison groups within their study design. For each of the four QOL domains, Figure 4.3 summarizes the proportion of studies that found patients' post-transplantation QOL to be similar to, or better than, that of nonpatient samples. Across the six transplant types, most studies did not find that recipients' QOL equalled that of normative samples for physical functional, mental health, and social functioning QOL domains.

It is important to bear in mind that the number of studies examining this issue has tended to be much smaller than the number addressing the other questions raised in this review. For physical functional QOL, one of the two lung/heart–lung transplant studies found no differences between recipients and healthy norms. For other transplant types, where studies were more numerous, recipient QOL outcomes were generally poorer than healthy norms. Interestingly, however, for the three transplant types with the largest numbers of studies available – kidney, heart, and liver – it is once more noteworthy that transplant recipients' perceptions of global QOL tended to

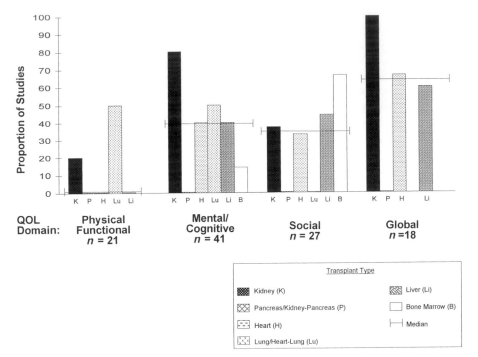

Figure 4.3. Proportion of studies in each type of transplantation that found recipients' quality of life (QOL) to be similar to, or better than, that of healthy people.

equal or surpass those of healthy samples.

Considering types of transplant separately, it can be seen that neither of the two pancreas studies found QOL in any domain to be as good as or better than healthy groups. Findings across QOL domains were quite variable for bone marrow and lung/heart–lung studies, possibly influenced by the small number of reports. However, the pattern of findings is also variable for kidney, heart, and liver, for which there were numerous studies.

In summary, the body of studies does not demonstrate that recipient QOL equals that of healthy nonpatient samples, suggesting that this may not be a realistic expectation for transplantation in the current era. Caution should be exercised, however, because there have been relatively few studies of this issue, particularly for some types of transplant.

Methodologic issues affecting study results

The six types of transplant often vary widely in the proportions of studies demonstrating QOL benefits. This variability no doubt reflects true differences across transplant types. Obviously, the various forms of transplantation are performed to treat different underlying illnesses, involve very different medical procedures, and have distinct long-term complications. However, methodologic differences are also likely to have contributed to this variability. Even within types of transplant, e.g., heart or liver, individual studies differ in their choice of QOL measures and QOL domains assessed. Clinical differences within and between samples in illness duration and severity before transplantation, and timepoints post-transplantation at which recipients are assessed are important also.

With regard to the latter issue, for example, recipients assessed in the first several months post-transplantation might have different QOL profiles than recipients several years post-transplantation. If QOL declines, for example, across the years post-transplantation, existing studies may have produced biased estimates of how positive QOL is during the post-transplantation lifespan. In general, however, longitudinal studies find QOL either to be stable or to improve over the first 1 to 7 years after transplantation (e.g., House 1987; Chao et al. 1992; Dew et al. 1994; Nakache et al. 1994; Matas et al. 1998; TenVergert et al. 1998). Reports of declining QOL post-transplantation are very rare, except in cases of graft failure. Thus, regardless of the timepoint(s) selected for assessment during the first several years post-transplantation, it is unlikely that the studies included in this review have seriously overestimated the differences between (a) post-transplantation QOL in recipients with functioning grafts and (b) either pre-transplantation QOL or QOL in comparison groups.

Differences in findings across studies may have been amplified by demographic and psychosocial differences in the samples studied. For example, certain variables including age, gender, personal history of psychiatric disorder, general coping style and specific coping strategies, and perceived and actual levels of social supports, have been shown to affect QOL ratings. However, although these factors may influence post-transplantation QOL, it is important to note that, even after their effects are controlled for, QOL benefits of transplantation are usually still observed. Individual reviews of these factors' unique effects in each of the six types of transplant provide an extended discussion of their contribution to QOL (e.g., Beidel 1987; Andrykowski 1994; Levy 1994; Surman 1994; Whedon and Ferrell 1994; Gross and Raghu 1997; Molassiotis, Van den Akker, and Boughton 1997; Cohen et al. 1998).

The issue of the influence of psychosocial factors – and social supports in particular – introduces the final question to be addressed in this review. Recipients' prime source of psychosocial support is their immediate family. However, the extent to which family members can provide emotional and tangible assistance to the patient is likely to be determined in part by these persons' reactions and adjustment to the transplantation experience.

What effect does transplantation have on the QOL of recipients' families?

This topic has been empirically examined in very few studies ($n < 25$), most of which have been conducted in North America since 1984. The majority focus on heart transplant recipients' families (Hyler, Corley, and McMahon 1985; Mishel and Murdaugh 1987; Busé and Pieper 1990; Baumann, Young, and Egan 1992; Grundböck, Bunzel, and Schubert 1992; Erdman et al. 1993; Canning, Dew, and Davidson 1996; Dew et al. 1998a; Konstam et al. 1998; Bunzel et al. 1999). Next most common are studies of families of kidney recipients (Gray, Brogan, and Kutner 1985; House 1987; Chowanec and Binik 1989; Frazier, Davis-Ali, and Dahl 1995), and then liver recipients (Tarter et al. 1988, 1990b; Benning and Smith 1994). There is only one study of QOL in bone marrow recipients' families (Zabora et al. 1992) and none in lung/heart–lung transplantation.

The earlier of the family studies focused heavily on patient concerns, while more recent work clearly recognizes that family members are also affected by the transplantation process. Of the four QOL domains addressed in this review, mental health, social functioning, and overall QOL have been studied in family members, but physical health QOL has rarely been considered. In addition to these QOL domains, the domain of family burden is prominent in the literature.

All studies focused on adult family members, although occasionally adults acted as informants for children of the transplant recipient as well. The mean age of family respondents is generally 40 to 46 years (Chowanec and Binik 1989; Busé and Pieper 1990; Tarter et al. 1990b; Baumann et al. 1992; Erdman et al. 1993; Canning et al. 1996; Frazier et al. 1995; Dew et al. 1998a; Konstam et al. 1998; Bunzel et al. 1999). The recipient's spouse is the most frequently studied family member. A few investigations described their samples in broader terms such as "partners," "significant others," "informants," or "caregivers" (e.g., Tarter et al. 1988; Baumann et al. 1992; Grundböck et al. 1992; Zabora et al. 1992; Erdman et al. 1993; Benning and Smith 1994; Canning et al. 1996; Dew et al. 1998a). Regardless of the recipient's gender, the studied family member was usually female. This overrepresentation of women has been noted in other studies of family caregivers to persons with medical illnesses (Biegel et al. 1991) and may limit the studies' generalizability to male family members.

Perceived burdens of the transplantation experience on family members

We discuss burden effects first, since many of these burdens may logically lead to QOL changes in the family. The literature suggests that there are four major categories of burden in transplant families: task performance, time management, transplant-related worries, and financial burdens.

The first category focuses on the tasks and roles family members assume in the wake of the patient's life-threatening illness and the transplant. Often, these roles were previously held by the patient (Mishel and Murdaugh 1987; Baumann et al. 1992; Zabora et al. 1992; Benning and Smith 1994; Busé and Pieper 1990). In one study of support groups, change in role and responsibility was among the most frequently mentioned topics (Hyler et al. 1985). Recipients' spouses have commented on increased responsibilities for home maintenance, fiscal management, and household chores, as well as becoming the major wage earner (Baumann et al. 1992; Zabora et al. 1992). On the basis of adult informants' reports, role change was also an issue for adolescent children, who had to assume new, previously parental responsibilities thereby affecting their own activities and schedules (Hyler et al. 1985; Zabora et al. 1992). As discussed below, these task/role changes appear to affect family members' QOL, especially in the social functioning domain.

Family members also share responsibility for the transplant recipient's health maintenance. Health maintenance tasks – such as assisting the recipient to remember and take medications, recipient care and household care to prevent infections, and scheduling and attending routine clinical follow-up visits – were the most frequently noted concern of one sample of spouses (Hyler et al. 1985). Another study found that spouses ranked the need to learn more about the transplant as a prominent task both before and after the transplantation surgery (Busé and Pieper 1990).

A second area of burden that is closely related to task responsibility is that of time burden. Here, the issue is not so much the difficulties of assuming or relinquishing roles, but rather the perceived time constraints in engaging in all work and leisure activities, whether or not they are related to the transplantation experience. Of the two investigations that have empirically addressed this issue, Busé and Pieper (1990) found that time constraints lessened from pre- to post-transplantation. Spouses indicated that the amount of time they had for themselves increased following the transplantation. Canning et al. (1996) found that during the initial year post-transplantation, burdens imposed by time constraints lightened as the months elapsed since transplantation. (See also Dew et al. (1998a), who report on a sample that partially overlaps with that of Canning et al.) Of particular importance, Canning et al. found that task performance itself was not burdensome, suggesting that it was the time requirements and not the tasks per se that were critical to perceived burden.

The third category of burden refers to family members' worries and concerns directly related to the transplant procedure and the recipient's health. Although it is clearly closely related to family member mental health QOL outcomes, this specific burden focuses on family members' experience with the transplant and with the recipient, rather than on their perceptions of their own well-being.

Several studies measured families' post-transplantation-related worries, including graft versus host disease, infections, the need for retransplantation, and fear that the recipient might die. Three investigations found that such concerns were prominent and major sources of transplant-related stress (Mishel and Murdaugh 1987; Busé and Piper 1990; Frazier et al. 1995). In contrast, Canning et al. (1996) found a lower overall level of worry among recipients' spouses, which was not related to spouse QOL outcomes. However, in the Canning et al. report, spouses' worries were measured at two months post-transplantation, while the other investigations focused on spouses either pretransplantation or 1 to 2 years post-transplantation. Thus, a possible explanation for the discrepancy in findings may lie in the choice of timepoint at which the transplant-related health worries were measured. During the initial post-transplantation period, spouses' feelings may be dominated by a sense of relief that the recipient survived the surgery and is recovering.

An indirect indicator of the burden of transplant-related worry in spouses is their frequent hesitancy to explicitly plan for the future. Even at 1 year post-transplantation, Zabora et al. (1992) found that spouses were unwilling to make long-range plans, and several studies suggest that fear of complications and continued uncertainty regarding the recipient's health may hamper families from making long-term future commitments (e.g., Busé and Pieper 1990).

The fourth major area of burden pertains to family finances. All studies investigating this issue in family members (and all focused on spouses) found budgetary matters to be a subject of great concern (Gray et al. 1985; Busé and Pieper 1990; Zabora et al. 1992). Indeed, financial burden is one area that has often been perceived to worsen rather than improve with the recipient's transplant (Gray et al. 1985). Financial concerns may arise from both medical and nonmedical (e.g., relocation) expenses, and families frequently report feeling ill-prepared by pretransplantation screenings for the expenses for which they are ultimately responsible (Gray et al. 1985).

Quality of life in transplant recipients' family members

Of the four domains of QOL considered in this review, physical functional QOL in family members has been evaluated least often, presumably under the assumption that these persons are healthy. It is noteworthy, then, that Canning et al. (1996) found that 20.5% of their sample of heart recipients' spouses had three or more chronic illnesses under ongoing medical care. Although many of these conditions began well prior to the transplantation, this study did not consider whether the transplantation experience exacerbates such conditions. However, in a later analysis of the same cohort, Dew et al. (1998a) found that distinct subgroups of caregivers could be identified whose health deteriorated post-transplantation. In some cases, the health decline could be directly linked to an elevated caregiving burden. Pre- to post-transplantation improvement of family members' general perceptions of their own physical health was noted in another study (Busé and Pieper 1990). The only other area of physical status specifically considered has been caregiver sleep difficulties, which have been found to be worse during the waiting period than post-transplantation. Sleep difficulties appear to persist, but at reduced levels, post-transplantation (Busé and Pieper 1990; Erdman et al. 1993).

Turning to mental health QOL, recipients' spouses show lower overall distress levels, depressive and anxiety-related symptom levels, and lower rates of diagnosable psychiatric disorder post-transplantation than the recipients themselves (House 1987; Erdman et al. 1993; Frazier et al. 1995). Nevertheless, spouses' distress levels are elevated above normative levels, at least in the early post-transplantation period, and their rates of clinically diagnosed psychiatric conditions are also high relative to norms (House 1987; Canning et al. 1996; Stukas et al. 1999). Although there has been little longitudinal examination of the course of distress post-transplantation, Canning et al. (1996) noted declining distress levels over the first postoperative year. Cross-sectional reports at later timepoints indicate that overall distress, depression and anxiety symptoms are in the range of normal comparison populations (Tarter et al. 1990b; Erdman et al. 1993; Frazier et al. 1995).

Informant reports suggest that very young children (less than 5 years old) often react to the transplantation experience with prolonged symptoms of depression, withdrawn behavior, and grief (Zabora et al. 1992). Older children are more likely to be confused about the experience, while adolescents may become depressed and resentful and angry over the family's overriding focus on the transplant recipient (Hyler et al. 1985; Zabora et al. 1992).

Of all QOL domains, social functioning QOL has received the most attention among family members. A large proportion of studies concentrated on family members' reactions to the task and role responsibility changes discussed above, some measuring perceptions of, and adaptation to, roles in both the recipient and his or her spouse (Mishel and Murdaugh 1987; Chowanec and Binik 1989; Grundböck et al. 1992; Bunzel et al. 1999). Grundböck et al. found that partners rated both their own and each other's role performance as poorer post-transplantation than they had rated it prior to transplantation. These declining perceptions appeared to be related to recipients' spouses' unwillingness to relinquish their new roles adopted during the illness and perioperative recovery periods. This, in turn, caused friction in their longer-term post-transplantation relationship. Changes and modifications in role responsibility and performance continued even at 1 year post-transplantation. Similar findings of long-term negative changes even at five years post-transplantation have been noted (Bunzel et al. 1999). Despite these difficulties, however, recipients' spouses have generally been found to carry out home and family responsibilities at an adequate level that did not differ from role performance evaluations in nontransplant families (Busé and Pieper 1990; Grundböck et al. 1992).

Indeed, though a concern for spouses and a source of conflict for the partnership, it is conceivable that role changes may, in the long run, be beneficial for family members. Role performance and related changes have been found to be related to increased self-esteem as a result of acquiring new skills, and to lower levels of psychological distress post-transplantation (Busé and Pieper 1990; Zabora et al. 1992; Canning et al. 1996). Similarly, although adolescents have felt that assuming roles and responsibilities caused disruption in their daily lives (Zabora et al. 1992), it is also possible that they might benefit from this early preparation for adult roles.

Beyond the issue of role performance, several studies considered the quality of the spouse's relationship with the recipient and with others. Busé and Pieper (1990) found that spouses rated feelings of closeness and tenderness as being one of the areas of the marital relationship most influenced, and most improved, by the transplantation experience. Canning et al. (1996) also found that, on average, spouses rated their relationship with the recipient as being of very high quality post-transplantation. Nevertheless, spouses have been found to rate the relationship as poorer than their respective recipients' ratings (Konstam et al. 1998). These three reports collected data only post-transplantation. In contrast, Grundböck et al. (1992) found in a prospective study that emotional involvement decreased significantly from pre- to post-transplantation. Although this decline is noteworthy, it is important to bear in mind that the pre-transplantation period does not provide a good "baseline" as to the preexisting quality of the relationship because families often undergo dramatic changes during the pre-transplantation waiting period.

In order to provide an external source of comparison, Frazier et al. (1995) compared the marital satisfaction of kidney transplant recipient–spouse pairs with that of non-transplant, married, adult couples. (The health status of these latter couples was not specified.) They found that transplant couples were quite similar to controls in their levels of marital satisfaction and perceived ability to offer support to each other. Moreover, several reports indicate that recipients' spouses do not perceive that their relationships with other close or extended family members or friends suffered after transplantation (Busé and Pieper 1990; Erdman et al. 1993). Ratings of these other relationships remain high post-transplantation (Frazier et al. 1995; Canning et al. 1996). In fact, some spouses even developed new relationships, particularly with other transplant families (Zabora et al. 1992).

Finally, the fourth domain of QOL, overall perceptions of one's life, has been found to be much improved post-transplantation in recipients' spouses, although these findings were based on a retrospective study design in which spouses were reflecting on their lives both before and after the transplantation (Busé and Pieper 1990). Level of satisfaction with life appears to remain relatively stable over time post-transplantation, at least during the first several years (Baumann et al. 1992).

In summary, relative to studies of transplant recipients, there is a paucity of research about their family members' QOL. The only family members to be empirically considered in any depth have been recipients' spouses. Study of family and caregiving burdens has generally taken precedence over the explicit study of QOL outcomes in these persons. With respect to both burden and QOL, the greatest emphasis has been on understanding change in role function and family relationships with the recipient. In contrast, family members' physical and mental health outcomes in the face of the transplantation experience have received relatively little attention.

General summary and conclusions

The sheer number of QOL studies in transplantation, plus the breadth and depth of coverage of QOL domains, are striking. Although research on family issues lags far behind the study of transplant recipients, this is somewhat understandable: the patient's QOL is intimately connected with judgments as to the efficacy of any given medical therapy, and constitutes a core element for judging the success and utility of the therapy. Effects on the family are difficult to determine until the effects of the therapy on the patient are understood. In addition to the fact that QOL research in transplant recipients is better established than in their family members, several other key conclusions can be drawn from our review.

First, the conceptualization and measurement of QOL is evolving in the direction of greater clarity and sophistication. Reliable measures that are sensitive to clinical change are available. Useful strategies have been developed for combining generic and disease-specific instruments in order to provide a broad assessment of the full range of outcomes encompassed by the term "quality of life". None of the measures or assessment strategies are infallible, but enough progress has been made that the study of QOL outcomes is becoming a routine feature, rather than an expensive novelty, in clinical trials.

Second, convergent evidence from a variety of transplant types, a variety of study designs, and demographically diverse study cohorts suggests that QOL is reliably improved by transplant. It is important to note that this is a general statement: QOL is not necessarily improved in every patient, or equally improved in every QOL domain, or equally improved across all types of transplantation. However, there is an impressive body of research demonstrating positive pre- to post-transplantation changes in multiple domains of specific functional and global QOL. There is also impressive evidence that transplant recipients show QOL advantages over similarly ill persons who have not received transplants.

Third, although transplantation can produce QOL benefits, transplant recipients do not have the QOL of essentially healthy nonpatient populations. This issue has clearly received the least consideration to date, and could benefit from continued, careful study. It is possible that surgical and immunosuppressive drug therapy innovations might boost future recipients' QOL to levels closer to norms. But it also may be the case that, to some extent, this issue matters less for recipients and their families than the issues of pre- to post-transplantation improvement and advantage over nontransplanted patients. Such a conclusion is suggested by our fourth, additional finding.

Fourth, regardless of any variations in QOL either as a function of the specific domain of QOL (e.g., physical functional, mental, social) or across the major types of transplant, transplant recipients overwhelmingly indicate that the global quality of their lives is high. Thus, among studies with the strongest research designs – prospective evaluations before and after transplantation – every investigation that considered global perceptions found improvement. The intriguing question now becomes, why did global QOL so consistently change, even in the face of more modest changes in specific health-related QOL domains?

This discrepancy may be due to measurement-related artefacts related to differences in scales or response categories used to assess specific versus global QOL. However, another explanation may be more accurate. As the late Roberta G. Simmons demonstrated so convincingly in her landmark study of kidney donors and recipients (Simmons et al. 1977), transplant patients have literally received the "gift of life" – or more accurately, the gift of an extension of a life that would otherwise be lost or severely constrained. This undoubtedly leads to a redefinition of "normal" life and what it entails. The studies considered in this review, as well as clinical case reports, frequently observe that transplant recipients live with many medication and treatment side effects and other health problems, yet feel that they value life more than ever before. Thus, what might appear to be a discrepancy between levels of improvement in domain-specific QOL and improvement in global QOL may simply reflect a revision in patients' standards of reference, and/or a revision in the way patients "add up" the components of their lives in order to arrive at its overall quality. This taps into a more spiritual, philosophical, or existential domain that has rarely been specifically addressed in QOL studies in transplant recipients (cf., Harris et al. 1995).

If we accept that, no matter what the flaws in any given investigation, the body of research on QOL in transplantation has demonstrated distinct benefits of transplantation for the patient, what directions are critical for future QOL work in this field? The continued evolution of transplantation is the first critical factor that will drive QOL work. Transplantation does not involve a static set of procedures. Innovative surgical techniques, immunosuppressive drugs and regimens, the development of mechanical devices to assist and/or replace failing organs, and the possibilities of xenografting will all require continued appraisal of patients' and their families' QOL.

Patient and family characteristics are the second set of critical factors that will drive future work. All of the QOL findings that we have discussed pertain to patients and families in general. Large differences in QOL are often observed, however, within specific transplant cohorts. A significant minority of any given sample may show relatively little or no QOL gains, even though the average gain for the sample as a whole is quite positive. In addition to continued attention to specific transplant-related factors that may account for within-sample QOL differences, one of the most important issues for the future is to specify more clearly the full range of other personal and environmental factors that reduce or enhance the QOL outcomes in transplantation. Better understanding of the roles of these factors is essential for the development of psychosocial interventions to maximize QOL in the context of transplantation and its continued evolution.

Acknowledgement

This work was supported in part by grants HL54326 and HL48883 from the National Heart, Lung and Blood Institute, Bethesda, MD.

References

Adams, P. C., Ghent, C. N., Grant, D. R., and Wall, W. J. (1995). Employment after liver transplantation. *Hepatology*, **21**, 140–4.

Al-Kattan, K., Tadjkarimi, S., Cox, A., Banner, N., Khaghani, A., and Yacoub, M. (1995). Evaluation of the long-term results of single lung versus heart–lung transplantation for emphysema. *J. Heart Lung Transplant*, **14**, 824–31.

Altmaier, E. M., Gingrich, R. D., and Fyfe, M. A. (1991). Two-year adjustment of bone marrow transplant survivors. *Bone Marrow Transplant*, **7**, 311–16.

Andrykowski, M. A. (1994). Psychosocial factors in bone marrow transplantation: a review and recommendations for research. *Bone Marrow Transplant*, **13**, 357–75.

Andrykowski, M. A., Altmaier, E. M., Barnett, R. L., Burish, T. G., Gingrich, R., and Henslee-Downey, P. J. (1990a). Cognitive dysfunction in adult survivors of allogeneic marrow transplantation: relationship to dose of total body irradiation. *Bone Marrow Transplant*, **7**, 269–76.

Andrykowski, M. A., Altmaier, E. M., Barnett, R. L., Otis, M. L., Gingrich, R., and Henslee-Downey, P. J. (1990b). The quality of life in adult survivors of allogeneic bone marrow transplantation. *Transplantation*, **50**, 399–406.

Andrykowski, M. A., Brady, M. J., Greiner, C. B. et al. (1995a). "Returning to normal" following bone marrow transplantation: outcomes, expectations and informed consent. *Bone Marrow Transplant*, **15**, 573–81.

Andrykowski, M. A., Greiner, C. B., Altmaier, E. M. et al. (1995b). Quality of life following bone marrow transplantation: findings from a multicentre study. *Br J Cancer*, **71**, 1322–9.

Andrykowski, M. A., Henslee, P. J., and Barnett, R. L. (1989a). Longitudinal assessment of psychosocial functioning of adult survivors of allogeneic bone marrow transplantation. *Bone Marrow Transplant*, **4**, 505–9.

Andrykowski, M. A., Henslee, P. J., and Farrall, M. G. (1989b). Physical and psychosocial functioning of adult survivors of allogeneic bone marrow transplantation. *Bone Marrow Transplant*, **4**, 75–81.

Angermann, C. E., Bullinger, M., Zellner, M., Kemkes, B. M., and Theisen, K. (1992). Quality of life in long-term survivors of orthotopic heart transplantation. *Z Kardiol*, **81**, 411–17.

Aravot, D. J., Banner, N. R., Khaghani, A. et al. (1989). Cardiac transplantation in the seventh decade of life. *Am J Cardiol*, **63**, 90–3.

Arria, A. M., Tarter, R. E., and Starzl, T. E. (1991). Improvement in cognitive functioning of alcoholics following orthotopic liver transplantation. *Alcohol Clin Exp Res*, **15**, 956–62.

Avis, N. E., Czajkowski, S. M., Dew, M. A. et al. (1995). Evaluation of an implantable ventricular assist system for humans with chronic refractory heart failure: measuring quality of life. *Am Soc Artificial Int Org Trans*, **41**, 32–41.

Baker, F., Curbow, B., and Wingard, J. R. (1991). Role retention and quality of life of bone marrow transplant survivors. *Soc Sci Med*, **32**, 697–704.

Baker, F., Wingard, J. R., Curbow, B. et al. (1994). Quality of life of bone marrow transplant long-term survivors. *Bone Marrow Transplant*, **13**, 589–96.

Barrett, B. J., Vavasour, H., and Parfrey, P. S. (1989). The relationship of affect to physical symptoms in renal transplant recipients. *Transplant Proc*, **21**, 3353–4.

Baruch, J., Benjamin, S., Treleaven, J., Wilcox, A. H., Barron, J. L., and Powles, R. (1991). Male sexual function following bone marrow transplantation. *Bone Marrow Transplant*, **7**, 52.

Baumann, L. J., Young, C. J., and Egan, J. J. (1992). Living with a heart transplant: long-term adjustment. *Transplant Int*, **5**, 1–8.

Beck, A. T., Steer, R. A., and Garbvin, M. G. (1988). Psychometric properties of the Beck Depression Inventory: twenty-five years of evaluation. *Clin Psychol Rev*, **8**, 77–100.

Beidel, D. C. (1987). Psychological factors in organ transplantation. *Clin Psychol Rev*, **7**, 677–97.

Belec, R. H. (1992). Quality of life: perceptions of long-term survivors of bone marrow transplantation. *Oncol Nurs Forum*, **19**, 31–7.

Belle, S. H. and Porayko, M. K. (1995). Improvement in quality of life after transplantation for recipients in the NIDDK liver transplantation database. *Transplant Proc,* **27**, 1230–2.

Benedetti, E., Mattas, A. J., Hakim, N. et al. (1994). Renal transplantation for patients 60 years of age or older: a single-institution experience. *Ann Surg,* **4**, 445–60.

Benning, C. R. and Smith, A. (1994). Psychosocial needs of family members of liver transplant patients. *Clin Nurs Specialist,* **5**, 280–8.

Bergner, M., Bobbitt, R. A., Carter, W. B., and Gilson, B. S. (1981). The Sickness Impact Profile: development and final revision of a health status measure. *Med Care,* **19**, 787–805.

Biegel, D. E., Sales, E., and Schulz, R. (1991). *Family Caregiving in Chronic Illness.* Sage Publications, Inc: Newbury Park, CA.

Binik, Y. M., Baker, A. G., Kalogeropoulos, D. et al. (1982). Pain, control over treatment, and compliance in dialysis and transplant patients. *Kidney Int,* **21**, 840–8.

Binik, Y. M. and Devins, G. M. (1986). Transplant failure does not compromise quality of life in end-stage renal disease. *Int J. Psychiatry Med,* **16**, 281–92.

Binik, Y. M., Devins, G. M., and Orme, C. M. (1989). Psychological stress and coping in end-stage renal disease. In *Advances in the Investigation of Psychological Stress,* ed. R. W. J. Neufeld, pp. 305–42. John Wiley & Sons: New York.

Bohachick, P., Anton, B. B., Wooldridge, P. J. et al. (1992). Psychosocial outcome six months after heart transplant surgery: a preliminary report. *Res Nurs Health,* **15**, 165–73.

Bombardier, C., Ware, J., Russell, I. J., Larson, M., Chalmers, A., and Read, J. L. (1986). Auranofin therapy and quality of life in patients with rheumatoid arthritis: results of a multicenter trial. *Am J Med,* **81**, 565–78.

Bonsel, G. J., Essink-Bot, M-L., de Charro, F. T., van der Maas, P. J., and Habbema, J. D. F. (1990). Orthotopic liver transplantation in the Netherlands: the results and impact of a medical technology assessment. *Health Policy,* **16**, 147–61.

Bonsel, G. J., Essink-Bot, M., Klompmaker, I. J., and Slooff, M. J. H. (1992). Assessment of the quality of life before and following liver transplantation. *Transplantation,* **53**, 796–800.

Bornstein, R. A., Starling, R. C., and Myerowitz, P. D. (1992). Neuropsychological function before and after cardiac transplantation. In *Quality of Life after Open Heart Surgery,* ed. P.J. Walter, pp. 419–24. Kluwer Academic Publishers: Dordrecht.

Bornstein, R. A., Starling, R. C., Myerowitz, P., and Haas, G. J. (1995). Neuropsychological function in patients with end-stage heart failure before and after cardiac transplantation. *Acta Neurol Scand,* **91**, 260–5.

Boudet, M.-J., Dousset, B., Calmus, Y. et al. (1995). Quality of life after liver transplantation for cancer. *Transplant Proc,* **27**, 1796–7.

Bradburn, N. M. (1969). *The Structure of Psychological Well-Being.* Aldine: Chicago.

Bremer, B. A., McCauley, C. R., Wrona, R. M., and Johnson, J. P. (1989). Quality of life in end-stage renal disease: a reexamination. *Am J Kidney Dis,* **13**, 200–9.

Brennan, A. F., Davis, M. H., Buchholz, D. J., Kuhn, W. F., and Gray, Jr., L. A. (1987). Predictors of quality of life following cardiac transplantation. *Psychosomatics,* **28**, 566–71.

Bullinger, M., Angermann, C. E., and Kemkes, B. M. (1992). Psychological well-being of heart transplant patients – cross-sectional and longitudinal results. In *Quality of*

Life After Open Heart Surgery, ed. P. J. Walter, pp. 445–55, Kluwer Academic Publishers: Dordrecht.

Bulpitt, C. J. (1997). Quality of life as an outcome measure. *Postgrad Med J*, **73**, 613–16.

Bunzel, B., Grundböck, A., Laczkovics, A., Holzinger, C., and Teufelsbauer, H. (1991). Quality of life after orthotopic heart transplantation. *J Heart Lung Transplant*, **10**, 455–9.

Bunzel, B., Grundböck, A., and Wollenek, G. (1992). Quality of life and satisfaction after heart transplantation. In *Quality of Life After Open Heart Surgery*, ed. P. J. Walter, pp. 501–6. Kluwer Academic Publishers: Dordrecht.

Bunzel, B., Laederach-Hofmann, K., and Schubert, M. T. (1999). Patients benefit – partners suffer? The impact of heart transplantation on the partner relationship. *Transplant Int*, **12**, 33–41.

Bunzel, B., Wollenek, G., Grundböck, A., and Schramek P. (1994a). Herztransplantation und Sexualität: Eine Erhebung bei 62 männlichen Patienten [Heart transplantation and its impact on sexual life: A retrospective inquiry of 62 male patients.] *Herz*, **18**, 294–302.

Bunzel, B., Wollenek, G., and Zuckerman, A. (1994b). Veränderung der lebensqualität nach Herztransplantation: Die subjektive Sicht der betroffenen Patienten – Teil I. [Quality of life after heart transplantation: the patients' perspective – Part I.] *Herz/Kreisl*, **26**, 41–6.

Busé, S. McG. and Pieper, B. (1990). Impact of cardiac transplantation on the spouse's life. *Heart Lung*, **19**, 641–8.

Bush, N. E., Haberman, M., Donaldson, G., and Sullivan, K. M. (1995). Quality of life of 125 adults surviving 6–18 years after bone marrow transplantation. *Soc Sci Med*, **40**, 479–90.

Busschbach, J. J. V., Horikx, P. E., van den Bosch, J. M. M., de la Rivière, A. B., and de Charro, F. T. (1994). Measuring the quality of life before and after bilateral lung transplantation in patients with cystic fibrosis. *Chest*, **105**, 911–17.

Buxton, M. J., Acheson, R., Caine, N., Gibson, S., and O'Brien, B. J. (1985). Costs and benefits of the heart transplant programmes at Harefield and Papworth Hospitals. *DHSS Research Report No. 12*. HMSO: London.

Caine, N. and O'Brien, V. (1989). Quality of life and psychological aspects of heart transplantation. In *Heart and Heart–Lung Transplantation*, ed. J. Wallwork, pp. 387–422, WB Saunders Co: Philadelphia.

Caine, N., Sharples, L. D., English, T. A. H., and Wallwork, J. (1990). Prospective study comparing quality of life before and after heart transplantation. *Transplant Proc*, **22**, 1437–9.

Caine, N., Sharples, L. D., Smyth, R., Scott, J., Hathaway, T., Higenbottam, T. W., and Wallwork J. (1991). Survival and quality of life of cystic fibrosis patients before and after heart-lung transplantation. *Transplant Proc*, **23**, 1203–4.

Caine, N., Sharples, L., and Wallwork, J. (1992). Quality of life before and after heart transplantation. In *Quality of Life after Open Heart Surgery*, ed. P. J. Walter, pp. 491–8. Kluwer Academic Publishers: Dordrecht.

Campbell, A., Converse, P. E., and Rodgers, W. L. (1976). *The Quality of American Life*. Russell Sage Foundation: New York.

Canadian Erythropoietin Study Group (1990). Association between recombinant human erythropoietin and quality of life and exercise capacity of patients receiving haemodialysis. *Br J Med*, **300**, 575–8.

Canning, R. D., Dew, M. A., and Davidson, S. (1996). Psychological distress among caregivers to heart transplant recipients. *Soc Sci Med*, **42**, 599–608.

Chao, N. J., Tierney, D. K., Bloom, J. R. et al. (1992). Dynamic assessment of quality of life after autologous bone marrow transplantation. *Blood*, **80**, 825–30.

Chen, C. L. and Sun, C. K. (1994). Quality of life following orthotopic liver transplantation. *Transplant Proc*, **26**, 2266–8.

Chowanec, G. D. and Binik, Y. M. (1989). End stage renal disease and the marital dyad: an empirical investigation. *Soc Sci Med*, **28**, 971–83.

Churchill, D. N., Torrance, G. W., Taylor, D. W. et al. (1987). Measurement of quality of life in end-stage renal disease: the time trade-off approach. *Clin Invest Med*, **10**, 14–20.

Cleary, P. D., Epstein, A. M., Oster, G. et al. (1991). Health-related quality of life among patients undergoing percutaneous transluminal coronary angioplasty. *Med Care*, **29**, 939–50.

Cohen, L., Littlefield, C., Kelly, P., Mauer, J., and Abbey, S. (1998). Predictors of quality of life and adjustment after lung transplantation. *Chest*, **113**, 633–44.

Collis, I., Burroughs, A., Rolles, K., and Lloyd, G. (1995). Psychiatric and social outcome of liver transplantation. *Br J Psychiatry*, **166**, 521–4.

Colonna II, J. O., Brems, J. J., Hiatt, J. R. et al. (1988). The quality of survival after liver transplantation. *Transplant Proc*, **20**, 594–7.

Commander, M., Neuberger, J., and Dean, C. (1992). Psychiatric and social consequences of liver transplantation. *Transplantation*, **53**, 1038–40.

Corry, R. J. and Zehr, P. S. (1990). Quality of life in diabetic recipients of kidney transplants is better with the addition of the pancreas. *Clin Transplant*, **4**, 238–41.

Craven, J. L., Bright, J., and Dear, C. L. (1990). Psychiatric, psychosocial, and rehabilitative aspects of lung transplantation. *Clin Chest Med*, **11**, 247–57.

Croog, S. H., Levine, S., Testa, M. A. et al. (1986). The effects of antihypertensive therapy on the quality of life. *N Engl J Med*, **314**, 1657–64.

Curbow, B., Somerfield, M. R., Baker, F., Wingard, J. R., and Legro, M. W. (1993). Personal changes, dispositional optimism, and psychological adjustment to bone marrow transplantation. *J Behav Med*, **16**, 423–43.

DeCampli, W. M., Luikart, H., Hunt, S., and Stinson, E. B. (1995). Characteristics of patients surviving more than ten years after cardiac transplantation. *J Thorac Cardiovasc Surg*, **109**, 1103–15.

Dennis, C., Caine, N., Sharples, L., Smiyth, R. et al. (1993). Heart–lung transplantation for end-stage respiratory disease in patients with cystic fibrosis at Papworth Hospital. *J Heart Lung Transplant*, **12**, 893–902.

De-Nour, A. K. and Shanan, J. (1980). Quality of life of dialysis and transplanted patients. *Nephron*, **25**, 117–20.

Derogatis, L. (1976). *Scoring and Procedures Manual for PAIS*. Clinical Psychometric Research: Baltimore, MD.

Derogatis, L. (1983). *SCL-90-R Administration, Scoring and Procedures Manual – II*, 2nd edn. Clinical Psychometrics Research: Towson, MD.

Devins, G. M., Binik, Y. M., Gorman, P. et al. (1982). Perceived self-efficacy, outcome expectations, and negative mood states in end-state renal disease. *J Abnorm Psychol*,

91, 241–4.

Devins, G. M., Binik, Y. M., Hollomby, D. J., and Barré, P. E. (1981). Helplessness and depression in end-stage renal disease. *J Abnorm Psychol*, **90**, 531–45.

Devins, G. M., Binik, Y. M., Hutchinson, T. A., Hollomby, D. J., Barré, P. E., and Guttmann, R. D. (1983–1984). The emotional impact of end-stage renal disease: importance of patients' perceptions of intrusiveness and control. *Int J Psychiatry Med*, **13**, 327–43.

Devins, G. M., Binik, Y. M., Mandin, H. et al. (1986–1987). Denial as a defense against depression in end-stage renal disease. *Int J Psychiatry Med*, **16**, 151–62.

Devins, G. M., Mandin, H., Hons, R. B. et al. (1990). Illness intrusiveness and quality of life in end-stage renal disease: comparison and stability across treatment modalities. *Health Psychol*, **9**, 117–42.

Dew, M. A. (1994). Behavioral factors in heart transplantation: quality of life and medical compliance. *J Appl Biobehav Res*, **2**, 28–54.

Dew, M. A. (1998). Quality-of-life studies: organ transplantation research as an exemplar of past progress and future directions. *J Psychosom Res*, **44**, 189–95.

Dew, M. A., Goycoolea, J. M., Stukas, A. A. et al. (1998a). Temporal profiles of physical health in family members of heart transplant recipients: predictors of health change during caregiving. *Health Psychol*, **17**, 138–51.

Dew, M. A., Harris, R. C., Simmons, R. G., Roth, L. H., Armitage, J. M., and Griffith, B. P. (1991). Quality-of-life advantages of FK 506 vs conventional immunosuppressive drug therapy in cardiac transplantation. *Transplant Proc*, **23**, 3061–4.

Dew, M. A., Kormos, R. L., Roth, L. H. et al. (1993). Life quality in the era of bridging to cardiac transplantation: bridge patients in an outpatient setting. *Am Soc Artificial Int Org J*, **38**, 145–52.

Dew, M. A., Roth, L. H., Schulberg, H. C. et al. (1996a). Prevalence and predictors of depression and anxiety-related disorders during the year after heart transplantation. *Gen Hosp Psychiatry*, **18**, 48S–61S.

Dew, M. A., Roth, L. H., Switzer, G. E. et al. (1996b). Gender differences in patterns of emotional distress following heart transplantation. *J Clin Psychol Med Settings*, **3**, 367–86.

Dew, M. A. and Simmons, R. G. (1990). The advantage of multiple measures of quality of life. *Scand J Urol Nephrol*, **131**, 23–30.

Dew, M. A., Simmons, R. G., Roth, L. H. et al. (1994). Psychosocial predictors of vulnerability to distress in the year following heart transplantation. *Psychol Med*, **24**, 929–45.

Dew, M. A., Switzer, G. E., and DiMartini, A. F. (1998b). Psychiatric morbidity and organ transplantation. *Cur Opin Psychiatry*, **11**, 621–6.

Dew, M. A., Switzer, G. E., Goycoolea, J. M. et al. (1997). Does transplantation produce quality of life benefits: a quantitative review of the literature. *Transplantation*, **64**, 1261–73.

Dubernard, J. M., Tajra, L. C. Lefrancois, N., Dawahra, M., Martin, C., Thivolet, C., and Martin, X. (1998). Pancreas transplantation: results and indications. *Diabetes Metab*, **24**, 195–9.

Duitsman, D. M. and Cychosz, C. M. (1994). Psychosocial similarities and differences among employed and unemployed heart transplant recipients. *J Heart Lung Transplant*, **13**, 108–15.

Edelson, J. T., Weinstein, M. C., Tosteson, M. A., Williams, L., Lee, T. H., and Goldman, L. (1990). Long-term cost-effectiveness of various initial monotherapies for mild to moderate hypertension. JAMA, 253, 407–13.

Eid, A., Steffen, R., Sterioff, S. et al. (1989). Long-term outcome after liver transplantation. Transplant Proc, 21, 2409–10.

Erdman, R. A. M., Horstman, L., Van Domburg, R. T., Meeter, K., and Balk, A. H. H. M. (1993). Compliance with the medical regimen and partner's quality of life after heart transplantation. Qual Life Res, 2, 205–12.

Eschbach, J. W., Abdulhadi, M. H., Browne, J. K. et al. (1989). Recombinant human erythropoietin in anemic patients with end-stage renal disease: results of a phase III multicenter clinical trial. Ann Intern Med, 992–1000.

Esmatjes, E., Ricart, M. J., Fernández-Cruz L., Gonzalez-Clemente, J. M., Sáenz, A., and Astudillo, E. (1994). Quality of life after successful pancreas–kidney transplantation. Clin Transplant 8, 75–8.

Evans, R. W. (1987). The economics of heart transplantation. Circulation, 75, 63–7.

Evans, R. W. (1990). Quality of life assessment and the treatment of end-stage renal disease. Transplant Rev, 4, 1–23.

Evans, R. W. (1991). Recombinant human erythropoietin and the quality of life of end-stage renal disease patients: a comparative analysis. Am J Kidney Dis, 18, 62–70.

Evans, R. W. (1992). Psychosocial aspects of heart transplantation: a comparative analysis. In Quality of Life after Open Heart Surgery, ed. P. J. Walter, pp. 469–82. Kluwer Academic Publishers: Dordrecht.

Evans, R. W., Manninen, D. L., Garrison, L.P. et al. (1985a). The quality of life of patients with end-stage renal disease. N Engl J Med, 312, 553–9.

Evans, R. W., Manninen, D. L., and Livak, C. (1990). The Kidney Transplant Health Insurance Study. Battelle Human Affairs Research Center: Seattle, WA.

Evans, R. W., Manninen, D. L., Maier, A., Garrison, L. P., and Hart, L. G. (1985b). The quality of life of kidney and heart transplant recipients. Transplant Proc, 17, 1579–82.

Evans, R. W., Manninen, D. L., Overcase, T. D. et al. (1984). The National Heart Transplantation Study: Final Report, Vols. 1–5. Battelle Human Affairs Research Centers: Seattle, WA.

Felser, I., Wagner, S., Depee, J. et al. (1991). Changes in quality of life following conversion from CyA to FK 506 in orthotopic liver transplant patients. Transplant Proc, 23, 3032–4.

Fisher, D. C., Lake, K. D., Reutzel, T. J., and Emery, R. W. (1995). Changes in health-related quality of life and depression in heart transplant recipients. J Heart Lung Transplant, 14, 373–81.

Fitzpatrick, R., Davey, C., Buxton, M. J., and Jones, D. R. (1998). Evaluating patient-based outcome measures for use in clinical trials. Health Technol Assess, 2914, i–iv, 1–74.

Foley, T. C., Davis, C. P., and Conway, P. A. (1989). Liver transplant recipients – self-report of symptom frequency, symptom distress, quality of life. Transplant Proc, 21, 2417–18.

Frazier, P. A., Davis-Ali, S. H., and Dahl, K. E. (1995). Stressors, social support, and adjustment in kidney transplant patients and their spouses. Soc Work Health Care, 21, 93–108.

Freedberg, K. A. Tosteson, A. N. A., Cohen, C. J., and Cotton, D. J. (1991). Primary prophylaxis for pneumocystis carinii pneumonia in HIV-infected people with CD4 counts below 200: a cost-effectiveness analysis. *J Acquired Immune Def Syndrome*, **4**, 521–31.

Freeman III, A. M., Folks, D. G., Sokol, R. S., and Fahs, J. J. (1988). Cardiac transplantation: clinical correlates of psychiatric outcome. *Cardiac Transplant*, **29**, 47–54.

Frisk, B., Blohmé, I., and Brynger, H. (1980). The social rehabilitation and quality of life in patients living with kidney transplants for more than 10 years. *Scand J Urol Nephrol*, **54**, 100–2.

Gaber, A. O., Hathaway, D. K., Abell, T. et al. (1994). Improved autonomic and gastric function in pancreas–kidney vs kidney-alone transplantation contributes to quality of life. *Transplant Proc*, **26**, 515–16.

Goff, J. S., Glazner, J., and Bilir, B. M. (1998). Measuring outcome after transplantation: a critical review. *Liver Transplant Surg*, **4**, 189–96.

Gorlén, T., Ekeberg, O., Abdelnoor, M., Enger, E., and Aarseth, H. P. (1993). Quality of life after kidney transplantation: a 10–22 years follow-up. *Scand J Urol Nephrol*, **27**, 89–92.

Gouge, F., Moore, Jr., J., Bremer, B. A., McCauley, C. R., and Johnson, J. P. (1990). The quality of life of donors, potential donors, and recipients of living-related donor renal transplantation. *Transplant Proc*, **22**, 2409–13.

Grant, D., Evans, D., Hearn, M., Duff, J., Ghent, C., and Wall, W. (1990). Quality of life after liver transplantation. *Can J Gastroenterol*, **4**, 49–52.

Grant, M., Ferrell, B., Schmidt, G. M., Fonbuena, P., Niland, J. C., and Forman, S. J. (1992). Measurement of quality of life in bone marrow transplantation survivors. *Qual Life Res*, **1**, 375–84.

Gray, H., Brogan, D., and Kutner, N. G. (1985). Status of life-areas: Congruence/noncongruence in ESRD patient and spouse perceptions. *Soc Sci Med*, **20**, 341–6.

Gross, C. R., Limwattananon, C., and Matthews, B. J. (1998). Quality of life after pancreas transplantation: a review. *Clin Transplant*, **12**, 351–61.

Gross, C. R. and Raghu, G. (1997). The cost of lung transplantation and the quality of life post-transplant. *Clin Chest Med*, **18**, 391–403.

Gross, C. R. and Zehrer, C. L. (1992). Health-related quality of life outcomes of pancreas transplant recipients. *Clin Transplant*, **6**, 165–71.

Gross, C. R. and Zehrer, C. L. (1993). Impact of the addition of a pancreas to quality of life in uremic diabetic recipients of kidney transplants. *Transplant Proc*, **25**, 1293–5.

Grundböck, A., Bunzel, B., and Schubert, M. T. (1992). Changes in partnership after cardiac transplantation. In *Quality of Life after Open Heart Surgery*, ed. P. J. Walter, pp. 483–90, Kluwer Academic Publishers: Dordrecht.

Gudex, C. M. (1995). Health-related quality of life in endstage renal failure. *Qual Life Rev*, **4**, 359–66.

Harris, R. C., Dew, M. A., Lee, A. et al. (1995). The role of religion in heart-transplant recipients' long-term health and well-being. *J Religion Health*, **34**, 17–32.

Hart, L. G., and Evans, R. W. (1987). The functional status of ESRD patients as measured by the Sickness Impact Profile. *J Chron Dis*, **40**, 117S–130S.

Harvison, A., Jones, B. M., McBride, M., Taylor, F., Wright, O., and Chang, V. P.

(1988). Rehabilitation after heart transplantation: the Australian experience. *J Heart Transplant*, **7**, 337–41.

Hathaway, D. K., Abell, T., Cardoso, S., Hartwig, M. S., El Gebely, S., and Gaber, A. O. (1994). Improvement in autonomic and gastric function following pancreas-kidney versus kidney-alone transplantation and the correlation with quality of life. *Transplantation*, **57**, 816–22.

Hauser, M. L., Williams, J., Strong, M., Ganza, M., and Hathaway, D. (1991). Predicted and actual quality of life changes following renal transplantation. *ANNA J*, **18**, 295–305.

Hengeveld, M. W., Houtman, R. B., and Zwaan, F. E. (1988). Psychological aspects of bone marrow transplantation: a retrospective study of 17 long-term survivors. *Bone Marrow Transplant*, **3**, 69–75.

Hicks, F. D., Larson, J. L., and Ferrans, C. E. (1992). Quality of life after liver transplant. *Res Nurs Health*, **15**, 111–19.

Hilbrands, L. B., Hoitsma, A. J., and Koene, R. A. P. (1995). The effect of immunosuppressive drugs on quality of life after renal transplantation. *Transplantation*, **59**, 1263–70.

Hlatky, M. A., Rogers, W. J., Johnstone, I. et al. (1997). Medical care costs and quality of life after randomization to coronary angioplasty or coronary bypass surgery. Bypass Angioplasty Revascularization Investigation (BARI) investigators. *N Engl J Med*, **336**, 92–9.

Hong, B. A., Smith, M. D., Robson, A. M., and Wetzel, R. D. (1987). Depressive symptomatology and treatment in patients with end-stage renal disease. *Psychol Med*, **17**, 185–90.

House, A. (1987). Psychosocial problems of patients on the renal unit and their relation to treatment outcome. *J Psychosom Res*, **31**, 441–52.

House, R., Dubovsky, S. L., and Penn, I. (1983). Psychiatric aspects of hepatic transplantation. *Transplantation*, **36**, 146–50.

Hunt, S. M., McEwen, J., and McKenna, S. P. (1985). Measuring health status: a new tool for clinicians and epidemiologists. *J R Coll Gen Pract*, **35**, 185–8.

Hyler, B. J., Corley, M. C., and McMahon, D. (1985). The role of nursing in a support group for heart transplantation recipients and their families. *Heart Transplant*, **4**, 453–6.

Jenkins, P. L., Lester, H., Alexander, J., and Whittaker, J. (1994). A prospective study of psychosocial morbidity in adult bone marrow transplant recipients. *Psychosomatics*, **35**, 361–7.

Jenkins, P. L., Linington, A., and Whittaker, J. A. (1991). A retrospective study of psychosocial morbidity in bone marrow transplant recipients. *Psychosomatics*, **32**, 65–71.

Johnson, J. L., Schellberg, J., Munn, S. R., and Perkins, J. D. (1990). Does pancreas transplantation really improve the patient's quality of life? *Transplant Proc*, **22**, 575–6.

Johnson, J. P., McCauley, C. R., and Copley, J. B. (1982). The quality of life of hemodialysis and transplant patients. *Kidney Int*, **22**, 286–91.

Jones, B. M., Chang, V. P., Esmore, D. et al. (1988). Psychological adjustment after cardiac transplantation. *Med J Aust*, **149**, 118–22.

Jones, B. M., Taylor, F., Downs, K., and Spratt, P. (1992a). Long-term follow-up of the emotional adjustment of patients after heart transplantation. In *Quality of Life after Open Heart Surgery*, ed. P. J. Walter, pp. 427–37. Kluwer Academic Publishers: Dordrecht.

Jones, B. M., Taylor, F., Downs, K., and Spratt, P. (1992b). Longitudinal study of quality of life and psychological adjustment after cardiac transplantation. *Med J Aust*, **157**, 24–6.

Jones, B. M., Taylor, F. J., Wright, O. M. et al. (1990). Quality of life after heart transplantation in patients assigned to double- or triple-drug therapy. *J Heart Transplant*, **9**, 392–6.

Joralemon, D. and Fujinaga, K. M. (1997). Studying the quality of life after organ transplantation: research problems and solutions. *Soc Sci Med*, **44**, 1259–69.

Julius, M., Hawthorne, V. M., Carpentier-Alting, P., Kneisley, J., Wolfe, R. A., and Port, F. K. (1989). Independence in activities of daily living for end-stage renal disease patients: biomedical demographic correlates. *Am J Kidney Dis*, **13**, 61–9.

Kalman, T. P., Wilson, P. G., and Kalman, C. M. (1983). Psychiatric morbidity in long-term renal transplant recipients and patients undergoing hemodialysis: a comparative study. *JAMA*, **250**, 55–8.

Karnofsky, D. A. and Burchenal, J. H. (1949). The clinical evaluation of chemotherapeutic agents in cancer. In *Evaluation of chemotherapeutic agents*. Symposium held at New York Academy of Medicine, New York 1948, ed. C. M. Macleod, pp. 191–205. Columbia University Press: New York.

Keegan, D. L., Shipley, C., Dineen, T., and Steiger, M. (1983). Adjustment to renal transplantation. *Psychosomatics*, **24**, 825–31.

Kiebert, G. M., van Oosterhout, E. C. A. A., van Bronswijk, H., Lemkes, H. H. P. J., and Gooszen, H. G. (1994). Quality of life after combined kidney–pancreas or kidney transplantation in diabetic patients with end-stage renal disease. *Clin Transplant*, **8**, 239–45.

Kober, B., Küchler, Th., Broelsch, Ch., Kremer, B., and Henne-Bruns, D. (1990). A psychological support concept and quality of life research in a liver transplantation program: an interdisciplinary multicenter study. *Psychother Psychosom*, **54**, 117–31.

Koch, U. and Muthny, F. A. (1990). Quality of life in patients with end-stage renal disease in relation to the method of treatment. *Psychother Psychosom*, **54**, 161–71.

Konstam, V., Surman, O., Hizzazi, K. H. et al. (1998). Marital adjustment in heart transplantation patients and their spouses: a longitudinal perspective. *Am J Family Therapy*, **26**, 147–58.

Küchler, Th., Kober, B., Broelsch, Ch., Kremer, B., and Henne-Bruns, D. (1991). Quality of life after liver transplantation. *Clin Transplant*, **5**, 94–101.

Kuhn, W. F., Brennan, A. F., Lacefield, P. K., Brohm, J., Skelton, V. D., and Gray, L. A. (1990). Psychiatric distress during stages of the heart transplant protocol. *J Heart Transplant*, **9**, 25–9.

Kuhn, W. F., Myers, V., Brennan, A. F. et al. (1988). Psychopathology in heart transplant candidates. *J Heart Transplant*, **7**, 223–6.

Kutner, N. G., Brogan, D., and Kutner, M. H. (1986). End-stage renal disease treatment modality and patients' quality of life: longitudinal assessment. *Am J Nephrol*, **6**, 396–402.

Lai, M.-K., Huang, C.-C., Chu, S.-H., Chuang, C.-K., and Huang, J.-Y. (1992a). Clinical analysis of 206 cases of kidney transplantation. *J Formosan Med Assoc*, **91**,

405–12.

Lai, M.-K., Huang, C.-C., Chu, S.-H., Chuang, C.-K., and Huang, J.-Y. (1992b). Two hundred and thirty cases of kidney transplantation: single-center experience in Taiwan 1992. *Transplant Proc*, **24**, 1452–4.

Leedham, B., Meyerowitz, B. E., Muirhead, J., and Frist, W. H. (1995). Positive expectations predict health after heart transplantation. *Health Psychol*, **14**, 74–9.

Lesko, L. M., Ostroff, J. S., Mumma, G. H., Mashberg, D. E., and Holland, J. C. (1992). Long-term psychological adjustment of acute leukemia survivors: impact of bone marrow transplantation versus conventional chemotherapy. *Psychosom Med*, **54**, 30–47.

Levy, M. F., Jennings, L., Abouljoud, M. S. et al. (1995). Quality of life improvements at one, two, and five years after liver transplantation. *Transplantation*, **59**, 515–18.

Levy, N. B. (1994). Psychological aspects of renal transplantation. *Psychosomatics*, **35**, 427–33.

Leyendecker, B., Bartholomew, U., Neuhaus, R. et al. (1993). Quality of life of liver transplant recipients: a pilot study. *Transplantation*, **56**, 561–7.

Litwins, N. M. and Rodrigue, J. R. (1994). Quality of life in adult recipients of bone marrow transplantation. *Psychol Rep*, **75**, 323–8.

Lough, M. E., Lindsey, A. M., Shinn, J. A., and Stotts, N. A. (1985). Life satisfaction following heart transplantation. *Heart Transplant*, **4**, 446–9.

Lough, M. E., Lindsey, A. M., Shinn, J. A., and Stotts, N. A. (1987). Impact of symptom frequency and symptom distress on self reported quality of life in heart transplant recipients. *Heart Lung*, **16**, 193–200.

Lowe, D., O'Grady, J. G., McEwen, J., and Williams, R. (1990). Quality of life following liver transplantation: a preliminary report. *J R Coll Physicians, Lond*, **24**, 43–6.

Magni, G. and Borgherini, G. (1992). Psychosocial outcome after heart transplantation. In *Quality of Life After Open Heart Surgery*, ed. P. J. Walter, pp. 457–65. Kluwer Academic Publishers: Dordrecht.

Mai, F. M., McKenzie, F. N., and Kostuk, W. J. (1986). Psychiatric aspects of heart transplantation: Preoperative evaluation and postoperative sequelae. *Br Med J*, **292**, 311–13.

Mai, F. M., McKenzie, F. N., and Kostuk, W. J. (1990). Psychosocial adjustment and quality of life following heart transplantation. *Can J Psychiatry*, **35**, 223–7.

Manninen, D. L., Evans, R. W., and Dugan, M. K. (1991). Work disability, functional limitations, and the health status of kidney transplantation recipients posttransplant. In *Clinical Transplants 1991*, ed. P. Terasaki, pp. 193–203. UCLA Tissue Typing Laboratory: Los Angeles.

Matas, A. J., McHugh, L., Payne, W. D. et al. (1998). Long-term quality of life after kidney and simultaneous pancreas-kidney transplantation. *Clin Transplant*, **12**, 233–42.

McAleer, M. J., Copeland, J., Fuller, J., and Copeland, J. G. (1985). Psychological aspects of heart transplantation. *Heart Transplant*, **4**, 232–3.

McMillem, C., Fiegl, P., Metch, B., Hayden, K. A., Meyskens, F. L., and Crowley, J. (1989). Quality of life end points in cancer clinical trials: review and recommendations. *J Nat Cancer Inst*, **81**, 485–95.

McNair, P. M., Lorr, M., and Droppelman, L. (1981). *POMS Manual*, 2nd edn.

Education and Industrial Testing Service: San Diego, CA.

Meister, N. D., McAleer, M. J., Meister, J. S., Riley, J. E., and Copeland, J. G. (1986). Returning to work after heart transplantation. *J Heart Transplant*, 5, 154–61.

Milde, F. K., Hart, L. K., and Zehr, P. S. (1992). Quality of life of pancreatic transplant recipients. *Diabetes Care*, 15, 1459–63.

Milde, F. K., Hart, L. K., and Zehr, P. S. (1995). Pancreatic transplantation: impact on the quality of life of diabetic renal transplant recipients. *Diabetes Care*, 18, 93–5.

Mishel, M. H. and Murdaugh, C. L. (1987). Family adjustment to heart transplantation: redesigning the dream. *Nurs Res*, 36, 332–8.

Molassiotis, A., van den Akker, O. B. A., and Boughton, B. J. (1997). Perceived social support, family environment and psychosocial recovery in bone marrow transplant long-term survivors. *Soc Sci Med*, 44, 317–25.

Moore, K. A., Jones, R. McL., Angus, P., Hardy, K., and Burrows, G. (1992). Psychosocial adjustment to illness: quality of life following liver transplantation. *Transplant Proc*, 24, 2257–8.

Morris, P. L. P. and Jones, B. (1988). Transplantation versus dialysis: a study of quality of life. *Transplant Proc*, 20, 23–6.

Morris, P. L. P. and Jones, B. (1989). Life satisfaction across treatment methods for patients with end-stage renal failure. *Med J Aust*, 150, 428–32.

Mulcahy, D., Fitzgerald, M., Wright, C., Sparrow, J., Pepper, J., Yacoub, M., and Fox, K. M. (1993). Long term follow up of severely ill patients who underwent urgent cardiac transplantation. *Br Med J*, 306, 98–101.

Mulligan, T., Sheehan, H., and Hanrahan, J. (1991). Sexual function after heart transplantation. *J Heart Lung Transplant*, 10, 125–8.

Mumma, G. H., Mashberg, D., and Lesko, L. M. (1992). Long-term psychosexual adjustment of acute leukemia survivors: impact of marrow transplantation versus conventional chemotherapy. *Gen Hosp Psychiatry*, 14, 43–55.

Nadel, C. and Clark, J. J. (1986). Psychosocial adjustment after renal retransplants. *Gen Hosp Psychiatry*, 8, 41–8.

Nakache, R., Tyden, G., and Groth, C. G. (1989). Quality of life in diabetic patients after combined pancreas–kidney or kidney transplantation. *Diabetes*, 38, 40–2.

Nakache, R., Tyden, G., and Groth, C. G. (1994). Long-term quality of life in diabetic patients after combined pancreas–kidney transplantation or kidney transplantation. *Transplant Proc*, 26, 510–11.

Nathan, D. M., Fogel, H., Norman, D. et al. (1991). Long-term metabolic and quality of life results with pancreatic/renal transplantation in insulin-dependent diabetes mellitus. *Transplantation*, 51, 85–91.

National Heart, Lung and Blood Institute (1995). *Health-related Quality of Life: A Review of Findings from NHLBI-supported Clinical Research*. U.S. Government Printing Office: Washington, DC.

Neitzert, C. S., Ritvo, P., Dancey, J., Weiser, K., Murray, C., and Avery, J. (1998). The psychosocial impact of bone marrow transplantation: a review of the literature. *Bone Marrow Transplant*, 22, 409–22.

Niset, G., Coustry-Degré, C., and Degré, S. (1988). Psychosocial and physical rehabilitation after heart transplantation: 1-year follow-up. *Cardiology*, 75, 311–17.

O'Brien, B. J., Banner, N. R., Gibson, S., and Yacoub, M. H. (1988). The Nottingham Health Profile as a measure of quality of life following combined heart and lung transplantation. *J Epidemiol Community Health*, **42**, 232–4.

O'Brien, B. J., Buxton, M. H., and Ferguson, B. A. (1987). Measuring the effectiveness of heart transplant programmes: quality of life data and their relationship to survival analysis. *J Chronic Dis*, **40**, 137S–153S.

Office of Technology Assessment (1990). *Recombinant Human Erythropoietin: Payment Options for Medicare*. Publication No. OTA-H-451. United States Government Printing Office: Washington, DC.

Ohkubo, M. (1995). The quality of life after kidney transplantation in Japan: results from a nationwide questionnaire. *Transplant Proc*, **27**, 1452–7.

Packa, D. R. (1989). Quality of life of adults after a heart transplant. *J Cardiovasc Nurs*, **3**, 12–22.

Pae, W. E., Copeland, J. G., McCarthy, P. M. et al. (1998). Bethesda Conference: conference for the design of clinical trials to study circulatory support devices for chronic heart failure. *Ann Thorac Surg*, **66**, 1452–65.

Parfrey, P. S., Vavasour, H., Bullock, M., Henry, S., Harnett, J. D., and Gault, M. H. (1989). Development of a health questionnaire specific for end-stage renal disease. *Nephron*, **52**, 20–8.

Parfrey, P. S., Vavasour, H. M., and Gault, M. H. (1988a). A prospective study of health status in dialysis and transplant patients. *Transplant Proc*, **20**, 1231–2.

Parfrey, P. S., Vavasour, H. M., Henry, S., Bullock, M., and Gault, M. H. (1988b). Clinical features and severity of nonspecific symptoms in dialysis patients. *Nephron*, **50**, 121–8.

Paris, W., Muchmore, J., Pribil, A., Zuhdi, N., and Cooper, D. K. C. (1994). Study of the relative incidences of psychosocial factors before and after heart transplantation and the influence of posttransplantation psychosocial factors on heart transplantation outcome. *J Heart Lung Transplant*, **13**, 424–32.

Paris, W., Woodbury, A., Thompson, S., Levick, M., Nothegger, S., Arbuckle, P., Hutkin-Slade, L., and Cooper, D. K. C. (1993). Returning to work after heart transplantation. *J Heart Lung Transplant*, **12**, 46–54.

Paris, W., Woodbury, A., Thompson, S. et al. (1992). Social rehabilitation and return to work after cardiac transplantation – a multicenter survey. *Transplantation*, **53**, 433–8.

Park, H., Bang, W. R., Kim, S. J. et al. (1992). Quality of life of ESRD patients: development of a tool and comparison between transplant and dialysis patients. *Transplant Proc*, **24**, 1435–7.

Patrick, D. L. and Deyo, R. A. (1989). Generic and disease-specific measures in assessing health status and quality of life. *Med Care*, **27**, S217–S232.

Patrick, D. L. and Erickson, P. (1993). *Health Status and Health Policy: Quality of Life in Health Care Evaluation and Resource Allocation*. Oxford University Press: New York.

Penn, I., Bunch, D., Olenik, D., and Abouna, G. (1971). Psychiatric experience with patients receiving renal and hepatic transplants. *Semin Psychiatry*, **3**, 133–44.

Petrie, K. (1989). Psychological well-being and psychiatric disturbance in dialysis and renal transplant patients. *Br J Med Psychol*, **62**, 91–6.

Piehlmeier, W., Bullinger, M., Nusser, J. et al. (1991). Quality of life in Type I (insulin-dependent) diabetic patients prior to and after pancreas and kidney transplantation in relation to organ function. *Diabetologia*, **34**, S150–S157.

Price, C. E., Lowe, D., Cohen, A. T. et al. (1995). Prospective study of the quality of life in patients assessed for liver transplantation: outcome in transplanted and not transplanted groups. *J R Soc Med*, **88**, 130–5.

Procci, W. R. (1980). A comparison of psychosocial disability in males undergoing maintenance hemodialysis or following cadaver transplantation. *Gen Hosp Psychiatry*, **2**, 255–61.

Procci, W. R., Hoffman, K. I., and Chatterjee, S. N. (1978). Sexual functioning of renal transplant recipients. *J Nerv Ment Dis*, **166**, 402–7.

Ramsey, S. D., Patrick, D. L., Albert, R. K., Larson, E. B., Wood, D. E., and Raghu, G. (1995a). The cost-effectiveness of lung transplantation: a pilot study. *Chest*, **108**, 1594–601.

Ramsey, S. D., Patrick, D. L., Lewis, S., Albert, R. K., and Raghu, G. (1995b). Improvement in quality of life after lung transplantation: a preliminary study. *J Heart Lung Transplant*, **14**, 870–7.

Rector, T. S., Ormaza, S. M., and Kubo, S. H. (1993). Health status of heart transplant recipients versus patients awaiting heart transplantation: a preliminary evaluation of the SF-36 Questionnaire. *J Heart Lung Transplant*, **12**, 983–6.

Revicki, D. A. and Ehreth, J. L. (1997). Health-related quality-of-life assessment and planning for the pharmaceutical industry. *Clin Ther*, **19**, 1101–15.

Riether, A. M., Smith, S. L., Lewison, B. J., Cotsonis, G. A., and Epstein, C. M. (1992). Quality-of-life changes and psychiatric and neurocognitive outcome after heart and liver transplantation. *Transplantation*, **54**, 444–50.

Robinson, L. R., Switala, J., Tarter, R. E., and Nicholas, J. J. (1990). Functional outcome after liver transplantation: a preliminary report. *Arch Phys Med Rehabil*, **71**, 426–7.

Rodin, G., Voshart, K., Cattran, D., Halloran, P., Cardella, C., and Fenton, S. (1985–1986). Cadaveric renal transplant failure: the short-term sequelae. *Int J Psychiatry Med*, **15**, 357–64.

Rogers, W. J., Johnstone, D. E., Yusuf, S. et al. (1994). Quality of life among 5,025 patients with left ventricular dysfunction randomized between placebo and enalapril: the studies of left ventricular dysfunction. *J Am Coll Cardiol*, **23**, 393–400.

Rosenblum, D. S., Rosen, M. L., Pine, Z. M., Rosen, S. H., and Borg-Stein, J. (1993). Health status and quality of life following cardiac transplantation. *Arch Phys Med Rehabil*, **74**, 490–3.

Russell, J. D., Beecroft, M. L., Ludwin, D., and Churchill, D. N. (1992). The quality of life in renal transplantation – a prospective study. *Transplantation*, **54**, 656–60.

Samuelsson, R. G., Hunt, S. A., and Schroeder, J. S. (1984). Functional and social rehabilitation of heart transplant recipients under age thirty. *Scand J Thor Cardiovasc Surg*, **18**, 97–103.

Schall, R. R., Petrucci, R. J., Brozena, S. C., Cavarocchi, N. C., and Jessup, M. (1989). Cognitive function in patients with symptomatic dilated cardiomyopathy before and after cardiac transplantation. *J Am Coll Cardiol*, **14**, 1666–72.

Schareck, W. D., Hopt, U. T., Geisler, F., Pfeffer, F., and Becker, H. D. (1994). Quality of life after combined pancreas-/kidney transplantation. *Transplant Proc*, **26**, 518–19.

Schmidt, G. M., Niland, J. C., Forman, S. J. et al. (1993). Extended follow-up in 212 long-term allogeneic bone marrow transplant survivors. *Transplantation*, **55**, 551–7.

Schron, E. B., Gorkin, L., and Garg, R. (1994). Evaluating quality of life in congestive heart failure: issues, progress, and recommendations. In *Congestive Heart Failure: Current Clinical Issues*, ed. G. T. Kennedy and M. H. Crawford. Futura Publishing Co., Inc: Armonk, NY.

Schron, E. B. and Shumaker, S. A. (1991). The integration of health quality of life in clinical research: experiences from cardiovascular clinical trials. *Prog Cardiovasc Nurs*, **7**, 21–8.

Scott, J. P., Dennis, C., and Mullins, P. (1993). Heart–lung transplantation for end-stage respiratory disease in cystic fibrosis patients. *J R Soc Med*, **86(20)**, 19–22.

Secchi, A., Di Carlo, V., Martinenghi, S. et al. (1991). Effect of pancreas transplantation on life expectancy, kidney function and quality of life in uraemic Type I (insulin-dependent) diabetic patients. *Diabetologia*, **34**, S141–S144.

Seedat, Y. K., Macintosh, C. G., and Subban, J. V. (1987). Quality of life for patients in an end-stage renal disease programme. *S Afr Med J*, **71**, 500–4.

Sensky, T. (1989). Psychiatric morbidity in renal transplantation. *Psychother Psychosom*, **52**, 41–6.

Shapiro, P. A. and Kornfeld, D. S. (1989). Psychiatric outcome of heart transplantation. *Gen Hosp Psychiatry*, **11**, 352–7.

Simmons, R. G. and Abress, L. (1990). Quality-of-life issues for end-stage renal disease patients. *Am J Kidney Dis*, **15**, 201–8.

Simmons, R. G., Abress, L., and Anderson, C. R. (1988). Quality of life after kidney transplantation. *Transplantation*, **45**, 415–21.

Simmons, R. G., Anderson, C. R., and Abress, L. K. (1990). Quality of life and rehabilitation differences among four end-stage renal disease therapy groups. *Scand J Urol Nephrol*, **131**(Suppl), 7–22.

Simmons, R. G., Anderson, C. R., and Kamstra, L. K. (1984). Comparison of quality of life of patients on CAPD, hemodialysis and transplantation. *Am J Kidney Dis*, **4**, 253–5.

Simmons, R. G., Kamstra-Hennen, L., and Thompson, C. R. (1981). Psychosocial adjustment five to nine years posttransplant. *Transplant Proc*, **13**, 40–3.

Simmons, R. G., Klein, S. D., and Simmons, R. L. (1977). *Gift of Life*. Wiley-Interscience: New York. Reprinted, 1987, Transaction Books: New Brunswick, NJ.

Sophie, L. R. and Powers, M. J. (1979). Life satisfaction and social function: post-transplant self-evaluation. *Dial Transplant*, **8**, 1198–202.

Spielberger, C. D., Gorsuch, R. L., and Lushene, R. E. (eds.) (1970). *STAI Manual for the State-Trait Anxiety Inventory*. Consulting Psychologists Press: Palo Alto, CA.

Spitzer, W. O., Dobson, A. J., and Hall, J. (1981). Measuring the quality of life of cancer patients. A concise QL index for use by physicians. *J Chronic Dis*, **34**, 587–97.

Stewart, A. L. and Ware, J. E. (eds.) (1992). *Measuring Functioning and Well-being: The Medical Outcomes Study Approach*. Duke University Press: Durham NC.

Stratta, R. J., Taylor, R. J., Ozaki, C. F. et al. (1993). A comparative analysis of results and morbidity in Type I diabetics undergoing preemptive versus postdialysis combined pancreas–kidney transplantation. *Transplantation*, **55**, 1097–103.

Strauss, B., Thormann, T., Strenge, H. et al. (1992). Psychosocial, neuropsychological and neurological status in a sample of heart transplant recipients. *Qual Life Res*, **1**, 119–28.

Stukas, A. A., Dew, M. A., Switzer, G. E., DiMartini, A., Kormos, R. L., and Griffith, B. P. (1999). Post-traumatic stress disorder in heart transplant recipients and their primary family caregivers. *Psychosomatics*, **40**, 212–21.

Surman, O. S. (1994). Psychiatric aspects of liver transplantation. *Psychosomatics*, **35**, 297–308.

Sutton, T. D. and Murphy, S. P. (1989). Stressors and patterns of coping in renal transplant patients. *Nurs Res*, **38**, 46–9.

Syrjala, K. L., Chapko, M. K., Vitaliano, P. P., Cummings, C., and Sullivan, K. M. (1993). Recovery after allogeneic marrow transplantation: prospective study of predictors of long-term physical and psychosocial functioning. *Bone Marrow Transplant*, **11**, 319–27.

Tarlov, A. R. (1992). Outcomes assessment and quality of life in patients with human immunodeficiency virus infection. *Ann Intern Med*, **116**, 166–7.

Tarter, R. E., Erb, S., Biller, P. A., Switala, J., and van Thiel, D. H. (1988). The quality of life following liver transplantation: a preliminary report. *Gastroenterol Clin North Am*, **17**, 207–17.

Tarter, R. E., Switala, J., Arria, A., Plail, J., and van Thiel, D. (1991). Quality of life before and after orthotopic hepatic transplantation. *Arch Intern Med*, **151**, 1521–6.

Tarter, R. E., Switala, J., Arria, A., Plail, J., and van Thiel, D. H. (1990a). Subclinical hepatic encephalopathy: comparison before and after orthotopic liver transplantation. *Transplantation*, **50**, 632–7.

Tarter, R. E., Switala, J., Kabene, M., and van Thiel, D. H. (1990b). Long-term psychosocial adjustment following liver transplantation: gender comparisons of patients and their spouses. *Fam Syst Med*, **8**, 359–64.

Tarter, R. E., Switala, J., Plail, J., Havrilla, J., and van Thiel, D. H. (1992). Severity of hepatic encephalopathy before liver transplantation is associated with quality of life after transplantation. *Arch Intern Med*, **152**, 2097–101.

Tarter, R. E., van Thiel, D. H., Hegedus, A. M., Schade, R. R., Gavaler, J. S., and Starzl, T. E. (1984). Neuropsychiatric status after liver transplantation. *J Lab Clin Med*, **103**, 776–82.

TenVergert, E. M., Essink-Bot, M. L., Geertsma, A., van Enckevort, P. J., de Boer, W. J., and van der Bij, W. (1998). The effect of lung transplantation on health-related quality of life: a longitudinal study. *Chest*, **113**, 358–64.

Testa, M. A., Anderson, R. B., Nackley, J. F., and Hollenberg, N. K. (1993). Quality of life and antihypertensive therapy in men: a comparison of captopril with enalapril. *N Engl J Med*, **328**, 907–13.

Testa, M. A. and Nackely, J. F. (1994). Methods for quality-of-life studies. *Annu Rev Public Health*, **15**, 535–59.

Their, S. O. (1992). Forces motivating the use of health status assessment measures in clinical settings and related clinical research. *Med Care*, **30**, MS15–MS22.

Voruganti, L. N. P. and Sells, R. A. (1989). Quality of life of diabetic patients after combined pancreatic-renal transplantation. *Clin Transplant*, **3**, 78–82.

Vose, J. M., Kennedy, B. C., Bierman, P. J., Kessinger, A., and Armitage, J. O. (1992). Long-term sequelae of autologous bone marrow or peripheral stem cell transplantation for lymphoid malignancies. *Cancer*, **69**, 784–9.

Walden, J. A., Stevenson, L. W., Dracup, K., Wilmarth, J., Kobashigawa, J., and Moriguchi, J. (1989). Heart transplantation may not improve quality of life for patients with stable heart failure. *Heart Lung*, **18**, 497–506.

Wallwork, J. and Caine, N. (1985). A comparison of the quality of life of cardiac transplant patients and coronary artery bypass graft patients before and after surgery. *Qual Life Cardiovasc Care*, Sept/Oct, 317–31.

Ware, J. E. and Sherbourne, C. D. (1992). The MOS 36-item Short-Form Health Survey (SF-36): I. Conceptual framework and item selection. *Med Care*, **30**, 473–83.

Whedon, M. and Ferrell, B. R. (1994). Quality of life in adult bone marrow transplant patients: beyond the first year. *Semin Oncol Nurs*, **110**, 42–57.

Williams, J. W, Vera, S., and Evans, L. S. (1987). Socioeconomic aspects of hepatic transplantation. *Am J Gastroenterol*, **82**, 1115–19.

Wilson, I. R. and Cleary, P. D. (1995). Linking clinical variables with health-related quality of life: a conceptual model of patient outcomes. *JAMA*, **273**, 59–65.

Wingard, J. R. (1994). Functional ability and quality of life of patients after allogeneic bone marrow transplantation. *Bone Marrow Transplant*, **14**, S29–S33.

Wingard, J. R. (1998). Quality of life following bone marrow transplantation. *Cur Opin Oncol*, **10**, 108–11.

Wingard, J. R., Curbow, B., Baker, F., and Piantadosi, S. (1991). Health, functional status, and employment of adult survivors of bone marrow transplantation. *Ann Intern Med*, **114**, 113–18.

Wingard, J. R., Curbow, B., Baker, F., Zabora, J., and Piantadosi, S. (1992). Sexual satisfaction in survivors of bone marrow transplantation. *Bone Marrow Transplant*, **9**, 185–90.

Wolcott, D., Norquist, G., and Busuttil, R. (1989). Cognitive function and quality of life in adult liver transplant recipients. *Transplant Proc*, **21**, 3563.

Wolcott, D. L., Wellisch, D. K., Fawzy, F. W., and Landsverk, J. (1986). Adaptation of adult bone marrow transplant recipient long-term survivors. *Transplantation*, **41**, 478–84.

World Health Organization (1948). *Constitution in Basic Documents.* WHO: Geneva.

Yoshimura, N., Ohmori, Y., Tsuji, T., and Oka, T. (1994). Quality of life in renal transplant recipients treated with cyclosporine in comparison with hemodialysis maintenance. *Transplant Proc*, **26**, 2542–3.

Zabora, J. R., Smith, E. D., Baker, F., Wingard, J. R., and Curbow, B. (1992). The family: the other side of bone marrow transplantation. *J Psychosom Oncol*, **10**, 35–46.

Zehr, P. S., Milde, F. K., Hart, L. K., and Corry, R. J. (1991). Pancreas transplantation: assessing secondary complications and life quality. *Diabetologia*, **34**, S138–S140.

Zehrer, C. L. and Gross C. R. (1991). Quality of life of pancreas transplant recipients. *Diabetologia*, **34**, S145–S149.

Zehrer, C. L. and Gross, C. R. (1994). Comparison of quality of life between pancreas/kidney and kidney transplant recipients: 1-year follow-up. *Transplant Proc*, **26**, 508–9.

Zung, W. (1965). A self-rating depression scale. *Arch Gen Psychiatry*, **12**, 63–70.

Quality of life of geriatric patients following transplantation: short- and long-term outcomes

Maria Paz González M.D., Ph.D.,
Abraham Sudilovsky M.D., Julio Bobes M.D., Ph.D.,
Andrea F. DiMartini M.D.

Introduction

In recent years there has been a considerable increase in the size of the elderly population (i.e., those over 64 years of age) in the USA, with this trend expected to continue into the twenty-first century (Anand et al. 1990). From 1900 to 1990, the number of elderly American citizens increased 10-fold, rising from 3.1 million to 31.4 million, and their proportion of the total population has tripled, rising from 4.1% to 12.6%. By 1996, 20% of the US population was older than 65 years of age (Latos 1996), while in developed countries overall those aged 65 or older make up 14% of the population (Gelbard, Haub, and Kent 1999). US men who survive to age 65 can expect to live another 16 years on average; US women who are age 65 can expect to live another 19 years (Gelbard et al. 1999).

The aging of the population will play an important and controversial role in the distribution and provision of health resources. On the one hand, the existing discrepancy between the percentage of elderly in the population and the high proportion of health care resources that they consume (Rowe, Grossman, and Bond 1987) will contribute to an increase in health care spending (Chelluri et al. 1993). On the other hand, the lack of information about the influence of age on outcomes suggests the need to readdress using age as a criterion for efficient distribution of health care resources (Callahan 1987; Veatch 1988; Hunt 1993).

In the field of organ transplantation, the distribution of resources based on measures of cost-effectiveness is of special interest. Over the last three decades, organ transplantation has developed from an experimental technique into the treatment of choice for end stage organ failure. Transplantation has a success rate that reaches 90% for adults for some organ types (Kluge 1993), and in the case of liver transplantation, a 5-year survival rate of 66% (Belle, Beringer, and Detre 1996). However, as result of clinical success, the increasing demand for organs, the high cost involved, and the low availability of donor organs, it is currently necessary to establish certain selection criteria in order to maximize cost-efficiency.

The choice of selection criteria is not an easy task and is, therefore, not free from controversy. Some of these criteria, including organ compatibility and probability of rejection, physiological fit, and urgency of the transplant are not usually debated. On the other hand, criteria that are widely debated and criticized from an ethical point of view include age and life style (e.g., alcohol and tobacco abuse) (Kluge 1993).

Employing advanced age as a criterion to contraindicate transplantation constitutes, in the opinion of some authors, a discriminatory attitude and is probably not a good criterion in clinical practice. Even though statistics indicate that certain age groups may benefit more than others, patients are not statistics and age is not a medical condition. According to Kluge (1993), the only selection criteria that should be used from an ethical point of view, should be those related to the health status of the patients. In addition, the elderly may have lower activity of their immunologic system, making rejection less likely (Calne 1994), and they have greater therapeutic compliance post-transplantation (Pirsch et al. 1991). On the other hand, Shaw (1994) suggests tempering the enthusiasm of some surgeons who give transplants to elderly patients with the realities of donor shortages, costs, and a desire to obtain good, long-term survival rates and a high quality of life. The elderly have more surgical complications, thereby using more resources, and the additional years of life saved in this age group are fewer. Transplantation in the elderly might be considered an irresponsible waste of economic and donor organ resources.

Thus, in the search for new indicators of cost-effectiveness, quality of life of the individual patient is emerging as an important parameter. In 1987 Katz stated, "The question of interest today is whether treatments result in a life of better quality – if not a longer life. In this respect, the effectiveness and cost-effectiveness of treatments must be measured in terms of quality of life."

From the database of the United Network for Organ Sharing (UNOS) ($n = 97\,587$ solid organs transplants performed in the USA), a report investigating risk factors affecting patient and graft survival rates found increased recipient age negatively affected survival for all organ types (Lin et al. 1998). However, other factors such as medical condition at the time of transplant and donor age were also consistently associated with worse survival (Lin 1998). This study combines data from centers across the USA, though the singular focus on survival does not provide sufficient details to understand the full dimensions of post-transplantation quality of life in these individuals. While there are increasing reports on survival and functional status in the elderly following transplantation, specific investigations of quality of life and comparisons to younger cohorts are lacking. This chapter reviews the available literature on transplantation in the elderly. Individually the studies are clinically informative, but it is difficult to make generalizations about giving the elderly transplants of various solid organs due to the differences between transplant centers, parameters studied, and the lack of standardized measures or variables. Future studies integrating and standardizing methods and measures are needed.

Quality of life of geriatric patients following transplantation

From the moment that post-transplantation survival rates reached acceptable and optimal levels, the prior measures of morbidity and mortality were replaced by more modern measures of outcomes to evaluate the success or failure of transplants. Dew et al. (1991) stated that "the quality of survival – defined not only by patients' general medical status but also by their long-term physical functional, psychological, and social adaptation following such efforts – is critical to the evaluation of the ultimate costs and consequences of biomedical innovations."

In general, in elderly people, the maintenance or reachievement of the highest level of independence possible becomes a crucial aspect regarding their quality of life and quality of care (Williams 1996). Health care in the elderly reflects the process of aging, with a greater emphasis on functional impairment than on the disease itself, and on the importance of the social environment. The maintenance of an independent life in the community, with sufficient resources and adequate social support, are currently considered to be the main aims in the care of the elderly. For transplantation in elderly patients, the focus has also been on maintaining a high level of functioning and independence. Elderly referred for transplantation tend to be a highly select group of those who are independent and high functioning, with minimal other systemic illnesses. Transplantation is not used to prolong life when overall functioning or quality of life is poor or the chance of recovery of functioning is poor.

Cardiac transplantation

The 1984 International Heart Transplant Registry reported data from 1968 to 1984 on 1076 patients from 44 heart transplant centers. The 6-year actuarial survival rates showed poorer survival for elderly patients; 28% for those > 50 years of age, 34% for those 40–49 years of age, and 51% for those 30–39 years of age (Kaye, Elcombe, and O'Fallon 1985). Age, the expertise of the center, and the use of cyclosporine were the most significant predictors of survival (Kaye et al. 1985). By the late 1980s, the issue concerning elderly patients (of over 50 years) in heart transplantation has been addressed frequently, as a result of the marked improvement in postoperative survival rates due to the advances in surgery, improved immunosuppressive agents, and the subsequent decreased incidence of rejection and infections. Miller et al. (1988) reported that the percentage of elderly (over 55 years) who underwent cardiac transplantation increased dramatically from 2% of the total number of patients who received heart transplants between 1973 to 1983, to 25% of the total in 1986.

Initial studies that referred exclusively to the issue of survival suggested that survival of elderly patients did not differ from that of other adult patients, demonstrating that the use of chronological age as a rigid criterion for cardiac transplant may be considered obsolete. However, current thinking is that survival and quality of life are both important, yet separate, issues that must be addressed when evaluating transplant outcomes. Despite increasing reports about liver and heart transplantation in the elderly (Shaw 1994), there is a paucity of specific information regarding the functional status and quality of life of geriatric cardiac transplant patients.

Carrier et al. (1986), retrospectively reviewed data from 13 patients over age 50 who had undergone cardiac transplantation at the University of Arizona between March 1979 and March 1985. Their mean age was 53 ± 1 years (range 50–57), two were women, and all patients were New York Heart Association functional class IV. They found a greater, though not statistically significant, 1-year actuarial survival rate for patients over 50 years of age compared to those patients under 50 ($72 \pm 14\%$ versus $66 \pm 7\%$). Early mortality (0 to 90 days) was also lower in the older patients compared to younger patients (16% versus 18%).

Frazier et al. (1988) studied the 1-year survival rate of 28 patients over 60 (mean age = 62.7 ± 2 years) who had received cardiac transplantation at the Texas Health Institute between July 1982 and August 1987, and compared this rate with that of younger patients who received cardiac transplantation during the same period. At the moment of admission, all patients were New York Heart Association class IV. These authors found "somewhat surprising results." The 1-year survival rate for the elderly was higher than that for the total heart transplant population at their center (83% versus 75%), even though these elderly patients also had numerous other high-risk factors (55% had previous cardiac surgery, all had renal dysfunction preoperatively, 35% had diabetes mellitus, etc.). Furthermore, the 23 surviving patients demonstrated good functional results and had resumed normal daily activities. The authors concluded that "advanced age should not be considered a major contraindication to heart transplantation." Nonetheless, they recommended considering transplantation of hearts from older donors, or from donors considered as undesirable, into elderly recipients.

Miller et al. (1988) retrospectively analyzed data from 30 patients who underwent orthotopic heart transplantation at St Louis University Hospital between May 1985 and October 1986. Eight patients (27%) were over 55 years of age (mean age = 57.0 years; oldest = 60.2 years). There were no females, and five of eight patients were in an intensive care unit at the time of transplantation. The average time in the intensive care unit after transplantation and the average time from transplantation to hospital discharge was not different between the older and younger groups. At follow-up (average of 10.4 months, range 7 to 22 months) no deaths occurred in the elderly group, whereas four patients died in the younger group. The risk of rejection was less in the elderly group (0.04 versus 0.11 rejection/patient month), though the risk of infection per patient month of follow-up was similar in both groups. All survivors were New York Heart Association functional class I within three months after transplantation, and all of the patients in the elderly group were able to return to work within four months of transplantation, with six of them working full-time.

Olivari et al. (1988) analyzed the results obtained in 23 patients over age 55 (mean age = 58.0 ± 2.6 years) who underwent heart transplantation from 1985 to 1986 at the University of Minnesota, and compared these results with those from younger patients ($n = 34$) who had received transplantations during the same time period. The 1-year actuarial survival was 96% for both groups. Actuarial freedom from rejection at 12 months was 94% for both groups. Complete rehabilitation after transplantation was achieved within six months, with 94% of the younger patients and 83% of the older active and having returned to a normal lifestyle. However, only 35% of the elderly group were able to return to their previous jobs, in contrast to 68% of the younger patients ($p < 0.05$). The authors stated that "heart transplantation not only prolongs survival in elderly recipients, but undoubtedly improves their life-styles."

Aravot et al. (1989) reported the results of 25 patients older than age 60 (mean age = 63 years, range 60 to 69 years) who underwent cardiac transplantation in their seventh decade of life at Harefield Hospital (England) and were followed up 5 to 59 months (mean 22 months) post-transplantation. Before transplantation 16 patients were New York Heart Association class IV and 9 were class III. The 1-year actuarial survival was 84%. Quality of life was assessed before transplantation and again at six months using the Nottingham Health Profile. The results showed an improvement in all dimensions, mobility showing the greatest improvement and energy the least. There was a reduction in symptoms and in perceived health problems. The authors concluded that these patients achieved a good quality of life and level of rehabilitation after transplantation.

Anguita et al. (1992) analyzed the influences of various theoretical contraindications for heart transplantation, one of these being age over 55 years. Twelve of 57 patients who underwent orthotopic heart transplantation at Reina Sofía University Hospital (Córdoba, Spain) between April 1986 and

April 1991 were over 55 years of age. The authors found that the probability of survival at 1 year was lower in elderly patients (60%) as compared with younger ones (78%), and that this difference reached statistical significance at 18 months (45% versus 68%). However, of the six deaths that occurred, three had additional concurrent risk factors.

Bourge et al. (1993) conducted a multicenter prospective study in which they attempted to identify the risk factors for death after heart transplantation. They analyzed data from 911 patients who underwent heart transplantation in 25 institutions between 1 January 1990 and 30 June 1991. Patients aged 60 years or older had a 1-year survival rate of 81%. Older age was identified as one of the independent pretransplantation risk factors for death during the first 18 months after transplantation ($p = 0.009$). Furthermore, using multivariate analysis they found that patients older than 50 had a slight, but progressive, increase in expected mortality rate. The authors recommended detailed screening for the elderly to select out other important risk factors also found to be associated with death (donor ischemic time, ventilator support at the time of transplantation, lower pretransplant cardiac output, etc.).

Heroux et al. (1993) retrospectively analyzed the postoperative outcome for elderly patients. They compared data from 12 patients 65 years or older (mean = 66.1 ± 0.9) with data from 57 patients aged 55 to 64 (mean = 59.3 ± 2.7 years) who underwent orthotopic heart transplantation at Loyola University Medical Center, between 1 January 1984 and 31 July 1991. In the older group the 1-year actuarial survival was poorer than (71%), but not significantly different from, those under 65 years (87%). Patients aged 65 years and older had a significantly higher number of hospital days ($p < 0.02$), and increased incidence of infections/month ($p < 0.03$) during the first postoperative year, but had a lower rate of rejection at one and six months post-transplantation ($p < 0.03$). Lower rejection and higher infection rates in patients over 65 years of age, suggest less intense immunosuppression for these patients. In addition, the functional capacity at six months after transplantation was significantly poorer in the older group: 62% showed severe functional limitation (i.e., difficulty in performing nonstrenuous daily activities) as compared with 11% of the younger group ($p < 0.002$). At 1 year this difference persisted (25% versus 5%), but did not reach statistical significance. Despite the retrospective nature of the study and small study sample, these authors could not advocate the use of age as the sole criterion for selecting heart transplant candidates.

Rosenblum et al. (1993) conducted a survey by post to over 200 patients, followed up at the Columbia Presbyterian Medical Center, who were at least six months post-transplantation. The instrument used for assessing quality of life was the Sickness Impact Profile (SIP). The response rate was 48%. The median age for those returning the survey was 53 years (range 27.1 to 68.7

years), and their median duration since cardiac transplantation was 2.3 years (range 0.5 to 9.7 years). The results showed a relatively better physical quality of life than a psychosocial one, many patients reporting difficulties similar to those recognized in patients with clinical depression. The most prevalent areas of dysfunction were sexual activity, housework, sleep patterns, and endurance. When these findings were compared with those from different populations, the patients had worse quality of life than normal, similar scores to survivors of cardiac arrest and postmyocardial infarction, and better scores than patients with low back pain of less than 1-year duration. No relationship was found between SIP scores and age. The authors concluded that global quality of life in their patients was better than one might have expected, though they did not separately report geriatric data.

Coffman et al. (1997) reported the results of the Cedars-Sinai Medical Center between December 1988 and August 1993. Of the 112 patients who underwent cardiac transplantation, 36% ($n = 40$) were age 60 or older (range 60 to 69 years). Older and younger recipients were demographically similar with respect to gender, race, functional class, left ventricular ejection fraction and pulmonary vascular resistance. The 1-year survival rate was similar between older and younger recipients. A Kaplan–Meier survival analysis at 4 years postoperatively still showed no statistical difference between the older and younger groups (75% versus 74%, respectively). In addition, quality of life was similar or better by several measurements. A comparable percentage of surviving patients were New York Heart Association functional class 1 at one year. Return-to-work rates were similar in older and younger recipients (50% versus 60%, respectively, $p = 0.48$). A slightly greater percentage of the older patients were alive and free from rejection at 1, 2, and 3 years postoperatively. Also, by subjective rating by their transplant coordinators and by self-rated Psychosocial Adjustment to Illness Scale (PAIS-SR), older recipients had greater improvement and better quality of life ($p = 0.004$). One year later repeated administration of the PAIS-SR continued to demonstrate this result, older recipients scoring significantly better on total quality of life ($p = 0.0005$), domestic environment ($p = 0.0001$), social environment ($p = 0.007$), and less psychological distress ($p = 0.0001$). Furthermore the younger group had a higher rate of alcohol and drug abuse/dependence and also more medical noncompliance pretransplantation.

Though individual centers report comparable survival, physical functioning, and quality of life for geriatric patients following heart transplantation, these data may reflect the particular selection practices or surgical experience of the programs involved. Overall, the International Heart and Lung Transplantation Registry consistently shows that recipient age greater than 60 years has a statistically significant impact on 1-year mortality (odds ratio 1.73, $p < 0.001$) (Hosenspud et al. 1995). The actuarial survival by age shows a statistically significant decrease in 3-year survival for those older than 65 years of age (65% versus 70%, $p=$ 0.006) (Hosenspud et al. 1995). Not surprisingly a heart donor older than 60 years of age carries a relative odds ratio equivalent in negative impact to repeat transplantation (odds ratio 3.49, $p < 0.001$) (Hosenspud et al. 1995).

Lung transplantation

For single-lung transplantation, the International Heart and Lung Transplantation Registry shows a trend toward worse survival in patients over the age of 60 years ($p=$ 0.190) and the 2-year actuarial survival is 51% compared with 61% for those over 60 years old (Hosenspud et al. 1995). However, recipient age did not appear to be an independent risk factor using multivariate analysis for 1-year survival in bilateral lung transplantation (Hosenspud et al. 1995).

Snell et al. (1993) reported the results of lung transplantation for older (defined as age > 50 years) compared to younger recipients at the Toronto Lung Transplantation Program. Between November 1983 and October 1991, 31 recipients aged 50 to 63 years (mean 55.3 years) underwent single-lung ($n=19$) or double-lung ($n=12$) transplants. Compared to their younger counterparts, older recipients had similar 1-, 3-, and 5-year actuarial survival. In fact, while the overall survival was similar, there was a tendency for older patients to do better when looking at the subgroup of single-lung transplant for restrictive lung disease ($p > 0.1$). Older patients had similar serum creatinine levels beyond 2 years post-transplantation, indicating renal functioning comparable to that of younger recipients ($p > 0.05$). In addition, for all recipients who survived 12 months post-transplantation, function of the transplanted lung was assessed by the six-minute walk test and modified Bruce Protocol Exercise Stress test and was found to be comparable between older and younger recipients ($p > 0.05$). At 1 year post-transplantation 8 of 40 surviving younger recipients were alive but functionally disabled from pulmonary symptoms, whereas only 1 of 16 surviving older recipients was functionally impaired ($p > 0.05$). In those patients who survived beyond six weeks post-transplantation the incidence of definite acute graft rejection was less in older recipients ($p < 0.05$). Younger recipients tended to die from graft rejection, while older recipients tended to die from sepsis (especially cytomegalovirus infections). These findings have been interpreted as evidence of the decreased immunologic responsiveness with age. In older recipients this may allow reduced immunosuppression, perhaps avoiding some of the long-term side effects of such medication use (i.e., nephrotoxicity, osteoporosis). Snell et al. concluded that isolated lung transplantation can be performed with acceptable results for well-selected patients in their sixth and seventh decades.

Liver transplantation

Several studies that focus on quality of life following liver transplantation report an increase in overall quality of life (Kober et al. 1990; Lundgren et al. 1994), marked improvement in well-being, return to work (Tarter et al. 1988; Lundgren et al. 1994), resumption and independence in daily living activities (Robinson et al. 1990), and improvement in the psychological profiles of the majority of patients (Kober et al. 1990; Tarter et al. 1991). Although very few studies address the impact of liver transplantation on the quality of life of geriatric patients, all of them report levels of improvement similar to those seen in adult populations.

Early in hepatic transplantation technology, age > 55 years was believed to be an absolute contraindication to liver transplantation, and elderly patients were felt to be at risk of dying of nonhepatic problems post-transplantation (Van Thiel et al. 1984). However, during that same time period Starzl et al. (1987) compared 363 adults younger than 50 years (mean age = 35.8 years) with 92 patients aged 50 to 77 years (mean age = 55.7 years) who had undergone orthotopic liver transplantation (OLTX) at the University of Pittsburgh Medical Center from 1980 to 1986. At both 1 and 5 years after OLTX, the actuarial patient survival was slightly more favorable among the younger patients (75% and 60%, respectively) than among the elderly (69% and 52%, respectively), though these differences were not statistically significant. Eighty-two percent of the surviving patients in the older age group were fully rehabilitated in the areas of domestic functioning, employment, and medical care.

Stieber et al. (1991) further described the original Pittsburgh sample of Starzl et al. from 1987. Of the 156 patients who were over 60, 45 (28.9%) were United Network of Organ Sharing (UNOS) class 3 (i.e., old UNOS criteria = hospitalized) or class 4 (urgent, in the intensive care unit). The authors reported actuarial survival rates for seniors with primary grafts of 71.3% after 1 year and 65.5% after 3 years compared to 78% and 71%, respectively, for non-senior (< 61 years) adults. Ninety-four percent of the survivors had either functional status I or II (i.e., fully functional or functional with some limitation). The authors concluded that, for elderly patients, liver transplantation assures them of a satisfactory quality of life post-transplantation. These results contrasted significantly with the statistics reported by UNOS for the calendar year 1988, in which the 1-year mortality rate was 50% for patients 65 years or older (UNOS 1990).

Later experience at the University of Pittsburgh (Alessiani et al. 1994) using tacrolimus (also called FK506) as the primary immunosuppressive agent showed better 1-year patient and graft survival for seniors compared to a prior group of senior patients (historical control) transplanted with cyclosporine-based immunosuppression. Compared to the previous reports from

Pittsburgh, all patients showed improved actuarial survival curves at 1 and 3 years post-OLTX. When their sample was compared with younger adults ($n = 747$), elderly patients ($n = 219$) had a statistically significant lower 1-year survival (75% versus 84%, $p = 0.0005$). Also, in patients over 60 years of age, the use of tacrolimus after liver transplantation seemed to be associated with advantages in terms of greater survival, lower incidence of rejection, and better quality of life; perhaps these factors accounted for the increase in adult survival overall.

Thus, as seen in the International Registry of Cardiac Transplant recipients, the number of elderly undergoing OLTX at the University of Pittsburgh nearly doubled from 10.6% in 1988 to 1989 to 19.3% in 1989 to 1992. Less rigid age criteria for both donor and recipient recruitment, improved surgical technique and post operative care, development of better immunosuppression, and overall progressively more positive experiences with OLTX and other solid organs contributed to the increase in numbers of elderly undergoing transplantation. A similar increase in the number of elderly undergoing OLTX was observed in the UK with the number of recipients ≥ 60 years of age increasing from 6.4% in 1991 to 10.2% in 1992 (Bromley et al. 1994).

Pirsch et al. (1991) described 23 patients of 60 years and older (mean age = 63.6 years, range = 60 to 72 years) who underwent OLTX at the University of Wisconsin Hospital between July 1984 and April 1990. The actuarial survival rate at 2 years was 83% in patients of ≥ 60 years compared with 76% in patients of 18 to 59 years (not statistically significant). There were no important differences in the initial transplantation hospitalization (pretransplantation complications, length of hospital stay, number of readmissions) or incidence of infection and rejection between older and younger patients. In addition, no patient over 60 years required retransplantation. The authors hypothesized that patients who survive into the seventh decade with liver disease may be a self-selected group such that other major medical complications are not present which could have caused earlier mortality. They concluded that advanced age should not be considered a contraindication for liver transplantation. However, this study did not report any data about quality of life in the elderly.

Fisher et al. (1995) reported that 1- and 3-year survival of liver transplant patients of ≥ 65 years ($n = 57$) was similar to that in younger patients ($n = 583$) at their center. Pretransplantation data (including UNOS status, age, presence of muscle wasting, fatigue, diabetes, primary liver malignancy), perioperative factors (including intraoperative use of blood products, need for dialysis, length of intensive care unit stay) or preoperative biochemical parameters (prothrombin time, bilirubin, creatinine and albumin) were not different between those of ≥ 65 years and others. No pretransplantation factors predicted outcome. Mean intensive care unit stay was 7.6 days in older patients and 10.3 days for younger adults, though this was not statistically significant. The authors conclude that elderly patients should not be routinely excluded from liver transplantation and that carefully selected older recipients can have survival rates equivalent to rates of younger recipients.

Bromley et al. (1994), using a retrospective case control analysis, reviewed the King's College Hospital experience with liver transplantation in patients ≥ 60 years old. Forty patients underwent liver transplantation between 1988 to 1993. There was no significant difference between elderly patients and younger patients in preoperative condition, interoperative interventions, or outcome as assessed by survival, complication rate (surgical, infection, or rejection episodes), and length of intensive care unit stay. Median length of hospital stay was slightly longer for elderly (24 versus 20 days, $p < 0.03$). With no difference in complication rate, longer length of stay may have reflected a longer recovery time for the elderly. The 1-year survival rate following liver transplantation for their patients over 60 years old was 78%, which was not different from the overall survival rate at their center. One month after transplantation these elderly patients did as well as their young counterparts.

González et al. (1995) studied all patients ($n = 73$) over 60 years old who had undergone OLTX at the University of Pittsburgh Medical Center from 1 January to 31 December 1990. The aim of the study was to describe the survival rate and the quality of life 4 years after OLTX. Information on quality of life included living conditions, functional status, pain, sleep complaints, and emotional and psychosocial status. This information was obtained from the transplant coordinators (staff who were directly involved in daily care of the patient and had interacted with the patients' relatives). At the time of OLTX, 35.6% of the patients were over 64 years old and 74% were UNOS class III (old classification = hospitalized). The actuarial survival rate was 67.1% after 4 years. When compared to the survival rate of adult patients (75.9%) who had undergone OLTX in the same year, survival was slightly more unfavorable in elderly patients, but the difference was not statistically significant. Of the elderly survivors, 68.3% were able to carry out normal physical activities and their activities of daily living were unaffected in at least 63.4%. Overall, emotional as well as psychosocial status was good in almost 70% of the survivors. Most of the patients showed high levels of quality of life after OLTX in a number of domains.

Zetterman et al. (1998) investigated the effect of recipient age on outcome using a multicenter, prospective database of 735 adults who received liver transplants in the USA. Older recipients were identified as those patients ≥ 60 years of age. Seven recipients were 70 years or older. At the time of transplantation the older recipients were similar to younger recipients with respect to overall clinical severity of liver disease but were more likely to have fair to poor nutritional status, muscle wasting, encephalopathy, and higher creatinine levels. Older recipients required a longer stay in an intensive care unit and total hospitalization compared to younger recipients. Acute cellular rejection was less common in older recipients (56% versus at 1 year, $p = 0.007$), whereas rates of cytomegalovirus infections were similar between the two groups. In the early post-transplantation phase quality of life assessed by a standardized, self-administered questionnaire was similar for both groups across most domains, though older recipients reported slightly lower personal functioning. However, by 1 year post-transplantation the older recipients' indices of quality of life were no longer significantly different than the younger recipients' and in fact their indices for well-being and scores for degree of psychological distress were better than those of the younger recipients. Similar to the UNOS database that reported a lower survival rate for older recipients, this study contained data from three US centers, controlled for factors that affected patient survival and outcome, and also found lower survival rates for older recipients (81% versus 90% at 1 year, $p = 0.004$). In contrast to patient survival, retransplant-free graft survival was not different between older and younger recipients. The excess mortality in the older recipients was mostly due to nonhepatic causes, including infections, cardiac, and neurologic disease occurring within the first six months post-transplantation. They concluded that older patients should not be excluded from transplantation if they are carefully selected for medical contraindications to transplantation (such as coronary or cerebral vascular disease). Future studies that include assessments of both medical and patient-rated outcomes are recommended to further our knowledge in this important area.

In a study extending the Liver Transplant Database, Wiesner et al. (1998) investigated the incidence and risk factors for acute allograft rejection in the first post-transplantation year for 762 liver transplant recipients. They used proportional hazards modeling and found that younger recipient age was independently associated with acute allograft rejection. The six-week incidence of acute rejection was lowest for those patients 60 years of age or older (34% cumulative percentages) as contrasted with those patients 16 to 29 years of age (65%). They believed this risk factor was indicative of healthier recipients who were more likely to have more aggressive immune system reactions.

Renal transplantation

The area of renal transplantation in the elderly for end stage renal disease (ESRD) has a history beginning with the advent of dialysis technology. ESRD is more common in patients over 60 years of age compared with any other age group (Tesi et al. 1994). Nevertheless, a few decades ago, people over the age of 60 with ESRD were often excluded from dialysis. By 1993 in the USA, patients older than 64 years undergoing dialysis or who had functional renal transplants numbered 69 937, representing a more than three-fold increase from 1984 (Latos 1996). Though the rates of elderly on dialysis were dramatically increasing, renal transplantation for the elderly was not. In the USA of the nearly 100 000 patients on dialysis as of June 1986, 48% were above the age of 60, but only 16% of those receiving renal transplantation were over the age of 55 (Pirsch et al. 1989). As of December 1992, the majority of ESRD elderly were undergoing hemodialysis (83%) and fewer than 5% had functioning renal transplants. These figures contrast with those ESRD patients aged 45 to 65 years who were more likely than elderly to be given transplants (27.4%) (Latos 1996).

The arguments against renal transplantation in the elderly have been similar to concerns over giving the elderly other types of solid organ transplant. Elderly patients were believed to be at higher risk for post-transplantation morbidity and mortality. Some nephrologists believe the risks of transplantation and immunosuppression are greater in the elderly or that organs should be used in patients with the greatest chance of long-term survival (Tesi et al. 1994). These biases may lead to fewer referrals of elderly for transplantation evaluation. Others suggest the long-term risks of transplantation, including cancer, cardiac disease, cerebrovascular disease, liver disease, and chronic infections, will be higher in the elderly (Santiago-Delpin 1996). Evidence to support these concerns comes from Scandinavian countries where ischemic heart disease is considered to be a major cause of death and graft loss (Santiago-Delpin 1996). In addition, the severity of cytomegalovirus infection increases with age and, in one study, infections were the leading cause of early death in the elderly (Santiago-Delpin 1996).

However, with the introduction of cyclosporine in 1983 and improved renal allograft survival rates, renal transplantation programs began to successfully include those "higher risk" patients (Pirsch et al. 1989). By the late 1980s several reports showed that by using cycloporine A (CYA) as the primary immunosuppression agent, older recipients could achieve similar patient and graft survival when compared to younger patients (Fehrman et al. 1989; Murie et al. 1989; Pirsch et al. 1989).

At the University of Wisconsin, between October 1983 and May 1988, 34 patients over 60 years of age (mean 62 years, range 60 to 73 years) underwent renal transplantation for ESRD. These patients had similar 3-year actuarial patient survival (91%) and graft survival (74%) compared to a group of patients 50 to 60 years old who were also given transplants at the University of Wisconsin (Pirsch et al. 1989). Post operative rejection was less frequent in older than younger recipients. They concluded that CYA had had a dramatic impact on patient and graft survival in the elderly. Prior to the use of CYA, for patients over 60 years of age, 1-year patient and graft survival averaged 62% and 57%, respectively (Pirsch et al. 1989).

In Sweden between 1975 and 1987, 55 patients between the ages of 65 and 75 years received kidney transplants (Fehrman et al. 1989). Primary immunosuppression was with prednisone and azathioprine (17 patients) prior to 1980 when CYA was then used in combination with corticosteroids. Though the 1- and 3-year survival rates improved dramatically in these patients from the azathioprine-treated patients to CYA-treated recipients (59% versus 65% patient and 41% versus 54% graft survival, respectively), the older CYA recipients had significantly lower graft survival compared to younger (ages 7 to 45 years) CYA-treated recipients who had 1- and 3-year graft survival of 83% and 70%, respectively ($p < 0.001$) (Fehrman et al. 1989). The frequency of rejection was similar in both groups. In the longer term, older patients had stable renal functions and lived an essentially normal life. After comparing these results with their data of 30% 3-year survival for dialysis patients, Fehrman et al. concluded renal transplantation was well justified in patients older than 65 years.

Howard et al. (1989) reported on the per-CYA experience at the University of Florida from December 1969 and December 1987. They performed 131 renal transplants in patients over 50 years of age (54 patients were 55 years or older). Prednisone and azathioprine were used for immunsuppression in most patients. Of first transplant recipients, the 2-year graft survival was 66.8% for patients at least 50 years old ($n = 92$) and 60.4% for patients younger than 50 years ($n = 399$) ($p > 0.05$). Patient survival 2 years after transplantation was 78.6% and 84.9%, respectively, for these two groups ($p > 0.05$). There were few differences between those older than 50 years of age and younger recipients, with respect to the incidence of post-transplantation complications or in causes of death. In fact the only statistical difference for the entire series was that older recipients of kidneys from related donors had lower patient survival (83% versus 93%) than recipients who were less than 50 years old.

Renal transplantation in patients of > 70 years of age was investigated over a 10-year period in Norway (Albrechtsen et al. 1995). All patients beginning renal replacement therapy from 1983 to 1993 were prospectively studied. Ninety-one percent of all renal replacement therapy patients younger than 70 years of age were considered for transplantation, but only 45% of older patients were considered to be viable candidates for transplantation. Grafts were provided to 53% of older patients in need versus 81% of those patients younger than 70 years. One hundred and twenty-six older patients, aged 70 to 83 years (mean age 73 years), were first-graft recipients. Initial graft function and the rate of rejection was comparable between those > 70 years old and a control group of patients 55 to 70 years old. Patient and graft survival rates for 5 years post-transplantation were comparable between these two groups. However, more grafts were lost in the older group due to patient death (83% died with functioning grafts versus 66%) compared with more deaths from rejection in the control group (29% versus 15%) ($p < 0.05$). In the older group, early and late death following transplantation was predominantly due to cardiac and cerebrovascular disease. An earlier study from this center reported inferior patient and graft survival in patients older than 55 years compared to younger patients in their national sample (Albrechtsen et al. 1992). However, on the basis of these data, the authors concluded that for patients older than 55 years there are no data to support the use of age per se as a selection factor for transplantation.

Summary and Conclusions

Review of the available literature indicates that quality of life improves in both adults and elderly after organ transplantation, though not always to the same degree. The survival rates in both age groups are often similar. Thus, it appears that age alone should not be a contraindication for organ transplantation, though any additional medical risk factors in the elderly might contribute to somewhat poorer outcomes. In addition, physiological effects of aging may vary between individuals such that age alone may be overly simplistic to predict physical outcome. On the other hand, though heart transplant recipients older than 65 years have consistently poorer survival, their quality of life can be comparable to that of younger recipients. In addition, decreased immunologic responsiveness with age may result in less morbidity and mortality due to graft rejection and may allow reduction of immunosuppression, perhaps avoiding medication-induced side effects. Nevertheless, elderly patients who are transplant candidates and recipients are a highly select group and studies suggest that matching patients for parameters other than age (preoperative status, severity of disease, presence of other organ system disease) makes the different age groups comparable. In addition, advances in transplantation technology from improved surgical techniques, better immunosuppression medications and improved post-operative care have improved survival and outcome for all ages if not especially in the elderly. Therefore, future studies must look beyond merely survival to identify the value of transplantation in geriatrics.

Unfortunately, most studies examining post-transplantation outcomes in geriatrics have major methodological limitations. These limitations include the lack of a clear definition of outcome (specifically quality of life), lack of control groups, and inadequate use of objective measurement instruments (if any) to rate quality of life and its multidimensionality. The majority of studies used subjective ratings by the clinical staff to assess overall functional status. Most studies did not include patient-rated data. In addition, a clear definition of geriatrics is needed as studies used an age criterion cutoff that ranged from 50 to 70 years old to distinguish older from younger recipients.

For the future, large-scale multicenter international studies with validated measures related to quality of life will be necessary in order to demonstrate that quality of life indeed improves after transplantation in adults and elderly, and that this improvement may be in fact similar for both age groups. Elderly patients may have different post-transplantation expectations, such as retirement, rather than reintegration back to the work force. Therefore, measures of quality of life and post-transplantation outcomes must reflect these differences. Because certain medical and psychosocial issues differ between populations of elderly as compared with other adults, these quality of life instruments need to reflect demographic differences as well as assessing the patient's perceptions of their own post-transplantation quality of life. So far research on outcomes in elderly patients post-transplantation is encouraging and clearly demonstrates that elderly patients cannot categorically be considered poor transplant candidates.

References

Albrechtsen, D., Leivestad, T., Fauchald, P. et al. (1992). Results of the National Kidney Transplantation Program in Norway. In *Clinical Transplants*, ed. P. Terasaki and J. M. Cecka, pp. 207–13. UCLA Tissue Typic Laboratory: Los Angeles.

Albrechtsen, D., Leivestad, T., Sodal, G. et al. (1995). Kidney transplantation in patients older than 70 years of age. *Transplant Proc*, **27**, 986–8.

Alessiani, M., Jabbour, N., Irish, W., Fung, J., and Starzl, T.E. (1994). Liver transplantation under FK506 immunosuppression in elderly patients. *Acta Gerontol*, **44**, 216–21.

Anand, K. B., Wolf-Klein, G. P., Silverstone, F. A., and Foley, C. J. (1990). Demographic changes and their financial implications. *Clin Geriatr Med*, **6**, 1–12.

Anguita, M., Arizon, J. M., Calles, F. et al. (1992). Influence on survival after heart transplantation of contraindications seen in transplant recipients. *J Heart Lung Transplant*, **11**, 708–15.

Aravot, D. J., Banner, N. R., Khaghani, A. et al. (1989). Cardiac transplantation in the seventh decade of life. *Am J Cardiol*, **63**, 90–3.

Belle, S. H., Beringer, K. C., and Detre, K. M. (1996). Recent findings concerning liver transplantation in the United States. *Clin Transplant*, 15–29.

Bourge, R. C., Naftel, D. C., Costanzo-Nordin, M. R. et al. (1993). Pretransplantation risk factors for death after heart transplantation: a multi-institutional study. *J Heart Lung Transplant*, **12**, 549–62.

Bromley, P. N., Hilmi, I., Tan, K. C., Williams, R., and Potter, D. (1994). Orthotopic liver transplantation in patients over 60 years old. *Transplantation*, **58**, 800–3.

Callahan, D. (1987). Terminating treatment: age as a standard. *Hastings Cent Rep*, **17**, 21–5.

Calne, R. (1994). Contraindications to liver transplantation. *Hepatology*, **20**, 3S–4S.

Carrier, M., Emery, R. W., Riley, J. E., Levinson, M. M., and Copeland, J. G. (1986). Cardiac transplantation in patients over 50 years of age. *J Am Coll Cardiol*, **8**, 285–8.

Chelluri, L., Pinsky, M. R., Donahoe, M. P., and Grenvick, A. (1993). Long-term outcome of critically ill elderly patients requiring intensive care. *JAMA*, **269**, 3119–23.

Coffman, K. L., Valenza, M., Czer, L. S. C. et al. (1997). An update on transplantation in the geriatric heart transplant patient. *Psychosomatics*, **38**, 487–96.

Dew, M. A., Harris, R. C., Simmons, R. G., Roth, L. H., Armitage, F. K., and Griffith, B. P. (1991). Quality-of-life advantages of FK 506 vs. Conventional immunosuppressive drug therapy in cardiac transplantation. *Transplant Proc*, **23**, 3061–4.

Fehrman, I., Brattstrom, C., Duraj, F., and Groth, C. G. (1989). Kidney transplantation in patients between 65 and 75 years of age. *Transplant Proc*, **21**, 2018–19.

Fisher, A., Sheiner P., Bodenheimer H., Mun, A., Atillasoy, E., and Wolf D. C. (1995). Liver transplantation in recipients 65 years and older. *Liver Transplant Surg*, **1**, 451.

Frazier, O. H., Macris, M. P., Duncan, J. M., Van Buren, C. T., and Cooley, D. A. (1988). Cardiac transplantation in patients over 60 years of age. *Ann Thorac Surg*, **45**, 129–32.

Gelbard, A., Haub, C., and Kent, M. M. (1999). World population beyond six billion. *Population Bulletin*, **54**(1), 18–19.

González, M. P., Bobes, J., Sudilovsky, A. et al. (1995). Survival rate and quality of life in elders following liver transplantation. *Qual Life Res*, **4**, 433.

Heroux, A. L., Costanzo-Nordin, M. R., O'Sullivan, J. E. et al. (1993). Heart transplantation as a treatment option for end-stage heart disease in patients older than 65 years of age. *J Heart Lung Transplant*, **12**, 573–9.

Hosenspud, J. D., Novick, R. J., Breen, T. J., Keck, B., and Daily P. (1995). The Registry of the International Society for Heart and Lung Transplantation: twelfth official report – 1995. *J Heart Lung Transplant*, **14**, 805–15.

Howard, R. J., Pfaff, W. W., Salomon, D. et al. (1989). *Transplant Proc*, **21**, 2020–1.

Hunt, R. H. (1993). Quality of life – the challenges ahead. *Scand J Gastroenterol*, Suppl. **199**, 2–3.

Katz, S. (1987). The science of quality of life. *J Chron Dis*, **6**, 459–63.

Kaye, M. P., Elcombe, S. A., and O'Fallon, W. M. (1985). The International Heart Transplantation Registry. The 1984 report. *Heart Transplant*, **4**, 290–2.

Kluge, E. H. (1993). Age and organ transplantation. *Can Med Assoc J*, **149**, 1003.

Kober, B., Kuchler, T. H., Broelsch, C. H., Kremer, B., and Henne-Bruns, D. (1990). A psychological support concept and quality of life research in a liver transplantation program: an interdisciplinary multicenter study. *Psychother Psychosom*, **54**, 117–31.

Latos, D. L. (1996). Chronic dialysis in patients over age 65. *J Am Soc Nephrol*, **7**, 637–46.

Lin, H.-M., Kauffman, M., McBride, M. et al. (1998). Center specific graft and patient survival rates; 1997 United Network of Organ Sharing (UNOS) report. *JAMA*, **280**, 1153–60.

Lundgren, M., Kristiansson, M., Ericson, B. G., and Eleborg, L. (1994). Improved quality of life after liver transplantation. *Transplant Proc*, **26**, 1979.

Miller, L. W., Vitale-Noedel, N., Pennington, D. G., McBride, L., and Kanter, K.R. (1988). Heart transplantation in patients over age fifty-five years. *J Heart Transplant*, **7**, 254–7.

Murie, J. A., Lauffer, G., Gray, D., Ting, A., and Morris, P. J. (1989). Renal transplantation in the older patient. *Transplant Proc*, **21**, 2024–5.

Olivari, M. T., Antolick, A., Kaye, M. P., Jamieson, S. W., and Ring, S. (1988). Heart transplantation in elderly patients. *J Heart Transplant*, 7, 258–64.

Pirsch, J. D., Kalayoglu, M., D'Alessandro, A. M. et al. (1991). Orthotopic liver transplantation in patients 60 years of age and older. *Transplantation*, 51, 431–3.

Pirsch, J. D., Stratta, R. J., Armbrust, M. J. et al. (1989). Cadaveric renal transplantation with cyclosporine in patients more than 60 years of age. *Transplantation*, 47, 259–61.

Robinson, L. R., Switala, J., Tarter, R. E., and Nicholas, J. J. (1990). Functional outcome after liver transplantation: a preliminary report. *Arch Phys Med Rehab*, 74, 490–3.

Rosenblum, D. S., Rosen, M. L., Pine, Z. M., Rosen, S. H., and Borg-Stein, J. (1993). Health status and quality of life following cardiac transplantation. *Arch Phys Med Rehab*, 74, 490–3.

Rowe, J. W., Grossman, E., and Bond, E. (1987). Academic geriatrics for the year 2000. An Institute of Medicine report. *N Engl J Med*, 316, 1425–8.

Santiago-Delpin, E. A. (1996). Transplantation in the elderly: changing philosophy. *Transplant Proc*, 28, 3408–9.

Shaw, B. W. (1994). Transplantation in the elderly patient. *Surg Clin North Am*, 74, 389–400.

Snell, G. I., de Hoyos, A., Winton, T., and Maurer, J. R. (1993). Lung transplantation in patients over the age of 50. *Transplantation*, 55, 562–6.

Starzl, T. E., Todo, S., Gordon, R. et al. (1987). Liver transplantation in older patients. *New Engl J Med*, 316, 484–5.

Stieber, A. C., Gordon, R. D., Todo, S. et al. (1991). Liver transplantation in patients over sixty years of age. *Transplantation*, 51, 271–2.

Tarter, R. E., Erb, S., Biller, P. A., Switala, J., and Van Thiel, D. H. (1988). The quality of life following liver transplantation: a preliminary report. *Gastroenterol Clin North Amer*, 17, 207–17.

Tarter, R. E. Switala, J., Arria, A., Plail, J., and van Thiel, D. (1991). Quality of life before and after orthotopic hepatic transplantation. *Arch Intern Med*, 151, 1521–6.

Tesi, R. J., Elkhammas, E. A., Davies, E. A., Henry, M. L., and Ferguson, R. M. (1994). Renal transplantation in older people. *Lancet*, 343, 461–4.

UNOS (United Network for Organ Sharing), Health Care Financing Administration and the Division of Organ Transplantation. (1990). *Annual Report on the Scientific Registry and the Organ Procurement and Transplantation Network*. US Department of Health and Human Services: Washington, DC.

Van Thiel, D. H., Schade, R. R., Gavaler, J. S., Shaw, B. W., Iwatsuki, S., and Starzl, T. (1984). Medical aspects of liver transplantation. *Hepatology*, 4 (Supplement 1), S79–S83.

Veatch, R. M. (1988). Justice and the economics of terminal illness. *Hastings Center Rep*, 18, 34–40.

Wiesner, R. H., Demetris, A. J., Belle, S. H. et al. (1998). Acute hepatic allograph rejection: incidence, risk factors, and impact on outcome. *Hepatology*, 28, 638–45.

Williams, T. F. (1996). Geriatrics: perspective on quality of life and care for older people. In *Quality of Life and Pharmacoeconomics in Clinical Trials*, 2nd ed, ed. B. Spilker, pp. 803–7. Lippincott-Raven: Philadelphia.

Zetterman, R. K., Belle, S., Hoffnagle, J. et al. (1998). Age and liver transplantation: a report of the Liver Transplantation Database. *Transplantation*, 66, 500–6.

6

Cognitive assessment in organ transplantation

Ralph E. Tarter Ph.D. and JoAnn Switala M.P.A.

Introduction

Deficits on neuropsychologic tests have been reported in patients with acute and chronic pulmonary (Incalzi et al. 1993), hepatic (Tarter et al. 1991), renal (Hart and Kreutzer 1988), cardiac (Bornstein et al. 1995) and pancreatic (Ryan 1988) diseases. At first glance, it would appear that injury or disease to a vital organ directly causes an encephalopathy that is manifest in part as a cognitive impairment. Upon more careful inspection, however, it is evident that biologic, psychologic, and social contextual factors synergistically determine the pattern and severity of cognitive deficit. Specifically, a cognitive impairment is not invariably due to an encephalopathy caused by organ–system disease. Numerous factors must be taken into consideration, resulting in a variety of etiologic pathways, in determining the extent to which a cognitive deficit is causally related to the medical illness.

Integrity of brain functioning is entirely dependent on the metabolic efficiency of the other vital organs. Because the brain's metabolic reserve capacity is very limited, satisfying its high oxygen, energy, and nutritional needs depends on efficient functioning of other vital organs. Consequently, even slight perturbation, or a small reduction of metabolic efficiency, can disrupt brain functioning to the degree that an encephalopathy is manifest. Impaired cognitive functioning is typically a salient facet of the neuropsychiatric disorder.

This chapter examines the cognitive sequelae of medical disorders in which organ transplantation is a recommended treatment. There is justification for determining the cognitive capacity and efficiency of patients undergoing organ transplantation. Cognitive ability, for example, covaries with severity of encephalopathy; hence measuring cognition is a precise and unobtrusive method of quantifying severity of underlying neurologic disorder. Significantly, one of the most salient features of impaired cognition is poor judgment. Impaired judgment predisposes to suboptimal compliance with a treatment regimen and other maladaptive decisions pertinent to everyday living (Kennedy et al. 1987). Cognitive deficit is also associated with poor work and social adjustment and low educational achievement (Heaton, Chelune, and Lehman 1978; Heaton and Pendleton 1981). Furthermore, risk for accidental injury is augmented concomitant to psychomotor, visuo-spatial, or attentional incapacity. For these reasons, determining a patient's level of cognitive functioning provides information that is useful for guiding medical management, preventing injury, and maximizing psychosocial reha-bilitation.

Two principles guide the cognitive evaluation of patients with chronic disease. First, it must be shown that the cognitive impairment is the direct manifestation of disease to a particular organ or system. In effect, an associ-ation between cognitive capacity and biochemical or physiologic indicators of the disease should be demonstrated in order to conclude that the cognitive disturbances, reflecting one aspect of a metabolic encephalopathy, are causally related to the organ–system. Toward this end, serial assessments are desirable so as to delineate covariation between changes in medical and cognitive status. In principle, because the encephalopathy has a metabolic etiology, medical or surgical (i.e. transplantation) restoration of normal organ–system functioning should result in amelioration of cognitive deficit.

Second, while it is well established that acute organ–system failure pro-duces florid and severe cognitive disturbances, it is also important to recog-nize that a low-grade cognitive deficit commonly results from chronic medi-cal disease in the absence of neurologic signs or symptoms of encephalopathy (Adrian et al. 1988; Tarter et al. 1990). Thus, the absence of disturbance indicated from clinical examination does not necessarily imply that an encephalopathy is not present. Rather a subclinical or latent encephalopathy may be present. Although not florid, this condition is nonetheless associated with significant cognitive impairment (Tarter et al. 1987).

The specialized class of psychometric tests validated for identifying neur-ologic disturbance are referred to as "neuropsychological tests". Unlike other neurodiagnostic procedures (e.g., electroencephalography (EEG), computed tomography (CT), magnetic resonance imaging (MRI), etc.) that directly measure brain morphology or physiology, the aim of the neuropsychological assessment is to profile cognitive processes such that accurate inferences about the integrity of brain functioning can be derived. Therefore, using tests that have proven validity and sensitivity, it is possible to reveal the presence of neuropsychiatric disturbance in the lower ranges of encephalopathy severity. Hence, a neuropsychologic evaluation not only provides the opportunity to detect disturbance that is not otherwise identifiable using other neurodiag-nostic procedures but can do so in a fashion that enables describing the encephalopathy in the context of the patient's functional abilities.

Procedure for conducting a cognitive assessment

The neuropsychologic evaluation is necessarily time consuming and labor intensive. This is due to the need to measure a diverse range of cognitive processes. In order to reduce cost and maximize efficiency, it is necessary to prioritize time and allocation of resources. This can be accomplished by adhering to a three-stage assessment procedure (Tarter and Edwards 1986).

Screening

At the outset, it is valuable to determine whether a cognitive impairment is present using neuropsychologic tests that have high sensitivity. Tests that are most informative at this juncture are capable of determining whether there is a lesion or dysfunction but not necessarily its location in the cortex. The detection of impairment, therefore, apprises the examiner that a comprehensive evaluation is likely to be informative. Cognitive screening takes approximately 15 minutes. Typically, three or four tests encompassing the domains of attention, visuospatial capacity and psychomotor capacity are administered. Commonly used measures include the Symbol Digit Modalities Test (Smith 1973), Trailmaking Test (Reitan 1958), Grooved Pegboard (Costa et al. 1963), Finger Tapping Speed Test (Reitan 1958) and Rey–Osterrieth Complex Figure Test (Osterrieth 1944).

Comprehensive assessment

In the event that an impairment is indicated in the screening battery, the second stage of evaluation is to profile cognitive strengths and limitations. This is accomplished using one of the following strategies: (a) administer a standardized battery, (b) administer a specialized battery tailored to the particular circumstances of the population, or (c) combine a standardized battery with selected additional measures.

Standardized battery

The Halstead Reitan Battery (Reitan 1955) and Luria Nebraska Neuropsychological Battery (Golden, Berg, and Graber 1981) are currently the two most commonly used standardized batteries. Psychometric studies indicate that they have comparable validity. Both batteries tap the same general domains of cognitive functioning. An advantage of the Luria Nebraska Battery is that the scores are documented using a common metric; this standardization enables comparison of performance across different cognitive domains. It also takes somewhat less time to administer than the Halstead Reitan Battery. However, it is important to point out that both of these latter batteries were standardized on patients with pronounced cortical lesions and thus may not be sensitive enough to detect a subclinical encephalopathy associated with chronic medical illness.

Specialized battery

A battery of tests can be specially composed to respond to the characteristics of a particular population. For example, patients who are not ambulatory or can be tested only at bedside cannot be administered the Halstead Reitan Battery. Also, where the measurement emphasis is on performance efficiency, neither the Luria Nebraska Battery nor Halstead Reitan Batteries is useful. Based on an understanding of the patient population, and the conditions available for testing, it is thus necessary to compose a specialized battery suitable to the patient's circumstances and goals of the evaluation. One example of a specialized battery is the Pittsburgh Initial Neuropsychological Test System (PINTS) (Goldstein et al. 1983). This battery comprises a complement of instruments selected from several previously validated batteries. Intelligence, perception, visuospatial capacity, memory, psychomotor efficiency, language and abstracting ability are evaluated in about 90 minutes. It is also noteworthy that a specialized battery has been developed for treating the cognitive capacities of human immunodeficiency virus (HIV) infected individuals (Maj et al. 1993). The point to be made, however, is that, depending on the goals of the assessment and the special characteristics of the patient population, it may be advisable to compose a test battery that satisfies the main considerations of sensitivity, breadth of coverage, and feasibility of obtaining valid information.

Combined standardized and specialized batteries

The number of processes comprising the cognitive architecture is too extensive to be evaluated by one battery. Under circumstances where the goal is to be very inclusive, a common procedure is to add tests to a standardized protocol. For example, the Halstead Reitan Battery only minimally evaluates learning and memory capacity. Thus, to fully evaluate these capacities, it is necessary to add tests of learning and memory to the evaluation protocol. In general practice, the Benton Visual Retention Test (Benton 1963), Wechsler Memory Scale (Wechsler 1945) and California Verbal Learning Test (Delis et al. 1987) are among the most common tests added to standardized batteries in order to obtain information about memory processes.

Modality-specific evaluation

The third stage of assessment is to obtain detailed information in a specific cognitive domain (e.g., language, memory, etc.). This is necessitated by the fact that comprehensive batteries do not fully detail the range of cognitive processes encompassed within a particular modality. Where information is required regarding a specific cognitive domain, it is necessary to administer a modality-specific battery. Thus, this stage of the neuropsychologic evaluation involves delineating within a particular modality the range and specificity of deficit.

With the exception of tests validated to assess language, modality-specific standardized batteries have yet to be developed. Consequently, a modality-specific battery can be created only by selecting specific tests from the existing armamentarium of validated tests. For example, while psychomotor visuo-spatial deficits are commonly observed among patients presenting for liver transplantation (Tarter et al. 1987), a modality-specific battery would encompass tests capable of determining the extent to which attentional, perceptual, and abstracting impairments contribute to the spatial deficit and the particular circumstances in which the deficit is manifest (e.g., visual, auditory, haptic (touch) modality). In this manner, a thorough understanding of the neurobehavioral causes and the manifestation of psychomotor disturbance can be understood.

Cognition in relation to psychopathology

A comprehensive neuropsychologic assessment encompasses the documentation of emotional and behavioral disturbances in addition to cognitive deficits. Neuropsychiatric disorder caused by medical illness is associated in varying degree with disturbances in these three facets of psychological functioning. The combined impairment impacts adversely on adjustment in the domestic, work, and social spheres such that overall quality of life is diminished (Tarter, Switala, and Van Thiel 1994).

Because a neuropsychiatric disturbance reflects the end-point confluence of cognition, emotion and behavior, the type, severity, and chronicity of medical illness determine in large part the clinical presentation. However, the individual's premorbid personality, motivation, social context, and cultural identity also strongly influence the neuropsychiatric profile. Hence, in order to fully understand the cognitive component of neuropsychiatric disorder, it is essential to take into account the other facets of the patient's psychological functioning and sociocultural context.

Psychopathology, independent of organ–system disease, is associated commonly with disturbed cognitive functioning. For example, patients receiving dialysis experience dysphoric mood and manifest impairment in cognitive capacity as measured by event-related potentials and neuropsychologic tests (Brown et al. 1991). The adverse life changes concomitant with chronic disease, and awareness by the patient that the disease may be fatal, commonly lead to severe psychiatric disturbance which, in turn, is featured by impaired cognitive functioning. Significantly, patients with pre-transplantation psychiatric disorder have a poorer postsurgery prognosis, including depression and organic mental syndrome (Phepps 1991).

Depression is the most common psychopathologic disturbance observed in patients before and after organ transplantation. It is not uncommon for depression to be so severe as to produce a pseudodementia. Thus, it is important to comprehensively evaluate psychopathology and determine its time course covariation with the particular disease and the cognitive impairment. For example, depression that is reactive to a perception of futility requires intervention that is different from depression which is a direct correlate of the neuropsychiatric disorder. Other correlated disturbances besides depression include anxiety, anger, apathy, and fear. These latter emotional and behavioral reactions are common responses to life-threatening disease and also comprise symptoms of encephalopathy. Furthermore, because emotional disturbances, where severe, are also associated with impairments in attention, memory, and judgment, it is informative to partition the sources of cognitive impairment where there is associated psychopathology. This is a rather difficult task that requires administration of structured psychiatric interviews that document the time course of symptoms (e.g., before or after onset of disease), their relationship to medical status, and their covariation with severity of cognitive deficit. Where it is not possible to administer a structured diagnostic interview or self-report questionnaire to determine severity of emotional distress medical histories are also informative for correlating the cognitive and psychiatric facets of encephalopathy.

Alcohol and drug abuse effects on cognition

Chronic and excessive alcohol abuse produces significant neurologic injury with accompanying cognitive deficits (Tarter and Van Thiel 1985; Ellis and Oscar-Berman 1989). Drug abuse has also been shown to be associated with cognitive impairment; however, the evidence in this regard is less conclusive (Spencer and Boren 1991). The neuropsychologic profile in alcoholism or drug abuse reflects a mild to moderate dementia, the most prominent features consisting of abstracting, memory, and visuospatial impairments. Thus, it is important to be cognizant of a history of substance abuse as a contributory factor in understanding cognitive functioning in patients with medical illness.

Related to this issue is the need to rule out neurologic disorder that results indirectly from alcohol or drug abuse. For example, Wernicke–Korsakoff syndrome, having its etiology in thiamine deficiency (Langlais 1995), is almost always associated with alcoholism. Dementia in drug abusers can ensue from acquired immune deficiency syndrome (AIDS) acquired either from infected needles or through sexual transmission. The point to be made is that a thorough examination of the person's history, behavior, and lifestyle is required in order to determine the impact of substance abuse on neuropsychologic test performance.

Neurodevelopmental disorder

A substantial proportion of the adult population has a neurodevelopmental disorder persisting since childhood. Dyslexia (reading disability) and attention deficit disorder with hyperactivity are featured by a variety of cognitive limitations. Hence, a systematic examination of the patient's developmental history that also includes documenting significant gestational and perinatal history needs to be conducted in order to exclude or otherwise account for these factors on test results.

Neurologic disease effects on cognition

It is essential to document and evaluate neurologic disorder that may be concurrent with medical illness. Neurospychologic test performance is affected by chronic neurologic disease (e.g., seizure disorder, multiple sclerosis), historical events (e.g., traumatic brain injury, hypoxic episodes), and normal aging. These factors need to be taken into consideration to prevent misinterpretation of test results.

Iatrogenic effects on cognition

Psychotropic medications such as benzodiazepenes have been frequently documented to impair attention and memory capacity. If possible, the neuropsychologic examination should, therefore, be conducted while the patient is not receiving psychotropic drugs. Less is known about the cognitive sequelae of medications used for treatment of organ-system disease. Effective treatment, by improving organ–system functioning, theoretically should result in amelioration of brain dysfunction and ultimately restore the person to normal neuropsychologic capacity. Empirical evidence is, however, lacking; thus, the potential confound of pharmacologic treatment should at least be recognized, since the impact on neuropsychologic test results cannot be determined. Moreover, it is important to be aware of the trade-off between the benefits gained in medical management of disease and the effects of pharmacologic therapy. For example, corticosteroids at high doses adversely impact on cognition and emotional stability but yet may be a necessary medical intervention. Also, empirical evidence has been accrued indicating that immunosuppressant drugs such as cyclosporine have transient neurotoxic effects. Inasmuch as their neurotoxic effects may be reversible, it would appear advisable to delay neuropsychologic examination until acute toxicity has subsided. It should also be noted that treatment may augment cognitive functioning. In a study of bone marrow recipients, Parth et al. (1989) observed a transient improvement following chemotherapy. These findings underscore the importance of determining as best as possible the influence of treatment on neuropsychologic test results.

Motivation effects on cognition

Impairment on cognitive tests can be manifest concomitant with low motivation. This is particularly evident on tasks that require sustained effort such as problem solving, attention, and the organization and implementation of a sequence of motor responses. In its most extreme form, low motivation can be expressed as apathy whereby the person has little, if any, capacity to initiate and sustain goal-directed behavior. Low motivation or apathy can have a multifactorial etiology. Feelings of hopelessness coexistent with a life-threatening medical illness, severe depression, neurologic injury (particularly in the prefrontal cortex) and early stage dementia all contribute to reduced motivation. It is important, therefore, to measure motivation and its impact on the results of a neuropsychologic evaluation.

Malingering and deception

Under circumstances where the patient believes a benefit can be obtained from poor performance, a conscious effort may be made to intentionally demonstrate a cognitive impairment. For example, the examinee may be under the mistaken impression that cognitive impairment will increase their priority ranking on a transplant candidacy list. It is important, therefore, for the examiner to inform the patient about the purpose of the evaluation and how the information will be used. Toward this end, the examiner should ensure that the testing environment and the test-taking instructions evoke maximum effort by the patient.

General physical fitness and cognition

The capacity to undergo neuropsychologic examination depends to a large degree on the physical fitness of the patient. The patient's ability to sit for a long period of time and use his or her hands in an unencumbered fashion and free from pain determines ultimately the validity of neuropsychologic test scores. One recently completed study demonstrates, for example, that isokinetic muscle strength covaries with level of neuropsychologic functioning (Tarter et al. 1997). The point is thus underscored that the assessment protocol should be tailored to the physical capacities of the patient in order to elicit valid information.

Cognitive capacity and cognitive style

There are two broad facets of cognition: *capacity* and *style*. Capacity refers to the ability to perform a particular cognitive task. Examples include whether the person can complete a crossword puzzle, learn a list of words, or put beads on a string. One aspect of cognitive capacity is *efficiency*; this parameter refers to the time it takes to complete a task correctly. Efficiency is measured by calculating the *rate* of performing correct responses. Because efficiency simultaneously entails both speed and accuracy, it is generally considered to be a more sensitive indicator of cognitive status than a measure of accuracy alone. This is particularly salient where the neuropsychiatric disorder is not in an advanced stage of deterioration or manifest as a florid syndrome. Typically, patients with chronic medical illnesses have more or less intact ability but reduced efficiency.

Cognitive style refers to how a task is performed rather than how well. The strategy employed in performing a task impacts on both accuracy and efficiency; thus, cognitive style and efficiency are not mutually exclusive. For example, in assembling a set of blocks to create a design, the person may organize the blocks one at a time to create the configuration; that is, the task ordering proceeds from part to whole. Alternatively, the person can adopt a "big picture" strategy or have a mental Gestalt in which, through the use of imagery, the blocks are assigned to positions based on perception of the whole picture. These two cognitive strategies are sometimes referred to as "analytical" and "holistic," respectively.

Figure 6.1 illustrates an example of analytic and holistic perception. As can be seen, it is possible to view the design as one "H" or alternatively as consisting of many Hs horizontally and vertically aligned. Injury to the brain can affect which cognitive style is adopted in performing a task inasmuch as the left hemisphere subserves primarily an analytic information-processing mode whereas the right hemisphere subserves primarily a holistic mode of information processing.

In summary, a comprehensive neuropsychologic assessment of cognition typically incorporates an evaluation of both cognitive capacity and cognitive style. It is important to learn how well cognitive processes are executed as well as the strategy adopted. Where neuropsychiatric disorder is not severe or even evident upon clinical examination, it is essential to measure efficiency. This facet of cognitive capacity is more sensitive to disruption from brain dysfunction or pathology than measures of performance accuracy.

Functional organization of the cortex

The human cerebral cortex is not equipotential. Rather, neuronal systems within and across specific cortical regions subserve specialized cognitive

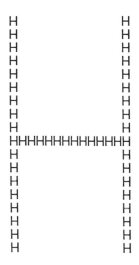

Figure 6.1. Analytic and holistic modes of cognitive processing.

functions. As a result, lesions in particular regions of the cortex are associated with unique cognitive deficits.

Neuropsychology is the discipline concerned with identification of lesions and their location using psychometric tests. With an understanding of functional neuroanatomy and specifically cortical organization of cognitive processes, it is possible to determine with a high degree of accuracy the location of a lesion lateralized within the left or right hemisphere and within a particular lobe (Walsh 1978). Significantly, neuropsychologic tests are capable of determining the presence of cerebral pathology in the absence of overt neurologic signs or symptoms such as in the early stages of dementia, psychiatric disorder, or concomitant to chronic medical illness (Grant and Adams 1986; Tarter and Edwards 1986). In these latter situations, a neuropsychologic evaluation is, however, typically utilized to detect diffuse cerebral pathology rather than a localized lesion.

Injury or pathology to the right hemisphere is associated primarily with cognitive deficits that involve visuospatial capacity. In contrast, a lesion in the left hemisphere is featured most saliently by a disruption of language processes. Specialization within each hemisphere is essentially homologous; that is, the occipital cortex subserves visual perception whereas the temporal cortex and parietal cortex subserve auditory and haptic perception, respectively. The region anterior to the motor cortex encompasses the prefrontal cortex. In humans, the prefrontal lobe comprises about 30% of brain mass. Unlike the other lobes, it does not encode sensory input. Rather, neuronal connections in the prefrontal cortex reciprocally innervate associated cortex and limbic structures. This high level of integrative communication among diverse brain regions comprises the substrate for cognitive functioning. Insofar as these higher-order cognitive processes exercise regulatory control over behavior, they are referred to as the "executive cognitive functions" (Luria 1966). They encompass a range of diverse cognitive processes such as judgment, formulation, and evaluation of plans or strategies to attain goals, self-monitoring behavior, working memory, and focused attention.

It is beyond the scope of this discussion to review in detail the functional organization of the brain. Suffice to point out that, regardless of cause (e.g., trauma, infection, etc.), a thorough evaluation of cognitive functioning requires administering a battery of tests that in aggregate can inform about the presence of a localized lesion, or alternatively, a diffuse lesion. Toward this objective, tests measuring abstracting, language, learning, memory, attention, visuospatial and psychomotor capacity are typically administered as part of a thorough examination in conjunction with standardized tests of intelligence and, where appropriate, tests of academic achievement. Before describing the process and content of neuropsychologic assessment, it is important to first discuss the factors that need to be considered in order to accurately interpret the results of a neuropsychologic assessment.

Organ–system interactions

Because of the synergy and interaction among organs and systems, disease or injury can have disruptive effects beyond the condition of interest. In effect, it is not justified to assume that the particular disease is the primary cause of the encephalopathy and accordingly the manifest cognitive impairment. For instance, renal disease is commonly associated with systemic hypertension; both of these latter conditions produce a cognitive deficit. Also, liver disease commonly results in a hepatorenal syndrome. Both liver disease and renal failure can lead to cognitive deficits concomitant to an encephalopathy. The point to be made is that disease of one organ or system can have far reaching effects on other organ–systems which may, in fact, be the proximal cause of the observed neuropsychologic deficits.

In summary, cognitive impairments observed in medical patients commonly have a multifactorial etiology. A major task, therefore, of the neuropsychologic evaluation either before or after transplantation is to disaggregate as best as possible the various sources of influence. Figure 6.2 depicts a model for partitioning the causes of cognitive deficit.

Cognitive deficit in patients presenting for organ transplantation

A review of the empirical literature indicates that there is a high degree of similarity among patients presenting for organ transplantation. The results

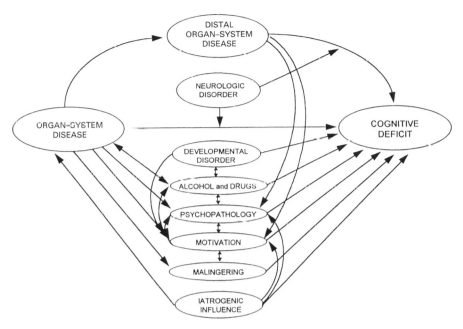

Figure 6.2. Etiologic pathways for cognitive impairment.

indicate that the affected organ or system does not produce a unique pattern of cognitive impairments. The reasons for this remain unclear but probably reflect the fact that the encephalopathy is associated with a diffuse cerebral lesion. The following discussion describes the traditional domains of neuro-psychologic assessment.

Intelligence

Adjustment in a variety of environments (work, school, social) depends to a large degree on the person's capacity to process complex information and adopt a successful strategy for a course of action. This capacity in totality is referred to as intelligence. Its constituent components comprise dozens of different cognitive functions (Reed 1982). There is evidence that some patients experience an improvement in general intellectual functioning following heart transplantation, although the extent to which this is due to severity of delirium during the presurgical assessment remains unknown. Schall et al. (1989) observed a modest four-point average improvement in overall IQ score following cardiac transplantation. In this latter study, the verbal IQ score on the Wechsler Adult Intelligence Scale did not change whereas the performance IQ score improved by an average of six points.

These findings suggest that transplantation does not improve the aspect of intelligence involved with accessing stored information (crystallized intelligence) but instead affects the facet of intelligence involving responding to new situations (fluid intelligence).

Attention and concentration

A disruption of attentional capacities is typically the first manifestation of neurologic disease or dysfunction. At first glance, attentional problems may mask as forgetfulness. For example, not remembering where an object was placed may in fact be due to the person not attending to their behavior. Thus, to ensure accurate interpretation of test findings, it is essential to differentiate a memory impairment from attentional deficit.

Attentional mechanisms regulate incoming sensory information. This regulatory process has both active and passive qualities. With respect to passive attentional control, sensory stimulation traverses a gating mechanism such that only relevant information reaches cognitive awareness. For example, a person who lives near a highway habituates to the sound of passing vehicles so that this noise does not penetrate conscious awareness on a moment to moment basis. In effect, passive attentional mechanisms selectively regulate sensory input. Active attentional mechanisms on the other hand involve intentional mental effort. Two types of focused effort involve *continuous* and *divided* attention. These two facets are not necessarily mutually exclusive; however, continuous attention; primarily involves selecting relevant from irrelevant stimuli occurring in an uninterrupted manner whereas divided attention entails responding to a relevant stimulus while simultaneously performing more than one task. Playing bingo involves continuous attention, while reading a book and listening to the radio involve divided attention.

Disruption of attentional mechanisms is associated with significant cognitive impairment. Deficits in virtually all cognitive domains can emerge concomitantly with attentional impairment. In other words, information that does not achieve conscious awareness will produce failure at tasks that have higher cognitive processing requirements. At a practical level, it is crucial to thoroughly evaluate attentional capacities inasmuch as deficiency is associated with injury risk in all facets of daily living.

Patients presenting as candidates for organ transplantation commonly manifest attentional deficits (Farmer 1994). This impairment has not, however, been systematically analyzed with respect to type of attentional processes, its covariation with severity of encephalopathy, and the extent to which it is moderated by other biopsychosocial processes.

Memory

The ability to retrieve information to guide behavior is integral to adaptive functioning. This capacity encompasses a set of interrelated functions occurring at different stages of information processing. Considered within a multistage framework, memory can be viewed as immediate (remembering a string of digits after their presentation), short term (recalling information for up to about an hour after the input) and long term. The level of retrieval difficulty may be easy (e.g., recognition of previously received information), or demanding (e.g., recall of information without memory-assisting cues).

There are different types of memory. One typology distinguishes declarative from procedural long-term memory. Declarative memory involves knowledge of information (e.g., remembering a spouse's birthday), whereas procedural memory involves remembering how to perform a task (e.g., driving a car). Declarative memory is further subdivided into semantic memory and episodic memory. Semantic memory involves the organization of the person's knowledge about the world (e.g., number of days in a week), whereas episodic memory pertains to the recollection of specific personalized events (e.g., what the person ate for breakfast). Working memory refers to an ability to hold information in temporary storage while performing a task (e.g., remembering a phone number while dialing), and it overlaps short-term memory.

Cerebral lesions do not affect all facets of memory in the same fashion. For example, Korsakoff syndrome is associated with profound episodic memory disturbance, whereas procedural memory is essentially intact. Systematic investigation has yet to be undertaken that is directed at elucidating the facets of memory impaired by organ–system disease. The available findings indicate that short-term memory is impaired (Hecker, Norvell, and Hills 1989; Tournes et al. 1989; Tarter, Van Thiel, and Edwards 1989). However, it needs to be emphasized that this deficit is in all likelihood exacerbated by poor attentional capacity, which in turn is influenced by severity of encephalopathy and a host of other medical, psychiatric, and psychosocial factors. Furthermore, it should be pointed out that organ transplant candidates do not as a rule manifest procedural memory disturbance. When a memory deficit is manifest, it is rather subtle and linked to numerous factors besides the specific organ–system disease.

Language

Comprehension of written and oral information having symbolic properties, and the ability to retrieve words from memory and express oneself fluently are integral to optimal functioning in all spheres of daily living. Language capacity is an especially important cognitive capacity with respect to management of patients with chronic disease because the patient as the primary informant of symptoms must be able to communicate effectively with physicians and ancillary professions. Moreover, the patient must be able to comprehend instructions in order to comply with a complicated treatment regimen and schedule of medications. Evidence accrued to date does not implicate a disorder in language capacities among patients having a metabolic encephalopathy (Tarter, Edwards and Van Thiel 1988; Farmer 1994). Nonetheless, the clinician should be sensitive to the impact of the encephalopathy on other cognitive functions, which in turn impede efficient communication. For example, impaired attentional capacities are likely to result in word-finding difficulties, and dysfluency can mistakenly be interpreted to reflect a dysphasia.

Perception

Perception is the elaboration of sensory input into meaningful information (e.g., words, objects). Whereas primary cortex analyzes and encodes sensory input, the surrounding association area elaborates on this information to enable perception in the visual, haptic, and auditory modalities. At the most basic level, perception consists of the recognition of stimulus features. For example, in the visual modality, salient features include size, shape, and angularity. More complex facets of perception involve the integration of features such as lines and angles to form shape, or pitch and notes to form melody.

From the neuropsychologic perspective, systematic analysis of perceptual processes enables determining with a high degree of precision the location of a lesion and, from a practical standpoint, the specificity of cognitive disorder. With respect to analysis of causes of disorder, it is important to recognize that the endpoint deficit could be due to a variety of factors. For example, reading involves perceptual analysis of complex stimuli (letters) and their sequential composition (words). A deficiency in letter recognition can be due to a perceptual incapacity in letter orientation (e.g., "b" versus "d"), shape (e.g., "u" versus "v") or feature detection ("e" versus "c"). Moreover, the source of deficit can reside at an integrative level such as connecting letters into morphemes, or linking the visual display of letters to the correct phoneme. In these latter types of impairment, involving intra- and intermodality, perceptual integration ultimately prevents the person from deriving meaning from a perceptual array. The endpoint disorder is dyslexia; however, as can be seen there are manifold causal pathways to this outcome stemming from a specific perceptual deficit.

Patients with chronic medical illness have been found in numerous studies to manifest perceptual deficits (Tarter et al. 1988). The available information indicates that the impairments are most pronounced on complex tasks requiring spatial analysis and integration rather than at the level of feature extraction and recognition. To date, the evidence also indicates that the impairments are confined to the visual and to lesser extent the haptic modality (Tarter et al. 1988). In view of the integral role of perception in all aspects of daily living, its measurement is an essential and core feature of any comprehensive cognitive evaluation.

Abstracting

The ability to plan a course of action and solve problems as well as reason inductively and deductively are increasingly required for successful social adaptation and vocational adjustment. As society becomes increasingly technologically sophisticated, greater cognitive demands are placed on the individual. Indeed, even relatively simple and routine tasks (e.g., using a telephone, driving a car, operating automatic teller bank machines) require a high level of cognitive ability.

An abstracting impairment has been reported in patients with a variety of different chronic medical illnesses (Tarter et al. 1988). To date, however, it remains unknown whether the deficits are pervasive or circumscribed to particular facets of abstracting capacity. Also, the extent to which the deficits are limited to verbal or nonverbal information processing is not known. Whereas investigations have identified the presence of abstracting deficit in a variety of diseases using different types of test, the causal determinants remain to be specified. One especially important task is to evaluate whether the manifest abstracting impairment is one facet of a more basic disorder in executive cognitive capacity (Luria 1966).

Psychomotor integration

Integration of perceptual and motor processes is essential for efficient execution of behavior. This aspect of the neuropsychologic examination is especially informative as part of overall patient management (e.g., preventing injury at work or caused by driving a car). Numerous investigations have revealed that patients with organ–system disease have reduced psychomotor efficiency (Tarter et al. 1988; Farmer 1994). Virtually all of the studies conducted to date have, however, been confined to visual–motor processes. Eye–hand coordination, fine motor control, and motor speed have been shown in many studies to be impaired in patients with chronic medical illness who present as candidates for organ transplantation.

Academic achievement

Evaluation of academic achievement level in the basic skills (reading, arithmetic, spelling) is recommended in order to gauge the magnitude of decline concomitant with medical illness. Used in conjunction with measures of crystallized intelligence (e.g., vocabulary level), tests of academic achievement inform about the extent to which the severity of encephalopathy measured neuropsychologically is concomitant with organ–system disease in relation to premorbid level. For example, average level of performance on neuropsychologic tests does not reflect intact capacity among individuals who have postgraduate university education and presumably a very high premorbid level of intellectual functioning. Hence, academic achievement level and crystallized intelligence level provide a reference for interpreting magnitude of impairment on neuropsychologic tests. The most commonly used measures of academic achievement are the Wide Range Achievement Test (Jastak and Jastak 1965) and the Peabody Individual Achievement Test (Dunn and Markwardt 1970).

Ecologically valid neuropsychologic assessment

The traditional psychometric approach to neuropsychologic assessment is based on the premise that the sample of behavior measured under controlled conditions informs about how well the person would perform in the natural environment. Whether or not this assumption is justified depends on the degree to which the tests have been shown to have concurrent and predictive validity. For example, the impairment index of the Halstead Reitan Battery has been shown to correlate with social and vocational adjustment (Heaton et al. 1978; Heaton and Pendleton 1981). Less confidence, however, can be attached to other commonly used psychometric measures.

Recently, neuropsychologic assessment procedures have been introduced which simulate "real life" situations. So far, these measures have been confined to tasks that primarily evaluate memory (Wilson, Cockburn and Baddeley, 1989). These types of test have not been widely adopted, even though they have obvious value and clear advantage over existing procedures. With the exception of one study demonstrating that psychomotor impairment in cirrhotic individuals correlates with performance on a task involving simulation of driving an automobile (Schomerus et al. 1981) these procedures have not been applied to the medically ill population.

Computer interactive evaluation

Neuropsychologic evaluation is rooted in the psychometric tradition of a skilled examiner administering and scoring tests in a standard manner. The tests typically involve either answering questions, performing mental operations upon command, performing tasks on paper, or requiring simple manual operations.

The availability of inexpensive and powerful microcomputers has ushered in a new era of neuropsychologic evaluation. Rather than a clinician or technician, personal computers can be used to administer neuropsychologic tests, thereby making cognitive assessment widely available. Significantly, computer interactive testing affords the opportunity more precisely to quantify cognitive processes than is possible using traditional methods. At present, a large number of standard neuropsychologic tests have been redesigned for computer administration and scoring, and a variety of new batteries has been developed (for a review, see Kane and Kay 1992). As yet, they have not been employed for routine assessment of encephalopathy concomitant with medical disorder. Inasmuch as computer interactive neuropsychologic assessment is inexpensive and largely automated, it provides an excellent method for serial assessment of patients during the course of their illness and following medical/surgical intervention. In this manner, neuropsychologic test performance can be used to accurately index the severity of encephalopathy to monitor patient status.

Neuropsychologic change associated with organ transplantation

As previously mentioned, the encephalopathy concomitant to organ–system disease has a metabolic etiology. Either toxins (e.g. ammonia) or insufficient resources (e.g. oxygen, glucose) affect the brain adversely. Assuming that chronic metabolic disruption does not produce permanent morphological damage, it is plausible to expect that restoration of optimal organ–system function is associated with amelioration of the encephalopathy.

The limited available findings indicate that patients undergoing heart (Bornstein et al. 1995) and liver (Arria et al. 1991) transplantation experience substantial recovery. The results further suggest that level of functioning does not return to normal. Whether the persisting deficit post-transplantation is due to residual neurologic impairment caused by the disease or due to manifold other factors has not been investigated. Most likely, the reasons differ among individuals when recovery is not complete. For example, older patients tend to manifest more severe cognitive impairment pretransplantation (Schall et al. 1989), which may mitigate improvement postsurgery. Also, the type of organ disease interacting with severity and chronicity of illness most probably influences the magnitude of postsurgery recovery. Furthermore, as noted previously, post-transplantation medications and psychiatric disorder impact on cognitive functioning. Finally, it should be pointed out that the temporal course of recovery has not been systematically researched. Indeed, studies have yet to be conducted beyond a 1-year postsurgery interval. It may be that transplantation effects full cognitive recovery after sufficient time has elapsed. Clearly, long-term prospective studies of recipients need to be conducted using the same assessment protocol across various diseases. Until such time that studies are conducted which inform about the pattern and extent of improvement and the factors influencing improvement following transplantation, our understanding of cognitive prognosis will remain uncertain.

Cognition and development

Brain injury or disease among adults is associated with the loss of established cognitive capacities. In contrast, children who are born with genetically determined metabolic diseases, or acquire disease before cognitive maturation is complete, do not develop cognitively in an age-concordant fashion (Stewart et al. 1994). The limited available findings on children do not allow for unequivocal conclusions about the effectiveness of transplantation in children. A recent review of the literature indicates that deficits on neuropsychologic tests are present before and after transplantation; however, it is recognized that there is substantial heterogeneity within and between disease groups (Stewart et al. 1992). Davis, Chang and Nevins (1990) found that 12 of 18 renal transplant patients who underwent surgery before the age of 30 months experienced improvement in mental and intellectual development. The findings in this latter study suggest that transplantation resulted in accelerated development in some individuals. With respect to heart and heart–lung transplantation, it appears that most children function within the normal ranges after surgery, although test scores are lower than those of healthy children (Wray et al. 1994). Persisting cognitive deficits having a pronounced level of severity appear to be present in some children following transplantation surgery; however, other children appear to undergo full recovery of cognitive capacities. This variability in cognitive improvement may be determined by multiple factors including absence from school, restriction of mobility, and reduced opportunity to participate in social interactions. Whether cognitive rehabilitation methods are effective in accelerating cognitive development remains unknown. Clearly, organ–system diseases adversely impact on cognitive development. Monitoring cognitive development through serial assessments before and after surgery can thus inform about the need for rehabilitation.

Conclusions

Cognitive impairment, demonstrated in many medical disorders, has a multifactorial etiology. The burgeoning field of medical neuropsychology is concerned with delineating the cognitive manifestations of brain pathology or dysfunction in patients with acute and chronic organ–system disease. Obtaining information about cognitive status has wide ranging ramifications. As discussed, cognitive capacity is intimately connected to social and vocational adjustment as well as risk for injury and compliance with a medical regimen. Employing cognitive assessment procedures routinely in clinical settings has, therefore, the potential to augment clinical prognosis and protection of patient safety. Ultimately, these benefits manifest as improved cost-effectiveness of the medical and surgical treatment of patients with organ–system diseases.

Acknowledgment

J.S. is supported by a grant from the University of Pittsburgh Institute of Alcohol Abuse and Alcoholism.

References

Adrian, J., Crankshaw, D., Tiller, J., and Stanley, R. (1988). Affective, cognitive and subjective changes in patients undergoing cardiac surgery – a preliminary report. *Anesth Intens Care*, **16**, 144–9.

Arria, A., Tarter, R., Starzl, T., and Van Thiel, D. (1991). Improvement in cognitive functioning of alcoholics following orthotopic liver transplantation. *Alcoholism Clin Exp Res*, **15**, 956–62.

Benton, A. (1963). *The Revised Visual Retention Test*. Psychological Corporation: New York.

Bornstein, R., Starling, R., Myerowitz, P., and Haas, G. (1995). Neuropsychological function in patients with end-stage heart failure before and after cardiac transplantation. *Acta Neurol Scand*, **91**, 260–5.

Brown, W., Marsh, J., Wolcott, D. et al. (1991). Cognitive function, mood and P3 latency: effects of the amelioration of anemia in dialysis patients. *Neuropsychologia*, **29**, 35–45.

Costa, L., Vaughn H., Levita E., and Farber, N. (1963). Purdue Pegboard as a predictor of the presence and laterality of cerebral lesions. *J Consult Psychol*, **27**, 133–7.

Davis, I., Chang, P., and Nevins, T. (1990). Successful renal transplantation accelerates development in young uremic children. *Pediatrics*, **86**, 594–600.

Delis, D. C., Kramer, J. H., Kaplan, E., and Obver, B. A. (1987). *California Verbal Learning Test*. The Psychological Corporation, Harcourt Brace Jovanovich, Inc: New York.

Dunn, L. and Markwardt, F. (1970). *Manual for the Peabody Individual Achievement Test*. American Guidance Service: Circle Pines, MN.

Ellis, R. and Oscar-Berman, M. (1989). Alcoholism, aging and functional cerebral asymmetries. *Psychol Bull*, **106**, 128–47.

Farmer, M. (1994). Cognitive deficits related to major organ failure. The potential role of neuropsychological testing. *Neuropsychol Rev*, **4**, 117–60.

Golden, C., Berg, R., and Graber, B. (1981). Test–retest reliability of the Luria–Nebraska Neuropsychological Battery. *J Consult Clin Psychol*, **50**, 452–4.

Goldstein, G., Tarter, R., Shelly, C., and Hegedus, A. (1983). The Pittsburgh Initial Neuropsychological Testing System (PINTS): a neuropsychological screening battery for psychiatric patients. *J Behav Assess*, **5**, 227–38.

Grant, I. and Adams, K. (1986). *Neuropsychiatric Assessment of Neuropsychiatric Disorder*. New York: Oxford University Press.

Hart, R. and Kreutzer, I. (1988). Renal system. In *Medical Neuropsychology: The Impact of Disease on Behavior*, ed. R. Tarter, D. Van Thiel, and K. Edwards, pp. 99–120. Plenum Press: New York.

Heaton, R., Chelune, G., and Lehman, R. (1978). Using neuropsycholgoical and personality tests to assess the likelihood of patients' employment. *J Nerv Ment Dis*, **166**, 408–16.

Heaton, R. and Pendleton, M. (1981). Use of neuropsychological tests to predict adult patients' everyday functioning. *J Consult Clin Psychol*, **49**, 807–21.

Hecker, J., Norvell, N., and Hills, H. (1989). Psychologic assessment of candidates for heart transplantation: toward a normative data base. *J Heart Transplant*, **8**, 171–6.

Incalzi, R., Gemma, A., Marra, C., Muzzulon, R., Capparella, O., and Carbonin, P. (1993). Chronic obstructive pulmonary disease. An original model of cognitive decline. *Am Rev Respir Dis*, **148**, 412–24.

Jastak, J. and Jastak, S. (1965). *The Wide Range Achievement Test Manual*. Guidance Associates: Wilmington, DE.

Kane, L. and Kay, G. (1992). Computerized assessment in neuropsychology. A review of tests and test batteries. *Neuropsychol Rev*, **3**, 1–117.

Kennedy, G., Hofer, M., Cohen, D., Shindledecker, R., and Fisher, J. (1987). Significance of depression and cognitive impairment in patients undergoing programmed stimulation of cardiac arythmias. *Psychosom Med*, **49**, 410–21.

Langlais, P. (1995). Alcohol-related thiamine deficiency: impact on cognitive and memory functioning. *Alcohol, Health Res World*, **19**, 113–21.

Luria, A. (1966). *Higher Cortical Functions in Man*. Basic Books: New York.

Maj, M., D'Elia, L., Satz, P., Janssen, R. et al. (1993). Evaluation of two neuropsychological tests designed to minimize cultural bias in the assessment of HIV-1 seropositive persons: a WHO study. *Arch Clin Neuropsychol*, **2**, 123–36.

Osterrieth, P. (1944). Le test de copie d'une figure complexe. *Arch Psychol*, **30**, 206–356.

Parth, R., Dunlap, W., Kennedy, R., and Lane, N. (1989). Motor and cognitive testing of bone marrow transplant patients after chemotherapy. *Percept Motor Skills*, **68**, 1227–41.

Phepps, L. (1991). Psychiatric aspects of heart transplantation. *Can J Psychiatry*, **36**, 563–8.

Reed, S. (1982). *Cognition: Theory and Applications*. Brook-Cole Publishing Company: Pacific Grove, CA.

Reitan, R. (1955). Investigation of the validity of Halstead's measures of biological intelligence. *Arch Neurol Psychiatry*, **73**, 28–35.

Reitan, R. (1958). Validity of the trailmaking test as an indicator of organic brain damage. *Perceptual Motor Skills*, **8**, 271–6.

Ryan, C. (1988). Neurobehavioral disturbances associated with disorders of the pancreas. In *Medical Neuropsychology: The Impact of Disease on Behavior*, ed. R. Tarter, D. Van Thiel, and K. Edwards, pp. 121–58. Plenum Press: New York.

Schall, R., Petrucci, R., Brozena, S., Cavarocci, N., and Jessup, M. (1989). Cognitive function in patients with symptomatic dilated cardiomyopathy before and after cardiac transplantation. *J Am Coll Cardiol*, **14**, 1666–72.

Schomerus, H., Hamster, W., Blunck, H., Reinhard, U., Mayer, K., and Dalle, W. (1981). Latent portosystemic encephalopathy. 1. Nature of cerebral functional deficits and their effects on fitness to drive. *Dig Dis Sci*, **26**, 622–30.

Smith, A. (1973). *Symbol Digit Modalities Test*. Western Psychological Services: Los Angeles, CA.

Spencer, J. and Boren, J. (eds.) (1991). *The Residual Effects of Abused Drugs on Performance*. US Superintendent of Documents, Public Health Service: Washington, DC.

Stewart, S., Campbell, R., McCallon, D., Waller, D., and Andrews, W. (1992). Cognitive patterns in school age children with end stage liver disease. *J Dev Behav Pediatr*, **13**, 331–4.

Stewart, S., Kennard, B., Waller, D., and Fixler, D. (1994). Cognitive function in children who receive organ transplantation. *Health Psychol*, **13**, 3–13.

Tarter, R. and Edwards, K. (1986). Neuropsycholgoical batteries. In *Clinical Application of Neuropsychological Test Batteries*, ed. T. Incagnoli, G. Goldstein, and C. Golden. Plenum Press: New York.

Tarter, R., Edwards, K., and Van Thiel, D. (1988). *Medical Neuropsychology*. New York: Plenum Press.

Tarter, R., Hegedus, A., Van Thiel, D., Edwards, N., and Schade, R. (1987). Neurobehavioral characteristics of cholestatic and hepatocellular disease: differentiation according to disease specific characteristics and severity of identified cerebral dysfunction. *Int J Neurol*, **32**, 901–10.

Tarter, R., Van Thiel, D., and Edwards, K. (1989). *Medical Neuropsychology: The Impact of Disease on Behavior*. Plenum Press: New York.

Tarter, R., Moss, H., Arria, A., & Van Thiel, D. (1991). Cognitive impairment in substance absuers. In *The Residual Effects of Abused Drugs on Performance*. ed. J. Spencer. US Superintendent of Documents: Washington, DC.

Tarter, R., Panzak, G., Lu, S., Simkevitz, H., and Switala, J. (1997). Isokinetic muscle strength and its association with neuropsychological capacity in cirrhotic alcoholics. *Alcoholism: Clin Exp Res*, **21**, 191–6.

Tarter, R., Switala, J., Arria, A., Plail, J., and Van Thiel, D. (1990). Subclinical hepatic encephalopathy: comparison before and after transplantation. *Transplantation*, **50**, 632–7.

Tarter, R., Switala, J., and Van Thiel, D. (1994). Psychosocial factors of organ transplantation. In *Anesthetic Principles for Organ Transplantation*, ed. D. Cook and P. Davis. Raven Press: New York.

Tarter, R. and Van Thiel, D. (eds.) (1985). *Alcohol and the Brain: Chronic Effects*. Plenum Press: New York.

Tournes, D., Bashein, G., Hornbein, T. et al. (1989). Neurobehavioral outcomes in cardiac operations. *J Thorac Cardiovasc Surg*, **98**, 774–82.

Walsh, K. (1978). *Neuropsychology: A Clinical Approach.* Churchill Livingston: New York.

Wechsler, D. (1945). A standardized clinical scale for clinical use. *J Psychol,* **19**, 87–95.

Wilson, B., Cocburn, J., and Baddeley, A. (1989). *The Rivermead Behavioral Memory Test.* Thames Valley Test Company: Reading.

Wray, J., Pot-Mees, C., Zeitlin, H., Radley-Smith, R., and Yacoub, M. (1994). Cognitive function and behavioral status in pediatric heart and heart-lung transplant recipients: the Harefield experience. *Br Med J,* **309**, 837–41.

7

Pharmacologic issues in organ transplantation: psychopharmacology and neuropsychiatric medication side effects

Paula T. Trzepacz M.D.,
Babu Gupta M.D., Andrea F. DiMartini M.D.

Introduction

Organ transplant candidates and recipients pose special pharmacologic problems because of organ–system insufficiency or failure, often multisystem, and the medical need for polypharmacy. The use of immunosuppressant agents post-transplantation complicates psychiatric assessment because of associated neuropsychiatric side effects. Because patients are also at risk for unusual infections that require aggressive treatment, neuropsychiatric syndromes resulting both from the medications and the infections further complicate psychiatric differential diagnosis (Trzepacz et al. 1991). The potential for drug–drug interactions is high, and can result in drug toxicity and delirium.

The psychologic stresses of undergoing organ transplantation are also high. Clinically significant depression or anxiety may be difficult to distinguish from secondary psychiatric symptoms, e.g., due to medications (e.g., ganciclovir, cyclosporine, prednisone) or to medical disorders (e.g., hypoxia, cytomegalovirus infection). Identification and treatment of primary psychiatric disorders in organ transplant patients is covered in detail elsewhere (Trzepacz et al. 1991; Trzepacz, DiMartini, and Tringali 1993b).

General issues in organ insufficiency

Some of the organs that are transplanted also play important roles in drug metabolism and clearance (for a review, see DiMartini and Trzepacz 1999). The liver is the most involved in detoxification and metabolism, with the kidneys responsible for excretion of some drugs (e.g., digoxin, lithium, gabapentin) and many metabolites of hepatically altered drugs. The heart is responsible for movement of blood that transports drugs and oxygen to all tissues. Third spacing of drugs into peritoneum (ascites) or interstitial tissues (edema) in the context of hepatic, cardiac, or renal failure may lower effective levels in the bloodstream, requiring adjustment of doses.

The liver not only chemically alters or deactivates drugs, but it is also responsible for producing plasma proteins (e.g., albumin) that bind a number of drugs. Enzymes of the smooth endoplasmic reticulum of the liver are present in smaller amounts in other tissues, e.g., lung, kidney, and gastrointestinal epithelium. Cytochrome P_{450} isoenzymes in the lungs may contribute a minor part to drug metabolism (Paine et al. 1996). Both hepatic and renal insufficiency can result in reduced levels of serum albumin, thereby increasing the unbound fraction of protein-bound drugs and increasing the risk of side effects or intoxication due to increased drug availability (Levy 1990). Reduced protein binding during renal failure is most significant for drugs whose normal binding is high (Bennett et al. 1983). Most psychotropic drugs are highly protein bound (see Table 7.1) and lipophilic, except lithium (Levy 1990) and methylphenidate. In addition, a recent report describes a serotonin transporter similar to that in brain and platelets that is expressed on human pulmonary membranes (Suhara et al. 1998). In this report tricyclic and selective serotonin reuptake inhibiting antidepressants were found trapped in the lung tissue in high concentration. It was hypothesized that the lungs may function as a reservoir for antidepressants with high affinity for serotonin binding sites (Suhara et al. 1998). However, the effect of lung insufficiency on these mechanisms is unknown.

Due to decreased excretion during renal failure, it is generally recommended that dosing intervals be increased (Bennett et al. 1983; Levy 1990). However, somewhat surprising is that reduced elimination is not the rule for all drugs in renal insufficiency, with phenytoin the notable exception. In uremia, drug oxidation is normal or accelerated, reduction and hydrolysis are slowed, and glucuronide and glycine conjugations are normal while acetylation may be slowed (Reidenberg 1977).

Absorption

For orally administered drugs, absorption is the initial step to adequate drug delivery. Alterations in gastrointestinal absorption occur as a result of a variety of situations: reduced gastric emptying or motility (e.g., diabetic gastroparesis); graft-versus-host disease in gut; portal hypertension with portal–systemic shunting from cirrhosis; and changes in transit time (e.g., bowel disease) (Leipzig 1990). Small intestinal transplantation adds a new level of psychopharmacologic complexity and has not been widely studied. Most patients requiring small intestinal transplantation have short-gut syndrome, which creates significant administration difficulties for drugs requiring small intestinal absorption. Unfortunately, few psychotropic drugs are available in parenteral forms, which would be the preferred route of administration (Thompson and DiMartini, 1999). Post-transplantation rejection, infection, cellular infiltration, graft-versus-host disease or post-transplantation lymphoproliferative disorder in the transplanted intestine can decrease absorption of medications (DiMartini et al. 1996a). If possible, selecting psychotropic medications that can be monitored by blood levels provides clinical data at least to guide medication adjustments in these patients.

Hepatic drug metabolism

Hepatic biotransformation of drugs occurs in two phases: phase I for oxidation, reduction, or hydrolysis; and phase II for conjugation. Each phase involves a large number of enzymes. For example, phase I enzymes (monooxygenases), also called the cytochrome P_{450} families, are located pericentrally in the smooth endoplasmic reticulum and are important for oxidation, dealkylation, reduction or hydrolysis (e.g., deamination, deesterification) of molecules (Howden, Birnie, and Brodie 1989). Phase I enzymes are affected mostly by acute viral hepatitis, alcoholic hepatitis, and active cirrhosis (Leipzig 1990). Metabolites from phase I can be active or inactive. Drugs are metabolized by specific cytochrome P_{450} isozymes and there is genetic heterogeneity for some of these isozymes such that some persons may be "slow metabolizers" (see below).

Phase II enzymes act on parent drugs (e.g., lorazepam) or metabolites generated from phase I activity, to conjugate molecules to a more polar compounds (Howden et al. 1989). Usually the conjugated compound is inactive, with a few exceptions, such as morphine 6-glucuronide. Phase II enzymes, located periportally in the liver, are involved in reactions for glucuronidation, sulfation, acetylation, and amino acid conjugation with glycine, glutamine, and glutathione (Leipzig 1990; Pacifici et al. 1990).

In cirrhosis, glucuronidation (a conjugation pathway) is actually preserved (Pacifici et al. 1990), so that choosing medications that require only glucuronidation (e.g., oxazepam, lorazepam, morphine) is advantageous. Choosing agents that do not require hepatic metabolism (e.g., methylphenidate, gabapentin) is also recommended, but, unfortunately, there are few such medications from which to choose.

Drugs can be characterized as being "high" or "low" clearance drugs, depending on whether blood flow or enzyme saturation are the rate-limiting factors for hepatic metabolism, at therapeutic doses. Enzyme affinities determine whether drugs are enzyme or flow dependent. Low clearance drugs (e.g., diazepam, quinidine, phenytoin) have low enzyme affinity and saturate the enzymes, and are therefore metabolized more slowly than high clearance drugs (e.g., beta-blockers, morphine, tricyclics, ketoconazole) that have a

Table 7.1. Commonly used psychotropic agents and metabolic issues[a] (active metabolites in square brackets)

Agent [active metabolite]	$T_{1/2}$ (h)	Protein binding (%)	Hepatic metabolism Cytochrome	Conjugation	Renal excretion
Alprazolam	12	71	$P_{450}IIIA$		Yes
Bupropion [threo-amino] [morphinol]	21 24 24	82–88	Unknown (?IID6)	Likely	Yes
Venlafaxine [O-desmethyl-venlafaxine]	5	27	$P_{450}IID6$ (weak inhibitor)	Yes	Yes
Buspirone [1-pyrimidinyl-piperazine]	11 2–3	30 95	$P_{450}IIIA4$	No	Yes
Carbamazepine [CBZ-10,11-epoxide]	15 (35 h single dose) 7.5	75 50	$P_{450}IID6$ (Induces)	Yes	Yes
Clonazepam	18–50	85	Nitroreduction and oxidative hydroxylation		Yes
Diazepam [nordazepam] [oxazepam]	30–60 ±100 5–10	98	$P_{450}IIIA$ and S-mephenytoin hydroxylase	Yes	Yes Yes
Fluoxetine [norfluoxetine]	96–144 96–384	95	$P_{450}IID6$ (potent inhibitor; ?also inhibits IIIA3/4 and IIC19) (also inhibits IID6)	Yes	Yes Yes
Fluvoxamine	15	80	$P_{450}IIIA4$ (inhibits IIIA4 and IA2)		Yes
Gabapentin	6.5 (6.2 in renal insufficiency)	<3	No	No	Yes (Renal failure affects serum levels)
Haloperidol [reduced haloperidol in "reversible metabolism" to parent][b]	10–36 67	92	N-dealkylation and reduction	Yes	Yes

Drug	Half-life (hrs)	% Protein binding	Metabolism		Dialyzable [a]
Lithium	14–28	0	No	No	Yes (Renal failure; no affect on serum levels)
Lorazepam	9–16	90	No	Yes	Yes
Methylphenidate	2.5	0	(deesterification to ritalinic acid in blood)	No	Yes
Nefazodone	2–4	> 99	P$_{450}$IIIA4 and IID6 (inhibits IIIA4 > IID6)		Yes
[hydroxy-NEF]	1.5–4				
[triazoledione]	18				
[mCPP]	4–8				
Nortriptyline	18–93	95	P$_{450}$IID6	Yes	Yes
[10-hydroxy-nortriptyline]				No	
Olanzapine	21–54	93	P$_{450}$IA2 (Minor pathway IID6)	Yes	Yes (also fecal) (Renal failure; no affect on serum levels)
Paroxetine	21	95%	P$_{450}$IID6	Yes	Yes
Risperidone	3	90	P$_{450}$IID5	Yes	Yes
[9-OH-risperidone]		70			
Sertraline	26	98	P$_{450}$IID6 (modest inhibition)	Yes	Yes
[desmethyl-sertraline]	62–104				
Temazepam	10–17	98	No (not IID6)	Yes	Yes
Trazodone	6 (biphasic – then 5–9)	93			
[m-chlorophenyl-piperazine]					
Valproic acid	15	90	P$_{450}$IID6 (and mitochondrial beta-oxidation)	Yes	Yes
[2-en-valproate]					
Zolpidem	2.6 (in cirrhosis: 9.9 hrs)	92.5	(no interactions with cimetidine)		Yes

[a] Information for oral preparations only.   [b] Inactive metabolite; glucuronidation is major metabolic pathway in humans.

high enzyme affinity and quicker metabolism. Metabolism of high clearance drugs depends on the rate of their delivery to the liver (by perfusion), which determines their metabolism rates. Drugs whose metabolism is such that serum levels increase linearly with increasing doses are categorized as having first-order kinetics (e.g., sertraline); when enzyme saturation or inhibition prevents rapid metabolism, then zero order (also called nonlinear or dose-dependent) kinetics occur. Some drugs (e.g., paroxetine and fluoxetine) have zero-order kinetics even at therapeutic doses. Metabolism that occurs with linear or first-order kinetics can become zero order when enzymes become saturated, such as at higher doses, during illness, or during competition with other drugs for enzyme sites.

In addition to characteristics of individual drugs and their enzyme affinities determining kinetics of metabolism, organ insufficiency also plays a role. Congestive heart failure and beta blockade can reduce blood flow to the liver, thereby lowering the metabolism rate of high clearance drugs. For example, even the short-acting benzodiazepine midazolam has reduced clearance in congestive heart failure (Patel et al. 1990). In cirrhosis, portal–systemic and intrahepatic shunting reduces perfusion so that high clearance drugs are handled more slowly and mimic low clearance drugs, changing their kinetics from first- to zero-order kinetics. Similar to physiologic shunting, surgical shunts also reduce total blood flow to the liver and slow metabolism of high clearance drugs. Low clearance drugs will not be affected by blood flow shunting, but may accumulate due to the decrease in metabolizing enzymes from loss of functional liver parenchyma.

In heart failure, there is a reduced volume of distribution of drugs due to third spacing into interstitial tissues, as well as hypoperfusion of organs, including kidneys and liver, so that drug metabolism and clearance decreases (Shamas and Dickstein 1988). Passive congestion of liver and gut alter drug metabolism and absorption. Doses should be reduced and dosing increments made more gradually (Shamas and Dickstein 1988). Because of reduced perfusion of muscle, intramuscular injection should be avoided.

Hepatic isozymes

Recently, a family of cytochrome (cyt) P_{450}-related isozymes have been identified and are important for understanding drug–drug interactions. These isozymes undergo oxidation and reduction, and can bind and transfer oxygen and electrons to organic molecules (Pollock 1994). There are two main classes of cyt P_{450} isozymes: those catalyzing formation of endogenous compounds, such as steroids and prostaglandins, and those that metabolize exogenous drugs (Preskorn and Magnus 1994). Three families of cyt P_{450} enzymes have thus far been identified as being related to drug metabolism (Preskorn and Magnus 1994). Different drugs and their metabolites have different affinities for various isozymes (e.g., for IID6 or IIIA3/4). Some drugs induce or inhibit particular isozymes, thereby causing drug–drug interactions such that accelerated clearance with reduced efficacy or prolonged half-lives with increased risk of toxicity can result when one or more drugs interact at the same isozyme. Inhibition of cyt $P_{450}IID6$ can reduce the analgesic efficacy of codeine, which depends on conversion to morphine (Pollock 1994).

The rate of metabolism of a parent drug can greatly affect therapeutic efficacy or side effect occurrence, compounded by isozyme interactions. If a metabolite is more active than its parent compound, accelerated metabolism might increase its therapeutic effect while reduced metabolism might reduce efficacy. Cisapride's cardiotoxicity, which increases when its metabolism to its active metabolite is inhibited by ketoconazole or erythromycin, occurs via cyt $P_{450}IIIA3/4$ interaction. Tricyclic antidepressant toxicity occurs when fluoxetine is added, via cyt $P_{450}IID6$ inhibition. Fluoxetine also inhibits its own metabolism, further increasing its already long half-life (Preskorn and Magnus 1994). Carbamazepine's (CBZ) active metabolite, CBZ-10,11-epoxide, is responsible for much of its side effects and its level increases disproportionately as CBZ induces its own metabolism via cyt $P_{450}IID6$. When valproic acid is added to carbamazepine, CBZ-10,11-epoxide levels increase even further and valproic acid's (VPA) metabolites are also produced at a faster rate, including two toxic metabolites, 4-en-VPA and 2,4-en-VPA (Wilder 1992). Therefore, knowledge of which isozyme is responsible for a drug's metabolism can assist in predicting drug interactions, e.g., cimetidine increasing benzodiazepine levels.

Table 7.2 lists drugs commonly used in organ transplant patients and their known isozyme affinities (Brockmoller and Roots 1994; Pollock 1994; Preskorn and Magnus 1994). Unfortunately, this information is incomplete for many drugs. Even when a drug is not a potent inhibitor of an isozyme, competition for enzyme sites between concurrently administered drugs can reduce metabolism, especially when one drug has a higher affinity and saturates the isozyme. This reduced metabolism is exacerbated during hepatic or cardiac insufficiency, which reduces enzyme efficiency. Function of donor liver enzymes may be a factor in maintenance of stable cyclosporine A (CYA) serum levels; postoperative cyt $P_{450}IIIA3/4$ activity, assessed in liver biopsies of transplant recipients, using a midazolam probe strategy, was highly variable, possibly accounting for difficulty in achieving stable CYA levels (Thummel et al. 1994). A few drugs induce activity of certain enzymes (e.g., carbamazepine), potentially lowering levels of themselves and similarly metabolized drugs.

Cytochrome $P_{450}IID6$, which metabolizes drugs such as fluoxetine, mexiletine, paroxetine, encainide and carbamazepine, is genetically polymorphic. Most psychotropic drugs are metabolized by cyt $P_{450}IID6$. Certain families

Table 7.2. Hepatic cytochrome isozymes, including drugs commonly used in organ transplant patients

$P_{450}IID6$	$P_{450}IIIA3/4$ (in liver and GI mucosa; no genetic polymorphism)
alprenolol	alprazolam
amitriptyline (hydroxylation)	amitriptyline (demethylation)
brofaromine	astemizole
carbamazepine (induces)	barbiturates (induces)
chlorpromazine (inhibits)	buspirone
cimetidine	carbamazepine
clozapine	cimetidine (inhibits)
codeine	clomipramine (demethylation)
clomipramine (hydroxylation)	corticosteroids (induces)
debrisoquine	cyclosporine
desipramine	dapsone
dextromethorphan	dexamethasone
encainide	diazepam
flecainide	diltiazem
fluoxetine (potently inhibits)	erythromycin (inhibits)
fluphenazine (inhibits)	estradiol
haloperidol (reversible metabolic pathway)	ethosuximide
imipramine (hydroxylation)	FK506
maprotiline	fluoxetine (inhibits)
metoprolol	fluvoxamine (inhibits)
mexiletine	flurazepam
mianserin	glyburide
nefazadone (modestly inhibits)	imipramine (demethylation)
norfluoxetine (potently inhibits)	ketoconazole (inhibits)
nortriptyline	lidocaine
olanzapine (minor pathway)	lovastatin
paroxetine (strongly inhibits)	midazolam
perphenazine (inhibits)	nefazodone (inhibits)
phenobarbital	nifedipine
propafenone (inhibits)	norfluoxetine (inhibits)
phenytoin	propoxyphene
propranolol (minor pathway)	quinidine
quinidine (inhibits)	rapamycin
remoxapride	rifampin (induces)
risperidone	tacrolimus
sertraline (modestly inhibits)	tamoxifen
thioridazine	terfenadine
timolol	testosterone
valproate	triazolam
venlafaxine	(tricyclics and SSRIs inhibit somewhat)
vinblastine	venlafaxine (?)
	verapamil

Table 7.2. (*cont.*)

$P_{450}IA2$	hexobarbital
amitriptyline (demethylation)	ibuprofen
caffeine	imipramine (demethylation)
clomipramine (demethylation)	meclobemide
fluvoxamine (potent inhibitor)	mephenytoin
imipramine (demethylation)	methylphenobarbital (induces)
olanzapine	omeprazole
phenacetin	phenytoin
tacrine	propranolol
theophylline	tolbutamide
tolbutamide	warfarin
warfarin	$P_{450}IIE1$
$P_{450}IIC9/19$	chlorzoxazone
alprenolol	disulfiram (inhibits)
amitriptyline (demethylation)	enflurane
citalopram	ethanol (induces)
clomipramine (demethylation)	paracetamol
diazepam	phenol
N-desmethyldiazepam	
fluvoxamine (inhibits)	

GI, gastrointestinal; SSRI, serotonin selective reuptake inhibitor.

and races have genetically determined lower levels of this isozyme activity ("poor metabolizers"). The elderly also have lower activity levels. Risk of drug toxicity is higher in these persons. Drug half-lives will be prolonged in poor metabolizers, for example, risperidone's half-life is 3 hours in extensive metabolizers and 20 hours in poor metabolizers (Heykantz et al. 1984).

Cytochromes $P_{450}IIC19$ and IA2 also have genetic polymorphism (Pollock 1994), but $P_{450}IIIA3/4$ is not known to have genetic polymorphism. Interestingly, IID6 has been identified in the brain and may play a role in altering brain concentrations of many psychotropics (Pollock 1994).

Table 7.1 lists metabolic information for commonly used psychotropic drugs, including half-life, protein-binding, phase I and phase II hepatic metabolism, cyt P_{450} isozymes, and renal excretion of parent compounds and/or metabolites. Alternative pathways for some drugs and their metabolites (not listed in Table 7.1) may compensate when the main pathway is not as functional or available. Haloperidol, though reduced by IID6 into reduced-haloperidol, which is in reversible equilibrium with the parent drug, has glucuronidation as its main metabolic pathway in humans (Someya et al. 1992). Table 7.1 could serve as a useful reference during administration of psychotropic medications for pre- and post-transplantation periods, especially when cross-referenced with Table 7.2.

Table 7.3 describes certain clinical "tips" regarding drug interactions, clinical situations, and side effects for psychotropic agents when used in the transplant population.

Neuropsychiatric issues with immunosuppressants

Cyclosporine

Cyclosporine (CYA) is a lipophilic cyclic polypeptide derived from the fungus *Tolypocladium inflatum* Goma. First used for human organ transplantation in 1978, its effectiveness is well established and usage is widespread. Nontransplant immunosuppressive applications are also under investigation (Humphreys et al. 1993). CYA primarily affects helper T lymphocytes, although specific mechanisms may be numerous and complex (Craven 1991). Primarily metabolized in the liver by cyt P_{450}IIIA3/4, its pharmacokinetics can be highly variable and influenced by numerous drug interactions. Side effects include neurotoxicity, nephrotoxicity, and lymphoproliferative disease (Trzepacz et al. 1993a). A newer oral form, Neoral, does not require bile acids for absorption.

A wide range of neuropsychiatric symptoms have been documented through case reports, though few systematic studies have investigated side effect incidence. In general, milder symptoms predominate, but may be more severe in liver transplant patients (Tollemar et al. 1988). In a large prospective study of renal transplant patients treated with CYA, fine tremor (39%) was the most frequently reported neurological symptom (European Multicentre Trial Group 1983). Other common symptoms were paresthesias, headache, insomnia, anxiety/agitation, apathy, blurred vision, anorexia, and nausea (European Multicentre Trial Group 1983; de Groen et al. 1987; Surman, Dienstag, and Cosimi 1987; Craven 1991; Humphreys and Leyden 1993). Adams et al. (1987) reported a 33% incidence of serious neurotoxic side effects in 52 liver transplant cases, the most common being seizures (in 25%), which were usually responsive to phenytoin; less common were central pontine myelinolysis, cerebral abscess, psychosis, and delirium. Sensorimotor disturbances may include dysarthria, paresis/paralysis, spasticity, ataxia, and cortical blindness (Noll and Kulkarni 1984; de Groen et al. 1987; Lane et al. 1988). Bone marrow transplants are especially vulnerable to CYA neurotoxicity, with seizures, ataxia, drowsiness, quadriparesis, intention tremor, and delirium (Atkinson et al. 1984).

Psychotic symptoms, specifically paranoid delusions and auditory and complex visual hallucinations, have been reported in patients who were not delirious, although seizures were not ruled out in most cases (Noll and Kulkarni 1984; Craven 1991; Steg and Garcia 1991; Tripathi and Panzer

1993). These symptoms were either transient or resolved with reduction of serum CYA levels. Other reported neuropsychiatric syndromes include akinetic mutism associated with dystonia, dyskinesias, and pseudobulbar palsy during CYA initiation (Bird et al. 1990), and catatonic features during chronic treatment (Bernstein and Levin 1993).

Severe central nervous system (CNS) side effects include seizures, delirium, stupor/coma, and death (de Groen et al. 1987; Lane et al. 1988; Appleton et al. 1989; Bird et al. 1990; Craven 1991: Barbui et al. 1992; Humphreys and Leyden 1993). In 57 consecutive liver transplant patients, 6 had either delirium, seizures, or "confusion" during the first week, with resolution of symptoms upon CYA reduction/discontinuation (Azoulay et al. 1993).

Persistent somnolence in patients given CYA may be a warning of severer neurotoxicity (Craven 1991). Though dose reduction may improve symptoms, no "threshold" serum drug level has been firmly established above which neurotoxicity is likely to occur. Azoulay et al. (1993) found a strong relationship between severe CNS/renal toxicity within the first week posttransplantation and CYA blood levels 12 hours after the initial dose, though levels were in the normal range.

The etiology of CYA neurotoxicity remains unclear and may be multifactorial. Suspected predisposing factors include hypomagnesemia, hypocholesterolemia (≤ 120 mg/dl), high dose corticosteroids, aluminum overload, fever, infection, intravenous administration, advanced liver failure, and malignant hypertension (Bird et al. 1990; Craven 1991; Trzepacz et al. 1993a). CYA is bound largely to plasma lipoproteins (Lucey et al. 1990). Though CYA is highly lipophilic, animal studies show that transport across the blood–brain barrier is normally restricted (Cefalu and Pardridge 1985; Wagner et al. 1987). De Groen et al. (1988) and Tollemar et al. (1988) suggested that advanced liver insufficiency and associated blood–brain barrier abnormalities lead to increased CYA neurotoxicity in liver transplant recipients. De Groen et al. (1988) found a correlation between preoperative hepatic encephalopathy and postoperative CYA CNS toxicity. He also found an association between CNS toxicity and low serum cholesterol levels during the first week after liver transplantation and proposed several explanations, including low serum cholesterol leading to upregulation and increased CYA binding to lipoprotein receptors and subsequent increased intracellular transport in brain tissue (de Groen et al. 1987). In fact, some pathological studies of fatal cases of convulsions and coma revealed cerebral edema with evidence of disruption of the blood–brain barrier (Lane et al. 1988).

A direct toxic effect of CYA on the brain has also been postulated (Sloane et al. 1985), perhaps explaining reported magnetic resonance imaging (MRI) and computed tomography (CT) evidence of white matter changes, consistent with blood–brain barrier disruption in patients with CNS toxicity

Table 7.3. Special considerations for psychotropic use in organ transplantation

Organ System	Psychotropic	Consideration
All	Neuroleptics	Akathisia can be confused with restlessness/tremor from immunosupressants
All	Haloperidol	Rare Torsades de Pointes ventricular arrhythmia if i.v. May be more common if patient has dilated cardiomyopathy or a history of alcohol abuse
All	Haloperidol	Can be given intravenously in doses as high as 1000 mg/day for severe intractable delirium
All	Haloperidol	Glucuronidation is major metabolic route, not cyt P_{450}
All	Fluoxetine	Not slow metabolism of CYA (Strouse et al. 1996) or FK506
All	Nefazadone	Avoid concurrent use of terfenadine, astemizole cisapride due to possible prolonged QT_c and cardiotoxicity
All	SSRIs, carbamazepine	Hyponatremia and SIADH may occur
All	MAOI	Danger of hypertensive crisis if combined with other commonly used pre- and post-transplantation medications opioids, vasopressors, anesthetic agents)
All	Lithium	Tremor can be confused with that of immunosuppressants
All	Valproic acid	Hyperammonemia may occur in absence of LFT abnormalities, possibly in carnitine-deficient patients
All	Zolpidem	Not effective in presence of benzodiazepines
All	Lithium	Avoid in immediate postoperative period. Dose after dialysis and check serum levels prior to dialysis. Monitor CYA levels due to renal interaction. In ascites, fluid overload, or edema dose may need to be increased
All	Propofol	The vehicle of this drug is a good substrate for bacteria and may put patient at risk for infections
Bone marrow	Lithium	Increases white blood count after Tx (Greenberg et al. 1993)

Table 7.3. (cont.)

Organ System	Psychotropic	Consideration
Heart	Lithium	Can cause or exacerbate sick sinus syndrome
Heart	Tricyclics	Quinidine-like effects even in denervated heart. Monitor EKG and for orthostatic hypotension. Nortriptyline can be safely used in Tx (Shapiro 1991; Kay et al. 1991)
Heart	Trazadone	Pretransplantation in cardiac failure may increase ventricular irritability and arrhythmias
Heart	Venlafaxine	6% of patients have hypertension at higher dosages
Heart	Mirtazapine	15% of patients have increased cholesterol; peripheral edema may also occur. Good for sleep and antiemetic
Kidney	Methylphenidate	Probably no clinically significant problems in clearance during renal insufficiency/dialysis (Stiebel 1994)
Kidney	Tricyclics	Levels of conjugated active metabolites increase in renal insufficiency
Kidney	Benzodiazepines	Glucuronidated metabolites increase in renal insufficiency
Liver	Chlorpromazine	Primary biliary cirrhosis patients at increased risk for hepatotoxicity due to deficiency in sulfoxidation
Liver	Benzodiazepines	Increased sedation, increased delirium in cirrhosis; (via increased GABA?)

i.v., intravenous; CYA, cyclosporine A; cyt_{450}, cytochrome P_{450}; MAOI, monoamine oxidase inhibitor; SSRI, serotonin selective reuptake inhibitor; SIADH, Syndrome of inappropriate antidiuretic hormone; LFT, liver function test; Tx, transplantation; EKG, electrocardiogram; GABA, γ-aminobutyric acid.

following cardiac (Lane et al. 1988) and liver (Bird et al. 1990) transplantation. These imaging abnormalities resolved, as did symptoms, when CYA was tapered off or discontinued (Lane et al. 1988; Bird et al. 1990). CYA (and FK506) bind proteins that then inactivate calcineurin, a calcium-binding protein that interacts with calmodulin and is abundant in neurons (Hooper 1991). CYA-binding proteins have been found in brain neurons, potentially mediating side effects by influencing second-messenger systems (Niederberger et al. 1983; Columbani, Robb, and Hess 1985; Fairley 1990). Alteration of calcineurin activity affects phosphate interactions with cellular nuclear material (Hooper 1991), possibly causing CNS side effects. A genetically determined decrease in hepatic IIIA3/4 activity has been suggested in patients who experience side effects when CYA is in the therapeutic range (Lucey et al. 1990). Renal insufficiency increases CYA toxicity related to reduced elimination.

Multiple drug interactions with CYA have been reported. Phenytoin, phenobarbital, carbamazepine, and rifampin may decrease CYA levels through hepatic induction (Baciewicz and Baciewicz 1989). Intravenous sulfa drugs and trimethoprim combinations lower CYA levels (Kerr 1984). Sulfonamides reduce levels through unknown mechanisms (Baciewicz and Baciewicz 1989). Many medications, including high dose corticosteroids, erythromycin, calcium channel blockers, and ketoconazole, may increase CYA levels (Ptachcinski et al. 1985; Baciewicz and Baciewicz 1989), probably through interactions at the cyt P_{450}IIIA3/4 family. Though some psychotropics (e.g. fluoxetine, fluvoxamine, nefazodone, sertraline) inhibit cyt P_{450}IIIA3/4 and could potentially increase CYA levels, one study found no elevation in CYA levels or any increase in adverse events after adding fluoxetine to patients' medication regimen (Strouse et al. 1996). CYA increases lithium resorption by the proximal tubule, which may lead to higher lithium levels (Vincent et al. 1987). Cyclosporine is extensively metabolized presystemically by cyt P_{450}IIIA3/4 enzymes in the gut wall. When taken with grapefruit juice, which inhibits presystemic metabolism by cyt P_{450}IIIA3/4, CYA peak concentrations in the blood were significantly increased (Anon., 1995a). CYA nephrotoxicity is increased when used with amphotericin B, cefotaxime, cefuroxime, and aminoglycosides (Kerr 1984). Doxorubicin was implicated in causing CYA toxicity attributed to enhanced doxorubicin CNS penetration (Barbui et al. 1992). Theoretically, drugs that alter CNS dopamine activity and/or affect prolactin might interfere with the mechanisms of immunosuppression (Kast 1989); however, there is no clinical indication that this is a problem; e.g., while haloperidol might adversely affect CYA activity, its benefit in treating delirium outweighs this theoretical biochemical concern.

FK506

FK506 (tacrolimus, Prograft, Fujisawa Pharmaceutical Co.) is a macrolide produced by *Streptomyces tsukubaensis* and is being used in liver, heart, and kidney transplantation as the primary immunosuppressant, as well as in bone marrow transplantation, as rescue therapy for those who fail CYA, and for graft versus host disease. Unlike CYA it does not require bile acids for absorption and thus has been the immunosuppression agent of choice for small intestine transplant recipients. It is being investigated for other autoimmune diseases also. Like CYA, it interferes with the production of interleukin-2 and other lymphokines by lymphocytes (Kay et al. 1990). It is more potent and possibly less toxic than CYA, though neuropsychiatric side effects are similar (DiMartini et al. 1991). Though FK506 and CYA have similar frequencies for infections, CYA has significantly more cerebrovascular lesions (Lopez, Martinez, and Torre-Cisneros 1991). Lopez et al. found fewer cerebrovascular disorders and intracranial infections (neuropathological findings) in 20 adult liver transplant cases given FK506 as compared with 20 CYA cases. FK506 lesions included intracranial hemorrhages, ischemic infarcts, global cerebral ischemia with focal neuronal necrosis and axonal spheroids in cuneatus and gracilis nuclei.

In a prospective study of 294 patients, 5.4% had major neurological problems (akinetic mutism, seizures, psychosis, delirium, focal deficits, movement disorders) on FK506 (Eidelman et al. 1991), with heart and lung transplants at somewhat lower risk than those of liver. Trough plasma levels were greater than 3 ng/ml in the majority of patients with neurotoxicity, side effects improving as levels decreased. Delirium was the most frequent retrospective diagnosis, while akinetic mutism was the most common prospective diagnosis in a review of 23 consultations (Eidelman et al. 1991). Seizures, including partial complex status epilepticus, occurred in a few cases presenting as delirium (Eidelman et al. 1991). MRI in four patients with focal signs showed focal white matter changes that improved over time, corresponding with clinical improvement. Wilson et al. (1994) reported 3 of 1000 liver transplant cases who developed severe multifocal demyelinating sensorimotor polyneuropathy 2 to 10 weeks after starting FK506, which improved with plasmapherisis or intravenous immunoglubulin, consistent with an autoimmune neuropathy. Weakness and painful dysesthesias were noted. Wijidicks et al. (1994) found a 33% incidence of neurotoxicity in 44 consecutive liver transplant cases, most often postural hand tremors (in 23%) with generalized tonic-clonic seizures, speech apraxia, delirium, and agitation seen less often.

Neuropsychiatric symptoms may be more common with intravenous administration. Frequent symptoms of FK506 toxicity include tremulousness and sleep disturbance, severity of which is worse shortly after transplantation, a time during which patients may be maintained on higher FK506 levels with intravenous administration (Eidelman et al. 1991). Headache, dysesthesia, mood changes, visual symptoms, vivid dreams, and nightmares are also reported (Eidelman et al. 1991; Trzepacz et al. 1993a). A case of possible FK506-induced akathisia was reported (Bernstein and Daviss 1992) as responsive to propranolol, but was confounded by concurrent neuroleptic use. A prospective study of anxiety versus akathisia (DiMartini et al. 1996a; DiMartini, Trzepacz, and Daviss et al. 1996b) found no correlation between akathisia ratings and FK506 serum levels in 25 renal transplant patients, though serum levels did correlate with symptoms of anxiety. The neurotoxicity profile for FK506 is similar to that for CYA (Freise et al. 1991) and is reversible upon tapering off or discontinuation.

Erythromycin, fluconazole, and clotrimazole may increase FK506 serum levels after oral use (Venkataramannan et al. 1991), presumably due to common metabolism at cyt $P_{450}IIIA3/4$. FK506 levels can increase with psychotropic drugs that inhibit cyt $P_{450}IIIA3/4$ (i.e., fluoxetine, fluvoxamine, nefazodone, sertraline) and two case reports identified significant increases in FK506 levels when nefazodone was added to the patients' medication regimen (Campo, Smith, and Perel, 1998; Olyael et al. 1998). We have not observed this consistently in clinical practice. Perhaps the effect is due to the degree of cyt $P_{450}IIIA3/4$ inhibition, is idiosyncratic, or the pharmacokinetics are confounded by more complex factors. We suggest cautious addition of these medicines while paying close attention to FK506 levels.

Because FK506 has been identified in animal brain tissue, it is believed to cross the blood–brain barrier in humans. However, due to its lipophilicity it is not found in the aqueous cerebral spinal fluid (Venkataramanan et al. 1991). Recent identification of a family of FK506-binding proteins, which are homologous with receptors from a human hippocampal complementary DNA library (Hung and Schrieber 1992), suggests that FK506 may act at cells outside of the immune system. A possible mechanism for neuropsychiatric toxicity is FK506's interference with intracellular steps of signaling transduction mediated by receptor protein FKBP25 in the hippocampus (Hung and Schrieber 1992). Additionally, FK506 inhibits neuronal enzymes, calcineurin and nitric oxide synthase, thereby reducing nitric oxide levels (Dawson and Dawson 1994). While nitric oxide is important in both neurophysiologic and neurotoxic processes, it is unknown whether the neurotoxic effects of FK506 are mediated by this pathway.

OKT3

The monoclonal antibody OKT3 prevents and reverses allograft rejection following kidney, liver, and heart transplantation, as well as graft versus host disease. It is a "rescue therapy" usually reserved for steroid-resistant rejection. It has aggressive immunosupression and can result in sepsis. Though neuropsychiatric side effects are reported as generally mild (Capone and Cohen 1991), brief episodes of delirium can recur with OKT3, temporally related to each dose (Trzepacz, Brown, and Stoudemire 1995). Tremors may accompany a mild febrile syndrome during OKT3 initiation (Capone and Cohen 1991).

Aseptic meningitis occurs, with fever, headache, cerebrospinal fluid pleocytosis, and sometime delirium, usually occurring during the first three weeks of treatment (Adair et al. 1991). Symptoms usually resolve within 72 hours, without treatment or drug discontinuation (Martin et al. 1988; Adair et al. 1991). Overall incidence ranges from 5% to 14% (Martin et al. 1988; Adair et al. 1991). OKT3 is linked rarely to focal seizures, cerebritis, brain edema, and obtundation (Coleman and Norman 1990; Capone and Cohen 1991). The etiology of OKT3 neurotoxicity is unclear but may involve the release of lymphokines and lymphotoxins from T cells within the first day of treatment (Capone and Cohen 1991).

Corticosteroids

Modest doses of corticosteroids are frequently used as a part of immunosuppressive regimens, with higher "pulsed" doses used during acute rejection. Their utility in immunosuppression may relate to direct inhibition of antigen-driven T-cell proliferation (Lau et al. 1984). Behavioral side effects are common but conclusions regarding incidence and characteristics are not well studied. Females may be at higher risk for neuropsychiatric side effects, but age does not appear to be important (Lewis and Smith 1983). Side effect incidence may be higher in patients with systemic lupus erythematosus and pemphigus than for other medical illnesses (Lewis and Smith 1983). Whether transplant patients are at higher risk is unknown. Seizures occur when high dose methylprednisolone is combined with CYA in bone marrow transplant patients (Kerr 1984), possibly related to alterations in blood–brain barrier permeability (Sloane et al. 1985).

Lewis and Smith (1983) reviewed 29 reports of corticosteroid efficacy in medical illness and found a 6% overall incidence of neuropsychiatric side effects, with mania or depression the most frequent. Anxiety, irritability, and obessional thoughts were noted and emotional lability may be prominent (Hall et al. 1979). Psychosis is less common; delirium can occur (Kershner and Wang-Cheng 1989). Varney, Alexander, and MacIndoe (1984) detected cognitive deficits consistent with dementia in six males that was reversed with drug reduction or cessation. Median duration of corticosteroid treatment before the onset of neuropsychiatric symptoms is about 11 days, though symptoms may occur months after continuous treatment (Kershner and Wang-Cheng 1989). However, most side effects occur within the first three weeks of treatment (Hall et al. 1979); most recover within six weeks (Lewis and Smith 1983). While prior episodes of mental illness do not predict future episodes (Kershner and Wang-Cheng 1989) and a past psychiatric history is not a necessary risk factor, corticosteroids have been implicated in inducing mania in patients with a family history of affective disorder (Trzepacz et al. 1993b). Though less common, withdrawal from corticosteroids, if not gradually tapered, may cause psychiatric symptoms (Campbell and Schubert 1991).

Side effects may be dose related (Hall et al. 1979). The Boston Collaborative Drug Surveillance Program (1972) found a highly significant relationship between side effects and prednisone dosage, particularly for psychosis, with an increased incidence above 40 mg /day. Alternate day dosing may reduce risk and severity (Fauci 1978), though rapid mood cycling might occur using this strategy (Sharfstein, Sack, and Fauci 1982). Dosage, however, is not clearly related to time of symptom onset after initiation of treatment, to symptom type, or to symptom duration, (Lewis and Smith 1983). Reus and Wolkowitz (1993) warn about potential problems with patients self-increasing doses because of tolerance to its euphoriant effects.

Side effects are best handled by gradually reducing doses to prevent rebound psychiatric depression/anxiety or relapse of medical problems (Lewis and Smith 1983); electroconvulsive therapy (Lewis and Smith 1983) or low dose neuroleptics may be needed (Hall et al. 1979). Clonazepam has been used to treat steroid-induced mania in transplant patients (Viswanathan and Glickman 1989). While lithium pretreatment helped in a placebo-controlled study of multiple sclerosis patients (Falk, Mahnke, and Poskanser 1979), this is more complicated in transplant patients because of hepatorenal syndrome, electrolyte disturbances, and interactions with CYA. Anecdotally, we have used haloperidol prophylactically to pretreat a patient with bipolar disorder prior to steroid pulse dosing. Though he had become manic during prior steroid recycles, when pretreated with haloperidol he did not have a manic recurrence during following recycles.

Azathioprine

Azathioprine is a purine analog first used in organ transplantation in 1968. It is less widely used today due to the introduction of alternative agents. Specific neuropsychiatric side effects have not been reported for this agent, though CNS complications of immunosuppression are a mechanism to keep in mind.

Cellcept (mycophenolate mofetil)

Cellcept is a new immunosuppressant medication for organ transplantation that is being promoted as a improvement over azathioprine. It is approved for concurrent use with cyclosporine and corticosteroids as adjunct therapy but may have a broader application as a rescue therapy and in refractory rejection. Mycophenolate is rapidly metabolized into mycophenolic acid (the active immunosuppressive agent), which is then inactivated by glucuronidation (Bullingham, Nicholls, and Kamm 1998). Unlike CYA and FK506, mycophenolic acid is highly protein bound (about 97% bound to albumin) (Bulingham et al. 1998). Mycophenolic acid selectively suppresses T and B lymphocyte proliferation. Compared to azathioprine, mycophenolate is associated with slightly higher incidence of diarrhea, leukopenia and tissue-invasive infection with CMV (Anon., 1995b). Adverse effects were higher with higher dosage (3 g daily). Incidence of tremor and insomnia were similar between mycophenolate and azathioprine (Roche Laboratories 1995). Adverse nervous system events ($\geq$ 3% incidence) included anxiety, depression, hypertonia, parasthesia, and somnolence (Roche Laboratories 1995).

Neuropsychiatric issues with antiinfections agents

Infection is a common, often life-threatening, complication of immunosuppression in organ transplant recipients. Symptoms of infection as well as side effects of agents used to combat infection can cause neuropsychiatric side effects, making differential diagnosis difficult. Immunosuppressed patients may contract unusual infections or pathogens not commonly found in the nervous system. Common CNS infections include *Cryptococcus neoformans*, *Listeria moncytogenes*, and *Aspergillus fumigatus* (Conti and Rubin 1988). Rarely viruses such as herpes virus may invade the CNS in immunosuppressed patients. Other common, but non-CNS infections involve CMV, *Candida*, *Streptococcus*, and *Pneumocystis carinii* (Kusne et al. 1988).

Antivirals

Acyclovir
Acyclovir is a well-accepted treatment for herpesvirus infections. It might be useful in preventing CMV infection after bone marrow and renal transplant (Myers et al. 1988; Balfour et al. 1989). Acyclovir is eliminated largely unchanged by the kidneys, perhaps augmented by active tubular secretion (Davenport, Goel, and Mackenzie 1992). Metabolites, a small proportion, are inactive (Haefeli et al. 1993).

Though the drug is generally well tolerated, neuropsychiatric side effects occur occasionally. A review of 24 cases found tremor/myoclonus in 58%, confusion in 50%, agitation in 38%, lethargy in 25%, hallucinations in 25%, extrapyramidal symptoms in 21%, clouding of consciousness in 17%, dysarthria in 17%, and unilateral focal symptoms in 13% (Haefeli et al. 1993). Seizures and psychotic depression have also been reported (Trzepacz et al. 1993a). Symptoms usually develop early (in the first 24 to 72 hours), are reversible, and may be correlated to serum and cerebrospinal fluid (CSF) levels, though high serum levels preceded symptom onset by one to two days and subsequently normalize before symptoms disappear (Haefeli et al. 1993). There may also be a delay in equilibrium between serum and CSF levels (Haefeli et al. 1993). Patients with renal failure are at higher risk for neurotoxicity (Haefeli et al. 1993; Davenport et al. 1992) and hemodialysis should be considered for severe cases of toxicity (Davenport et al. 1992).

DHPG (ganciclovir)

DHPG is a second-generation nucleoside analogue structurally similar to acyclovir and primarily indicated for prophylaxis and treatment of CMV infections in immunocompromised patients. It might have a therapeutic effect in reducing rejection and graft versus host disease that is possibly initiated by CMV in kidney, heart, and bone marrow transplants (Frank and Friedman 1988). Neuropsychiatric side effects occasionally occur and include nightmares, visual hallucinations, agitation, delirium, and headache (Chen, Brocavich, and Lin 1992; Trzepacz et al. 1993a). Like acyclovir, renal impairment is a risk factor for side effects, and the manufacturer recommends lower doses for these patients (Chen et al. 1992). Symptoms usually develop soon after initiation, but have been reported as long as two weeks later (Chen et al. 1992). Temporary discontinuation with reintroduction at a lower dosage is appropriate. Low dose haloperidol may be useful (Chen et al. 1992). Symptoms subside after reduction or cessation of medication.

Alpha-interferon

Alpha-interferon is used in liver transplant patients for chronic viral hepatitis-C infection. Neuropsychiatric side effects are common and dose related (McDonald, Mann, and Thomas 1987). They include delirium and organic personality disorder (irritability), occurring at two to three months of treatment, and organic depression with prominent affective lability (Renault and Hoofnagle 1989). A flu-like syndrome occurs soon after initial doses, with fever, chills, lethargy, headache, decreased concentration, insomnia, and anorexia (McDonald et al. 1987; Renault and Hoofnagle 1989). Fatigue can be associated with marked psychomotor retardation and dulled cognition (Adams, Quesada, and Gutterman 1984) and mimic frontal lobe syndrome (McDonald et al. 1987). With chronic use (> 2 weeks), psychiatric side effects occurred in < 20% of patients in one study (Renault et al. 1987). Anxiety and irritability develop insidiously and may be misattributed to environmental or interpersonal stressors (Renault and Hoofnagle 1989). Frank depression may occur, accompanied by suicidal ideation and excessive tearfulness, similar to pseudobulbar palsy (Renault and Hoofnagle 1989). Delirium is more common in patients with predisposing factors, such as prior CNS insults, substance abuse, and hepatic insufficiency (Renault et al. 1987). Patients with previous substance abuse may be at risk for relapse (Renault et al. 1987).

Impairment of cognitive functioning without overt clinical impairment was induced within a week of starting treatment at a minimum dose of 3 million units/day (Renault et al. 1987). Psychiatric side effects may also be dose related and global cognitive dysfunction may underlie clinically overt psychiatric syndromes (Renult et al. 1987). Doses may need to be reduced, though symptoms may recur (Renault and Hoofnagle 1989). Methylphenidate may help to combat irritability (Renault and Hoofnagle 1989). In one study, quantitative electroencephalogram changes (39% of patients with increased slow wave activity and 6% of patients with paroxysmal discharges) were observed in patients after the initiation of alpha interferon therapy (Matsuzaki and Masumara 1998).

Antifungals

Amphotericin
Amphotericin B continues to be used three decades after its introduction. CNS toxicity is low because it does not penetrate the blood–brain barrier, but occurs with intrathecal administration (Walker and Rosemblum 1992). Delirium, confusion, and restlessness are reported (Trzepacz et al. 1993a). A febrile syndrome that includes headache and tremor occurs with acute administration. Three cases of fatal leukoencephalopathy associated with personality changes, akinetic mutism, and confusion have been reported, though a causal relationship was tentative (Walker and Rosenblum 1992).

Metronidazole
This drug can cause sensory peripheral neuropathy, with a stocking-glove distribution of paresthesias and hyperesthesias (Snavely and Hodges 1984) that is reversible following discontinuation of the drug, possibly related to axonal degeneration. Ataxia, dysarthria, and seizures occur as CNS side effects (Snavely and Hodges 1984). Metronidazole may also cause hallucinations, depression, or agitation (Giannini 1977).

Ketoconazole
This is a broad spectrum antifungal agent. It has important interactions with drugs utilizing cyt $P_{450}IIIA3/4$. It increases cardiotoxicity of terbutaline and it increases immunosuppressant activity of prednisolone (Ulrich et al. 1992).

Antibiotics

Penicillins and cephalosporins
Penicillins are excitotoxic and can cause seizures and delirium (Barrons, Murray, and Richey 1992), probably related to decreased CNS γ-aminobutyric acid (GABA) activity (Trzepacz et al. 1993a, 1995). Cephalosporins have a β-lactam ring that binds to GABA receptors and antagonizes them, and also can cause seizures and delirium. Renal failure increases the risk of cephalosporin-induced delirium (Snavely and Hodges 1984).

Quinolones
CNS side effects have been described for many of the quinolones, including norfloxacin, enoxacin, penfloxacin, and ciprofloxacin (Altes et al. 1989),

possibly due to interactions with the GABA-benzodiazepine receptor (Fenny and Mauas 1992). Ciprofloxacin was temporally associated with causing visual hallucinations, disorientation, changes in the sleep–wake cycle and impaired thinking (Altes et al. 1989), consistent with delirium. Overall, neuropsychiatric side effects are relatively uncommon with this class of antibiotics (Trzepacz et al. 1993a, 1995), but neurotoxicity may be increased during coadministration with nonsteroidal anti-inflammatory drugs (Iwamoto et al. 1993).

Aminoglycosides

Aminoglycosides are derived from *Streptomyces*. Delirium may occur as a result of therapeutic doses or from renal insufficiency, increasing serum levels (Trzepacz et al. 1993a, 1995). Neuromuscular blockade is a common side effect (Snavely and Hodges 1984) and can cause hypoactive deep tendon reflexes, flaccid paralysis, mydriasis, and respiratory weakness. Gentamicin may cause delirium, especially if given intrathecally, perhaps related to brainstem spongiosis (Snavely and Hodges 1984).

References

Adair, J. C., Woodley, S. L., O'Connell, J. B. et al. (1991). Aseptic meningitis following cardiac transplantation: clinical characteristics and relationship to immunosuppressive regimen. *Neurology*, **41**, 249–52.

Adams, D. H., Penfold, S., Gunson, B. et al. (1987). Neurological complications following liver transplantation. *Lancet*, **1**, 949–51.

Adams, F., Quesada, J. R., and Gutterman, J. U. (1984). Neuropsychiatric manifestations of human leukocyte interferon therapy in patients with cancer. *JAMA*, **252**, 938–41.

Altes, J., Gasco, J., de Antonio, J. et al. (1989). Ciprofloxacin and delirium. *Ann Intern Med*, **110**, 170–1.

Anon. (1995a). Grapefruit juice interactions with drugs. *The Medical Letter*, **37**(955), 73–4.

Anon. (1995b). Mycophenolate mofetil – a new immunosuppressant for organ transplantation. *The Medical Letter*, **37**(958), 84–6.

Appleton, R. E., Farrell, K., Teal, P. et al. (1989). Complex partial status epilepticus associated with cyclosporine A therapy. *J Neurol Neurosurg Psychiatry*, **52**, 1068–71.

Atkinson, K., Biggs, J., Darveniza, P. et al. (1984). CYA-associated central nervous system toxicity after allogenic bone marrow transplantation. *New Engl J Med*, **310**, 34–7.

Azoulay, D., Lemoine, A., Dennison, A. et al. (1993). Incidence of adverse reactions to cyclosporine after liver transplantation is predicted by the first blood level. *Hepatology*, **17**, 1123–6.

Baciewicz, A. M. and Baciewicz, F. A. (1989). Cyclosporine pharmacokinetic drug interactions. *Am J Surg*, **157**, 264–71.

Balfour, H. H., Choce, B. A., Stapleton, J. T. et al. (1989). A randomized placebo-controlled trial of oral acyclovir for the prevention of cytomegalovirus disease in recipients of renal allografts. *New Engl J Med*, **320**, 1381–7.

Barbui, T., Rambaldi, A., Parenzan, L. et al. (1992). Neurological symptoms and coma associated with doxorubicin administration during chronic cyclosporin therapy. *Lancet*, **339**, 1421.

Barrons, R. W., Murray, K. M., and Richey, R. M. (1992). Populations at risk for penicillin-induced seizures. *Ann Pharmacother*, **26**, 26–29.

Bennett, W. M., Aronoff, G. R., Morrison, G. et al. (1983). Drug prescribing in renal failure: dosing guidelines for adults. *Am J Kidney Dis*, **3**, 155–93.

Bernstein, L. and Daviss, S. R. (1992). Organic anxiety disorder with symptoms of akathisia in a patient treated with the immunosuppressant FK506. *Gen Hosp Psychiatry*, **14**, 210–11.

Bernstein, L. and Levin, R. (1993). Catatonia responsive to intravenous lorazepam in a patient with cyclosporine neurotoxicity and hypomagnesemia. *Psychosomatics*, **34**, 102–3.

Bird, G. L. A., Meadows, J., Goka, J. et al. (1990). Cyclosporine-associated akinetic mutism and epileptic syndrome after liver transplant. *J Neurol Neurosurg Psychiatry*, **53**, 1068–71.

Boston Collaborative Drug Surveillance Program (1972). Acute adverse reactions to prednisone in relation to dosage. *Clin Pharmacol Ther*, **13**, 694–8.

Brockmoller, J. and Roots, I. (1994). Assessment of liver function. Clinical implications. *Clin Pharmacokinet*, **27**, 216–48.

Bullingham, R. F., Nicholls, A. J., and Kamm, B. R. (1998). Clinical pharmacokinetics of mycophenolate mofetil. *Clin Pharmacokinet*, **34**, 429–55.

Campbell, K. M. and Schubert, D. S. (1991). Delirium after cessation of glucocorticoid therapy. *Gen Hosp Psychiatry*, **13**, 270–2.

Campo, J. V., Smith, C., and Perel, J. M. (1998). Tacrolimus toxic reaction associated with the use of nefazodone: paroxetine as an alternative agent (letter). *Arch Gen Psychiatry*, **55**, 1050–2.

Capone, P. M. and Cohen, M. E. (1991). Seizures and cerebritis associated with administration of OKT3. *Pediatr Neurol*, **7**, 299–301.

Cefalu, W. T. and Pardridge, W. M. (1985). Restrictive transport of a lipid-soluble peptide (cyclosporin) through the blood–brain barrier. *J Neurochem*, **45**, 1954–6.

Chen, J. L., Brocavich, J. M., Lin, A. (1992). Psychiatric disturbances associated with ganciclovir therapy. *Ann Pharmacother*, **26**, 193–5.

Coleman, A. E. and Norman, D. J. (1990). OKT3 encephalopathy. *Ann Neurol*, **28**, 837–8.

Columbani, P., Robb, A., and Hess, A., (1985). Cyclosporine A binding to calmodulin: a possible site of action on T-lymphocytes. *Science*, **228**, 337–9.

Conti, D. J. and Rubin, R. H. (1988). Infection of the central nervous system in organ transplant recipients. *Neurol Clin*, **6**, 241–60.

Craven, J. L. (1991). Cyclosporine-associated organic mental disorders in liver transplant recipients. *Psychosomatics*, **32**, 94–102.

Davenport, A., Goel, S., and Mackenzie, J. C. (1992). Neurotoxicity of acyclovir in patients with end-stage renal failure treated with continuous ambulatory peritoneal dialysis. *Am J Kidney Dis*, **20**, 647–9.

Dawson, T. M. and Dawson, V. L. (1994). Nitric oxide: actions and pathologic roles. *Neurosc Preview Issue*, 9–20.

de Groen, P. C., Aksamit, A. J., Rakela, J. R. et. al. (1987). Central nervous system toxicity after liver transplantation: the role of cyclosporine and cholesterol. *New Engl J Med*, **317**, 861–6.

de Groen, P. C., Aksamit, A. J., Rakela, J. et. al. (1988). Cyclosporine-associated central nervous toxicity (reply to letter). *New Engl J Med*, **318**, 789.

DiMartini, A. F., Fitzgerald, M. G., Magill, J. et al. (1996a). Psychiatric evaluations of small intestinal transplantation patients. *Gen Hosp Psychiatry*, **18**, 25S–29S.

DiMartini, A. F., Pajer, K., Trzepacz, P. T. et al. (1991). Psychiatric morbidity in liver transplant patients. *Transplant Proc*, **23**, 3179–80.

DiMartini, A. F. and Trzepacz, P. T. (1999). Psychopharmacologic issues in organ transplantation. In *Cutting-edge Medicine and Liason Psychiatry: Psychiatric Problems of Organ Transplantation, Cancer, HIV and Gene Therapy*, Proceedings of the 13th Tokyo Institute of Psychiatry International Symposium, Tokyo, 29–30 September 1998, International Congress series 1174, ed. M. Matsushita and I. Fukunishi, in press.

DiMartini, A. F., Trzepacz, P. T., and Daviss, S. (1996b). FK506 side effects: anxiety or akathisia. *Biol Psychiatry*, **40**, 407–11.

Eidelman, B. H., Abu-Elmagd, K., Wilson, J. et al. (1991). Neurologic complications of FK506. *Transplant Proc*, **23**, 3175–8.

European Multicentre Trial Group (1993). Cyclosporin in cadaveric renal transplantation: one-year follow-up of a multicentre trial. *Lancet*, **2**, 986–9.

Fairley, J. A. (1990). Intracellular targets of cyclosporine. *J Am Acad Dermatol*, **23** (Supplement), 1329–34.

Falk, W. E., Mahnke, M. W., and Poskanser, D. C. (1979). Lithium prophylaxis of corticotropin-induced psychosis. *JAMA*, **241**, 1011–12.

Fauci, A.S. (1978). Alternate-day corticosteroid therapy. *Am J Med*, **64**, 729–31.

Fenny, S. and Mauas, L. (1992). Ofloxacin-induced delirium. *J Clin Psychiatry*, **53**, 137–8.

Frank, I. and Friedman, H. M. (1988). Progress in the treatment of CMV pneumonia. *Ann Intern Med*, **109**, 769–71.

Freise, C. E., Rowley, H., Lake, J. et al. (1991). Similar clinical presentation of neurotoxicity following FK506 and cyclosporine in a liver transplant recipient. *Transplant Proc*, **23**, 3173–4.

Giannini, A. J. (1977). Side effects of metronidazole. *Am J Psychiatry*, **134**, 329–30.

Greenberg, D. B., Younger, J., and Kaufman, S.D. (1993). Management of lithium in patients with cancer. *Psychosomatics*, **34**, 388–94.

Haefeli, W. E., Schoenenberger, R. A. Z., Weiss, P. et al. (1993). Acyclovir-induced neurotoxicity: concentration–side effect relationship in acyclovir overdose. *Am J Med*, **94**, 212–15.

Hall, R. C. W., Popkin, M. D., Stickney, S. K. et. al. (1979). Presentation of the steroid psychosis. *J Nerv Ment Dis*, **167**, 229–36.

Heykantz, J., Hiang, M. L., Mannens, G. et al. (1984). The pharmacokinetics of risperidone in humans: a summary. *J Clin Psychiatry*, **55** (Supplement1), 13–17.

Hooper, C. (1991). Immune suppressants signal surprises in T cell activation. *J NIH Res*, **3**, 70–1.

Howden, C. W., Birnie, G. G., and Brodie, M. J. (1989). Drug metabolism in liver disease. *Pharmac Ther*, **40**, 439–74.

Humphreys, T. R. and Leyden, J. J. (1993). Acute reversible central nervous system toxicity associated with low-dose oral cyclosporine therapy. *J Am Acad Derm*, **29**, 490–2.

Hung, D. T. and Schrieber, S. L. (1992). cDNA cloning of human 25 kDa FK506 and rapamycin binding protein. *Biochem Biophys Res Communi*, **184**, 733–8.

Iwamoto, K., Naora, K., Katagiri, Y. et al. (1993). Comparative neurotoxicity study of ciprofloxacin and sparfloxacin after coadministration with fenbufen in rats. *Drugs*, **45** (Supplement 3), 290–1.

Kast, R. (1989). Blocking of CYA immunosuppression by neuroleptics. *Transplantation*, **47**, 1095–8.

Kay, J., Bienenfeld, D., Slomowitz, M. et al. (1991). Use of tricyclic antidepressants in heart transplant recipients. *Psychosomatics*, **32**, 165–70.

Kay, J. E., Moore, A. L., Doe, S. et al. (1990). The mechanism of action of FK506. *Transplant Proc*, **22**, 96–9.

Kerr, L. E. (1984). Drug interactions with cyclosporine. *Clin Pharmacol*, **3**, 345–6.

Kershner, P. and Wang-Cheng, R. (1989). Psychiatric side effects of steroid therapy. *Psychosomatics*, **30**, 135–9.

Kusne, S., Dummer, J. S., Singh, N. et al. (1988). Infections after liver transplantation: an analysis of 101 consecutive cases. *Medicine*, **67**, 132–43.

Lane, R. J. M., Roche, S. W., Leung, A. et al. (1988). Cyclosporine neurotoxicity in cardiac transplant recipients. *J Neurol, Neurosurg Psychiatry*, **51**, 1434–7.

Lau, N. C., Karin, M., Nguyen, T. et al. (1984). Mechanisms of glucocorticoid hormone action. *J Steroid Biochem*, **20**, 77.

Leipzig, R.M. (1990). Psychopharmacology in patients with hepatic and gastrointestinal disease. *Intl J Psychiatry Med*, **20**, 109–39.

Levy, N. B. (1990). Psychopharmacology in patients with renal failure. *Intl J Psychiatry Med*, **20**, 325–34.

Lewis, D. A. and Smith, R. E. (1983). Steroid-induced psychiatric syndromes. *J Affective Dis*, **5**, 319–32.

Lopez, O. L., Martinez, A.J., and Torre-Cisneros, J. (1991). Neuropathologic findings in liver transplantation: a comparative study of cyclosporine and FK506. *Transplant Proc*, **23**, 3181–2.

Lucey, M. R., Kolars, J. C., Merion, R.M. et al. (1990). Cyclosporin toxicity at therapeutic blood levels and cytochrome P_{450}IIIA. *Lancet*, **1**, 11–15.

Martin, M. A., Massanari, R. M., Dai, D. N. et al. (1988). Nosocomial aseptic meningitis associated with administration of OKT3. *JAMA*, **259**, 2002–5.

Matsuzaki, Y. and Matsumura, T. (1998). The influence of interferon therapy on CNS function – from aspects of quantitative EEG and biogenic amines. [In Japanese.] *Seishin Shinkeigaku Zasshi – Psychiatr Neurolog Japon*, **100**(2), 77–91.

McDonald, E. M., Mann, A. H., and Thomas, H. C. (1987). Interferons as mediators of psychiatric morbidity. *Lancet*, **2**, 1175–8.

Myers, J. D., Reed, E. C., Sheep, D. H. et al. (1988). Acyclovir for the prevention of cytomegalovirus infection and disease after allogenic marrow transplantation. *New Egnl J Med*, **318**, 70–5.

Niederberger, W., Lemaire, M., Maurer, G. et al. (1983). Distribution of cyclosporine in blood and tissues. *Transplant Proc*, **15** (Supplement) 203–5.

Noll, R. B. and Kulkarni, R. (1984). Complex visual hallucinations and cyclosporine.

Arch Neurol, **41**, 329–30.

Olyael, A. J., de Mattos, A. M., Norman, D. J. and Bennett, W. M. (1998). Interaction between tacrolimus and mefazodone in a stable renal transplant recipient. *Pharmacotherapy,* **18**, 1356–9.

Pacifici, G. M., Viani, A., Franchi, M. et al. (1990). Conjugation pathways in liver disease. *Br J Clin Pharmacol,* **30**, 427–35.

Paine, M. F., Shen, D. D., Kunze, K. L. et al. (1996). Pharmacokinetics and drug disposition: first-pass metabolism of midazolam by the human intestine. *Clin Pharmac Therapeut,* **60**, 14–24.

Patel, I. H., Soni, P. P., Fukuda, E. K. et al. (1990). The pharmacokinetics of midazolam in patients with congestive heart failure. *Br J Clin Pharmacol,* **29**, 565–9.

Pollock, B. G. (1994). Recent developments in drug metabolism of relevance to psychiatrists. *Harvard Rev Psychiatry,* **2**, 204–13.

Preskorn, S. H. and Magnus, R. D. (1994). Inhibition of hepatic P_{450} isozymes by serotonin-selective reuptake inhibitors: in vitro and in vivo findings and their implications for patient care. *Psychopharamacol Bull,* **30**, 251–9.

Ptachcinski, R. J., Carpenter, B. J., Burkhart, G. J. et. al. (1985). Effect of erythromycin on cyclosporine levels. *New Engl J Med,* **313**, 1416–17.

Reidenberg, M. M. (1977). The biotransformation of drugs in renal falure. *Am J Med,* **62**, 482–5.

Renault, P. F. and Hoofnagle, J. H. (1989). Side effects of alpha interferon. *Semin Liver Dis,* **9**, 273–7.

Renault, P. F., Hoofnagle, J. H., Park, Y. et. al. (1987). Psychiatric complications of long-term interferon alpha therapy. *Arch Intern Med,* **147**, 1577–80.

Reus, V. I. and Wolkowitz, O. M. (1993). Behavioral side effects of corticosteroid therapy. *Psychosom Ann,* **23**, 703–8.

Roche Laboratories (1995). *CellCept (mycophenolate mofetil capsules).* Monograph distributed by Hoffman-LaRoche Inc.

Shammas, F. V. and Dickstein, K. (1988). Clinical pharmacokinetics in heart failure, an updated review. *Clin Pharmacokin,* **15**, 94–113.

Shapiro, P. (1991). Nortriptyline treatment of depressed cardiac transplant recipients. *Am J Psychiatry,* **148**, 371–3.

Sharfstein, S. S., Sack, D. S. and Fauci, A. S. (1982). Relationship between alternate-day corticosteroid therapy and behavioral abnormalities. *JAMA,* **248**, 2987–9.

Sloane, J. P., Lwin, K. Y., Gore, M. E. et al. (1985). Disturbance of blood–brain barrier after bone-marrow transplantation. *Lancet,* **2**, 280–1.

Snavely, S. R. and Hodges, G. R. (1984). The neurotoxicity of antibiotics. *Ann Intern Med,* **101**, 92–104.

Someya, T., Shibasaki, M., Noguchi, T. et al. (1992). Haloperidol metabolism in psychiatric patients: importance of glucuronidation and carbonyl reduction. *J Clin Psychopharmacol,* **12**, 169–74.

Steg, R. E. and Garcia, E. G. (1991). Complex visual hallucinations and cyclosporine neurotoxicity. *Neurology,* **41**, 1156.

Stiebel, V. G. (1994). Methylphenidate plasma levels in depressed patients with renal failure. *Psychosomatics,* **35**, 498–500.

Strouse, T. B., Fairbanks, L. A., Skotzko, C., and Fawzy, F. I. (1996). Fluoxetine and cyclosporine in organ transplantation: failure to detect significant drug interactions or adverse events in depressed organ recipients. *Psychosomatics,* **37**, 23–30.

Suhara, T., Sudo, Y., Yoshida, K. et al. (1998). Lung reservoir for antidepressant in pharmacokinetic drug interaction. *Lancet*, **351**, 332–5.

Surman, O. S., Dienstag, J. L., and Cosimi, B. (1987). Liver transplantation: psychiatric considerations. *Psychosomatics*, **28**, 615–21.

Thompson, D. and DiMartini, A. F. (1999). Nonenteral routes of administration of psychiatric medications. *Psychosomatics*, **40**, 185–92.

Thummel, K. E., Shen, D. D., Podoll, T. D. et al. (1994). Use of midazolam as a human cytochrome P4503A probe. II: Characteristics of inter- and intraindividual hepatic CYP3A variability after liver transplant. *J Pharmacol Exp Ther*, **271**, 557–66.

Tollemar, J., Ringden, O., Ericzon, B. et al. (1988). Cyclosporine-associated central nervous system toxicity (letter). *New Engl J Med*, **318**, 788–9.

Tripathi, A. and Panzer, M. (1993). Cyclosporine psychosis (letter). *Psychosomatics*, **34**, 101–2.

Trzepacz, P. T., Brown, T. M., and Stoudemire, A. (1995). Substance-induced delirium. In *Treatments of Psychiatric Disorders*, vol, 1, 2nd edn, editor-in-chief G. O. Gabbard. American Psychiatric Press: Washington, DC.

Trzepacz, P. T., DiMartini, A. F., and Tringali, R (1993a). Psychopharmacologic issues in organ transplantation. Part 1: Pharmacokinetics in organ failure and psychiatric aspects of immunosuppressants and anti-infectious agents. *Psychosomatics*, **34**, 199–207.

Trzepacz, P. T., DiMartini, A. F., and Tringali, R. (1993b). Psychopharmacologic issues in organ transplantation. Part 2: Psychopharmacologic medications. *Psychosomatics*, **34**, 290–8.

Trzepacz, P. T., Levenson, J.L. and Tringali, R. A. (1991). Clinical problems in psychiatric treatment of the medically ill: psychopharmacology and neuropsychiatric syndromes in organ transplantation. *Gen Hosp Psychiatry*, **13**, 233–45.

Ulrich, B., Frey, F. J., Speck, F., and Frey, B. M. (1992). Pharmacokinetics/pharmacodynamics of ketoconazole-prednisolone interaction. *J Pharmacol Exp Ther*, **260**, 487–90.

Varney, N. R., Alexander, B., and MacIndoe, J. H. (1984). Reversible steroid dementia in patients without steroid psychosis. *Am J Psychiatry*, **141**, 369–72.

Venkataramanan, R., Jain, A., Warty, K. et al. (1991). Pharmacokinetics of FK 506 in transplant patients. *Transplant Proc*, **23**, 2736–40.

Vincent, H. H., Wenting, G. J., Schalekamp, M. A. D. H. et. al. (1987). Impaired fractional excretion of lithium: a very early marker of cyclosporine toxicity. *Transplant Proc*, **19**, 4147–8.

Viswanathan, R. and Glickman, L. (1989). Clonazepam in the treatment of steroid-induced mania in a patient after renal transplant. *New Engl J Med*, **320**, 319–20.

Wagner, O., Schreier, E., Heitz, F. et. al. (1987). Tissue distribution, disposition, and metabolism of cyclosporine in rats. *Drug Metab Dispos*, **15**, 377–83.

Walker, R. W. and Rosenblum, M. K. (1992). Amphotericin B-associated leukoencephalopathy. *Neurology*, **42**, 2005–10.

Wijidicks, E. F. M., Wiesner, R. H., Dahlke, L. J., and Kron, R. A. F. (1994). FK506-induced neurotoxicity in liver transplantation. *Ann Neurol*, **35**, 498–501.

Wilder, B. J. (1992). Pharmacokinetics of valproate and carbamazepine. *J Clin Psychopharmacol*, **12**, 64S–68S.

Wilson, J. R., Conwit, R. A., Eidelman, B. H. et al. (1994). Sensorimotor neuropathy resembling CIDP in patients receiving FK506. *Muscle Nerve*, **17**, 528–32.

8

Alcoholism and organ transplantation

Andrea F. DiMartini M.D and Paula T. Trzepacz M.D.

Epidemiology

The frequency of alcohol-related end stage organ disease is surprisingly low given the prevalence of alcoholism (nearly 9% of US adults) (Grant 1994) and the toxic effects of ethanol on the liver and heart. There is not a direct concordance between alcohol use, alcohol abuse or dependence and either the development of alcoholic cirrhosis (Simko 1983; Arria, Tarter, and Van Thiel 1991) or alcoholic cardiomyopathy (Hosenspud 1994). Evidence from the natural history of alcoholic liver disease suggests that the risk of alcoholic liver disease increases with habitual alcohol intake of 20 g ethanol/day for women and 80 g ethanol/day for men (Diehl 1997) (there are approximately 10 g of ethanol per standard drink). But, despite the amount of heavy drinking, the lifetime incidence of alcoholic cirrhosis only approaches 50% of people who drink excessively (i.e., consumption of 227 g pure ethanol or nearly one-fifth of a gallon of hard liquor per day) for over two decades (Lelbach 1975). Inconsistencies in the risk of cirrhosis by level of alcohol consumption may be due to lack of controlling for body size, gender, and alcohol consumption patterns (frequency and temporal patterns) (Parrish, Higuchi, and Dufour 1991). Nevertheless, alcohol related end stage liver disease results typically from 10 to 20 years of heavy drinking. Though a diagnosis of alcohol-induced liver disease can be supported by medical data (liver biopsy and liver enzyme profiles) in conjunction with a history of heavy alcohol consumption, a patient may not meet the criterion for alcohol abuse or dependence in the *Diagnostic and Statistical Manual of Mental Disorders*, 4th edition (DSM-IV). One study showed that alcohol dependence occurred in 79% of those with alcoholic cirrhosis who presented for liver transplant evaluation (Beresford and Lucey 1994). Thus a patient may not develop the behavioral, physiologic, or psychologic features of an addiction to alcohol, but nevertheless could develop end stage alcoholic liver disease. Even the pathology seen on liver biopsy may not be pathognomonic of alcoholic liver disease. Mallory's bodies, long believed to be a characteristic liver biopsy finding for alcoholic liver disease, have a prevalence of 51% in alcoholic cirrhosis and the presence of Mallory's bodies does not always imply alcoholic pathogenesis (Jensen and Gluud 1994). Nevertheless, alcoholic cirrhosis is the most common cause of end stage liver disease. Of the 50 000 people in the USA who die annually from end stage liver disease, alcohol-related liver disease accounts for up to 50% of these deaths (Grant, DeBakey, and Zobeck 1991).

The incidence of alcohol being identified as a significant risk factor in the development of cardiomyopathy is reported as 20% to 30% (Hosenspud 1994). Although alcoholic cardiomyopathy can occur after 10 years of heavy drinking (Fabrizio and Regan 1994), its development appears to be more related to the total lifetime dose of ethanol exerting its effect in a dose-dependent manner (kg ethanol/kg body weight) (Rubin and Urbano-Marquez 1994; Urbano Marquez et al. 1995). Alcohol may lead to clinical, hemodynamic, and pathologic findings identical with idiopathic cardiomyopathy, but should be a diagnosis of exclusion (Schwartz et al. 1984). In addition, there appears to be different organ susceptibility to the effects of alcohol because those individuals who develop cardiomyopathy are unlikely to develop alcoholic cirrhosis (Lefkowitch and Fenoglio 1983; Hosenspud 1994).

Women are more susceptible than men to the toxic effects of alcohol on both hepatocytes and the myocardium. Women develop cirrhosis at a more rapid rate than do men and with a lower total alcohol consumption (Blume 1986). This phenomenon may be due to smaller body size, lower volume of distribution, and lower activity levels of alcohol dehydrogenase, which lead to higher peak blood alcohol levels in women than in men following the same dose of alcohol per kilogram of body weight (Marshall et al. 1983; Arthur, Lee, and Wright 1984). The threshold dose of alcohol to develop alcoholic cardiomyopathy is considerably less in women than in men (Urbano-Marquez et al. 1995). An accelerated course of symptom severity in female alcoholics (Piazza, Vrbka, and Yeager 1989) and consistent differences between male and female alcoholics suggest that female alcoholics should be targeted as a population with special needs. Women become heavier drinkers at later ages, are often solitary drinkers, need psychiatric treatment, and often have polysubstance abuse (Blume 1986).

Though transplantation is increasingly becoming a treatment of choice for end stage organ disease, the need for organs greatly exceeds availability. Approximately 6000 people wait to receive one of only 3000 livers donated annually for transplantation. Approximately 3000 patients wait annually for 2000 donated heart transplants. According to the Pitt- United Network of Organ Sharing (UNOS) Liver Transplant Registry, in the USA alcoholic cirrhosis is the largest single diagnostic group receiving liver transplantation (26% of recipients in 1995) (Belle and Detre 1997). However this represents only 6% of those dying from alcohol-related liver disease (Keeffe 1997). In Europe, the numbers of patients receiving liver transplants for alcoholic liver disease are also increasing (Neuberger and Tang 1997). At the University of

Pittsburgh Medical Center (UPMC), patients undergoing liver transplantation for alcoholic cirrhosis were predominantly male (80%) (DiMartini et al. 1996), which is similar to the general alcoholic population, of which 75% are male.

In heart transplantation, exact numbers of patients receiving transplantation for alcoholic cardiomyopathy are not known, perhaps due to difficulty in distinguishing idiopathic cardiomyopathy from alcohol-induced cardiomyopathy or because these patients are denied cardiac transplantation (Schroeder and Hunt 1987). The 1995 International Heart and Lung Transplant Registry did not identify alcoholic cardiomyopathy among the diagnoses of the 30 297 patients who had received heart transplants between 1983 to 1995 (Hosenspud et al. 1995). Such patients may have been part of the group identified as having "cardiomyopathy" (44% of recipients) without a specific etiology.

As we enter an era of cost containment and managed health care, it is clear that advancing medical technology has exceeded our ability to provide this higher standard of care to all people. Medical resources and health care are being rationed. Organ transplantation is no exception. These factors significantly impact on the selection of transplant candidates and, within this climate, patients with alcohol induced end stage organ disease may not compete equally for donated organs. Social and moral debates about eligibility for alcoholics are argued. Beliefs about personal responsibility for self-induced disease and an assumption that drinking post-transplantation will be deleterious are common. Research is not yet able to support or refute these arguments nor to completely guide clinical decisions. However, early studies are beginning to shed some light on these issues. This chapter provides an overview of the existing data relevant to alcoholic cirrhosis and liver transplantation and the smaller body of data available on alcoholism and heart transplantation.

Pretransplantation issues

Pretransplant survival

Patients with end stage liver disease are not expected to survive long without orthotopic liver transplantation (OLTX). Advanced alcoholic liver disease carries a 5-year survival rate of only 50% (Schenker 1984), a prognosis further worsened by ascites, portal hypertension, bleeding varices, hepatic encephalopathy and hepatorenal syndrome (Kumar, Stauber, and Gavaler 1990). In a study of patients referred for transplantation, alcoholic cirrhotics with end stage liver disease and no transplant had significantly poorer survival than alcoholics given a transplant and followed up at 1 year (50%

versus 78%) and 2-years (30% versus 73%) (Lucey et al. 1992). The group without transplants included patients who were deemed "too well" to be given a transplant (Lucey et al. 1992); however, their survival declined to 59% at the 2-year follow-up (Lucey et al. 1992).

Abstinence from alcohol can have a favorable outcome on alcoholic cardiomyopathy. One-third of 64 alcoholic cardiomyopathy patients who were not heart transplant candidates and were drinking actively discontinued alcohol use. The 4-year mortality rate in that abstaining group was 9%, in contrast to a 57% mortality rate in those who continued drinking, though other factors besides abstinence (such as extent of myocardial damage) affected prognosis (Demakis et al. 1974). Similar survival data for abstainers was reported in another study of patients with alcoholic cardiomyopathy (Shugoll et al. 1972). Twelve of 31 patients who were drinking alcohol in excess stopped or significantly reduced their alcohol use. After being followed for a mean of 30 months, none of these 12 patients died, compared to 25% of those who continued to drink (Shugoll et al. 1972). Pretransplantation survival statistics are not reported for patients with alcoholic car-diomyopathy who are awaiting cardiac transplantation.

Selection for transplantation

Ethics and policies
Consideration of OLTX for patients with alcoholic cirrhosis presents clinical, ethical, legal, and financial challenges to the transplant team. There is little consensus among physicians, clinicians, transplant programs or insurance companies in this selection process. Physicians (Moss and Siegler 1991) and philosophers (Glannon 1998) argue that alcoholic cirrhotics should have lower priority for receiving a liver transplant than patients who develop other types of end stage liver disease "through no fault of their own" (Moss and Siegler 1991). Others believe that alcoholism prevents long-term survival due to redevelopment of liver disease (Atterbury 1986) or perceive alcoholics as a group that would be noncompliant (Cohen and Benjamin 1991; Sherman and Williams 1995). Though the moral model of addictions (i.e., a person is held responsible for both acquiring and solving the problem) has little support in the addictions literature (Marlatt et al. 1988), this moral argument against considering alcoholic cirrhotics for transplantation is widespread (Cohen and Benjamin 1991). In an extensive commentary on the moral arguments against giving transplants to patients with alcoholic liver disease, Shelton and Balint (1997) argued that alcoholism is a medical diagnosis and support fair treatment for these patients. Public awareness of increasing numbers of alcoholic cirrhotics being given transplants is believed to have an adverse effect on organ donation (Caplan 1994; Sherman and Williams 1995). A Harris public opinion poll showed that the public assigned the

lowest national health care priority for liver transplantation to alcoholic liver disease (Evans, Mannine, and Dong 1991). These issues may have an emotional impact on opinions in the medical community, but others challenge these notions and argue for further research (Atterbury 1986; Flavin, Niven, and Kelsey 1988; Cohen and Benjamin 1991; Beresford 1994a; Caplan 1994; Shelton and Balint 1997).

In December 1996, UNOS, the nonprofit policy making organization that administers the Organ Procurement and Transplantation Network in the USA, recommended the imposition of a mandatory six-month sobriety criterion for all alcoholic cirrhotic transplant candidates nationwide. UNOS also recommended that all alcoholic cirrhotics with less than six months demonstrated sobriety enter into a written contract with the transplant team. These and other changes in organ allocation policies were reviewed by the US Department of Health and Human Services but the policy for a mandatory length of sobriety was not implemented. Further research on risk factors and outcomes for patients with alcoholic cirrhosis is needed so that they are not categorically regarded as poor candidates or held to inflexible candidacy criteria.

Liver transplantation selection criteria and pre-transplantation length of sobriety requirements

Due to these various forces, transplant centers across the USA have very different selection criteria for these patients (Caplan 1989). Most centers mandate a period of sustained sobriety (commonly defined as more than six months sober), good social supports, and previous alcohol rehabilitation in order for alcoholic cirrhotics to be accepted as transplant candidates and many centers require these patients to undergo psychiatric or psychologic evaluations to assess their alcoholism. A 1992 survey of 14 US liver transplant centers revealed wide variations in candidate requirements for sobriety, ranging from one center willing to consider alcoholics who were drinking up until transplantation to other centers categorically refusing all alcoholic cirrhotics with less than six months of sobriety (Snyder, Drooker, and Strain 1996). In another survey of 41 US liver transplant centers, current heavy alcohol use (80% of programs) and alcohol abuse within the past six months (24% of programs) were viewed as absolute contraindications to transplantation (Levenson and Olbrisch 1993). By comparison, only 41% of renal transplant programs viewed current heavy alcohol use as an absolute contraindication (Levenson and Olbrisch 1993). In Canada, the Canadian Liver Transplant Study Group, in an attempt to standardize the selection process has recommended the adoption of basic principles for giving transplants to patients with alcoholic liver disease, including formalized written protocols and the patient's demonstration of abstinence and compliance with medical recommendations (Wall 1998). Patients with fulminant alcoholic hepatitis would be unable to demonstrate these abilities and are generally not considered to be suitable for liver transplantation (Wall 1998).

The philosophy at the UPMC has been that the imposition of an arbitrary period of abstinence prior to transplantation is medically unsound or even inhumane (Starzl et al. 1988). Since most patients' medical condition precludes a long wait, requesting alcoholics to achieve a certain length of sobriety would result in some candidates deteriorating into a poor risk category, and those at poor risk might not survive until transplantation (Starzl et al. 1988). However, an initial study from UPMC (Kumar et al. 1990) showed a higher relapse rate for patients with alcohol-related liver cirrhosis and short pre-OLTX durations of sobriety (< 6 months) than those with ≥ 6 months. Though the sample size was insufficient for statistical analysis, this report may have contributed to the establishment of the "six months sober" criterion, a benchmark now used by many programs (Beresford and Lucey 1995). In contrast, in long-term studies of alcoholism in the USA (not necessarily cirrhotics), sustained sobriety is measured in years, not in months, and abstinences of six months duration reveal little about long-term relapse outcome (Vaillant 1988).

Given the critical timing for OLTX, requirements for pre-OLTX rehabilitation and/or a required length of sobriety can be critical to an alcoholic cirrhotic patient's post-OLTX outcome and survival. At one center, chemically dependent patients had a pretransplantation death rate of 48% as compared to 34% for the nonchemically dependent patients (Currie, Jones, and Piedmont 1994). Of the chemically dependent patients whose pretransplantation cause of death was known, 48% died while in the process of meeting pretransplantation sobriety/rehabilitation requirements (Currie et al. 1994).

The imposition of an arbitrary waiting period is not supported by all medical data (Flavin et al. 1988). In 1986, a legal precedent was set in the USA with the *Allen vs Mansour*[1] case in which the United States District Court ruled that the Medicaid 2-year abstinence requirement for liver transplantation was "arbitrary and unreasonable," based on evidence that alcoholic cirrhotics could deteriorate into high operative risks or may not survive the waiting period. In addition, pre-OLTX duration of sobriety has been a poor predictor of post-OLTX alcohol relapse (Tringali et al. 1996; Foster et al. 1997) or long-term survival (DiMartini et al. 1995; Tringali et al. 1996).

Though duration of sobriety is commonly reported as a variable in the selection process, less is reported about definitions of alcoholism or alcohol-related behaviors such as diagnoses of alcohol abuse or dependence. Whether instituting a systematic and consistent national approach to the evaluation

---

[1] *Allen vs. Mansour* 86–73429. *Federal Supplement*, **681**, 1232–9. District Court for the Eastern District of Michigan, Southern Division, 1986.

and selection of alcoholic cirrhotics for liver transplantation would address inequities in the current system is uncertain.

Heart transplantation selection criteria

The earliest studies on psychopathology in cardiac transplant candidates identified a significant proportion of patients with a history of alcohol abuse (17% to 39%) (Kuhn et al. 1988; Maricle et al. 1989), though the use of this information in candidate selection was not specified. However, in contrast to liver, the selection of heart transplant candidates tends to follow more complex and stringent criteria. Compared to liver and renal programs, heart transplant programs are more likely to view negative lifestyle, behavioral or psychosocial factors as absolute contraindications to transplantation (Levenson and Olbrisch 1993). As of 1993, over 70% of the US heart transplant programs excluded patients with current heavy alcohol use, including considerable controversy about also excluding patients with recent alcohol use (Levenson and Olbrisch 1993). In one US study, the most common psychiatric diagnosis for patients who were refused a heart transplant on psychiatric grounds was alcohol or drug abuse (Frierson and Lippman 1987). Concerns over comorbid alcoholic liver disease is also frequently mentioned in the heart transplant literature and is generally screened for during the evaluation phase.

Candidate selection instruments

Since psychosocial selection criteria differ significantly among programs and organ transplant type, the development and use of structured evaluation instruments may help to direct and standardize future selection protocols in the USA. Though there are many instruments and measures for assessing alcoholism, none are tailored to transplant populations and many target the needs of treatment and rehabilitation goals rather than assessing appropriateness for transplantation. The Psychosocial Assessment of Candidates for Transplantation (PACT) was the first published psychosocial structured instrument for screening transplant candidates (Olbrisch, Levenson, and Hamer 1989). It includes an overall score and scale scores for psychologic health (psychopathology, risk for psychopathology, stable personality factors), lifestyle factors (healthy lifestyle, ability to sustain change in lifestyle, compliance, drug and alcohol use), social support (support system stability and availability), and educability about and understanding of the transplant.

Another instrument, the Transplant Evaluation Rating Scale (TERS), rates patients' level of adjustment in 10 areas of psychosocial functioning (Twillman et al. 1993): prior psychiatric history, DSM-III-R Axis I and Axis II diagnoses, substance use/abuse, compliance, health behaviors, quality of family support, prior history of coping, coping with disease and treatment, quality of affect, and mental status. In one study, the TERS was significantly correlated with several clinician-reported outcome variables (compliance, health behaviors, substance use) with particularly high correlations between pretransplantation TERS scores and post-OLTX substance use ($r = 0.64$), though the patients studied were not given transplants as a result of alcoholic liver disease (Twillman et al. 1993).

Both the PACT and TERS require administration by skilled clinicians, without which their predictive power could be diminished (Presberg et al. 1995), and neither instrument focuses only on alcohol use/abuse. For the PACT, the final rating for candidacy acceptability is decided by the clinician, with the freedom to weigh individual item ratings variably (Presberg et al. 1995). Thus, a single area, such as alcohol abuse, could carry higher weight and disproportionately impact on the final rating. The TERS summary score does not have this flexibility, being derived by a mathematical formula where individual item scores are multiplied by theoretical, predetermined weightings. (For further details on these instruments, see Chapter 2.)

Using variables selected from Vaillant's (1983) work on the natural history and treatment outcome of alcoholism (not necessarily cirrhotics), Beresford et al. (1990b; Beresford 1992) designed a decision algorithm as a quantifiable measure for candidate evaluation and prediction of post-OLTX outcome for alcoholic cirrhotics. This Alcoholism Prognosis Scale (APS) is the first published scale rating pre-OLTX prognostic features of alcoholism but is designed as a research tool rather than for use in making clinical recommendations for or against transplantation candidacy. The APS items include resolution of ambivalence, stable social groups, and two or more of Vaillant's good prognostic indicators (positive rehabilitative relationship, substituted activities, source of hope or improved self-esteem, negative behavioral reinforcement). Using the APS, Beresford studied 38 alcoholic liver transplant candidates who had been accepted for transplantation because they were considered to be at low risk for alcohol relapse in accordance with a low score on the APS prognostic scale and index. Though the APS did not reliably predict subsequent alcohol use post-OLTX (Beresford 1994b), it is the prototype for a scale to predict post-OLTX alcohol relapse from pre-OLTX variables.

The High-Risk Alcoholism Relapse (HAR) scale was designed and piloted in a group of male veterans to rate the risk of alcohol relapse following alcohol rehabilitation (mean age 42.8 ± 10.8 years) (Yates et al. 1992). This scale has also been used to compare the profiles of patients with end-stage liver disease undergoing liver transplantation evaluation with the male veterans population (Yates et al. 1993; DiMartini et al. 1997). The HAR uses daily alcohol consumption, drinking duration, and previous treatment history to grade the severity of alcoholism. The HAR has predictive validity for early relapse in the first six months after treatment, with a sensitivity of 69% and a specificity of 65%. From the HAR, using an estimated six-months relapse risk of 15% or less as suitable criteria for transplant listing for alcoholic cirrhotics, 48 patients met eligibility status for transplant listing compared with only 36 patients when using the six-months abstinence rule as the sole criteria (Yates 1996). Thus the 6-months abstinence criterion alone appears to have limitations in selecting transplant candidates with low alcoholism relapse risk (Yates 1996). The HAR is currently being tested as a model to predict risk for alcohol relapse in the general alcoholic population in the USA following treatment, but has yet to be validated with post-OLTX relapse or outcome data (Yates et al. 1992). In addition, the study population does not include women.

Post-transplantation issues

Post-transplantation outcome and survival

Liver transplantation – post-OLTX survival

In the first decade of liver transplantation, physicians believed that alcohol-associated medical problems would lead to higher perioperative mortality, a higher complication rate, and potentially poorer outcome in alcoholic cirrhotics (Van Thiel et al. 1984; Schenker, Perkins, and Sorrell 1990). These ideas seemed justified by initial reports of poor outcome statistics for alcoholic cirrhotic patients. In 1984, the survival rates of 540 liver transplant recipients from four centers in the USA and Western Europe were reported. Of the patients given transplants for end stage cirrhosis, patients with alcoholic cirrhosis had the poorest 3-year survival (20%) (Scharschmidt 1984). However, that cohort had been selected specifically because of the gravity of their medical conditions and were most likely very poor surgical candidates. Nevertheless, this statistic supported the US National Institutes of Health consensus opinion of the early 1980s that only a small number of alcoholic cirrhotics were chosen for OLTX after establishing abstinence and having clinical indicators of an otherwise expected fatal outcome (Bernstein 1983).

In contrast to those early findings, years of transplant experience show that liver transplantation is a viable option for alcoholic cirrhotics. The transplants can be successful and the recipients can achieve post-transplantation health status at 1 to 2 years post-OLTX that does not differ significantly from patients receiving transplants for other liver diseases (Kumar et al. 1990). Recent studies show that 1- to 5-year actuarial survival post-transplantation of alcoholic cirrhotics is comparable to (Bird et al. 1990; McCurry et al. 1992; Lucey et al. 1992; DiMartini et al. 1995) or better than (Gish et al. 1993; Belle, Berringer and Detre 1996) that for patients given transplants for other types of end stage liver disease. In addition, new evidence suggests that not only can alcoholic cirrhotics successfully undergo transplantation but their resource utilization (length of stay in intensive care units and in the hospital, number of days on a ventilator, number of readmissions in the first post-OLTX year) is comparable to that for nonalcoholic cirrhotics (McCurry et al. 1992). In one study the strongest predictor of post-OLTX patient and graft survival for alcoholic cirrhotics who were critically ill at the point of transplantation was renal functioning, rather than variables of the alcohol history or pre-OLTX length of sobriety (DiMartini et al. 1995). This finding is consistent with results from studies of critically ill patients given transplants for other types of end stage liver disease (Cuervas-Mons et al. 1986). However, those patients with the shortest length of sobriety ($\leq$ 1 month) were more likely to be in multiorgan failure and on dialysis prior to transplantation (DiMartini et al. 1995). Their short length of sobriety may have been due to their medical decline and inability to survive longer without transplantation.

Defining relapse in post-OLTX alcoholic cirrhotics

Definitions of alcohol relapse are inconsistent in the post-OLTX literature. Without standardized definitions, it is impossible to link post-OLTX medical events to alcohol exposure or to compare data across studies. Definitions of quantity, frequency, or pattern of post-OLTX alcohol use are not commonly reported. In addition, most studies report relapses as percentages over a specified period of time (i.e., percentage who relapsed by 1 year) without specific information on timing of alcohol use or behaviors across that time period. When defined as a percentage over time, liver transplant centers from the USA, England and the rest of Europe report 1- to 3-year post-transplantation relapse rates ranging from 0% to 30% (Bird et al. 1990; Kumar et al. 1990; Lucey et al. 1992; Gish et al. 1993; Knechtle et al. 1993; Beresford 1994b; Krom 1994; Howard et al. 1994; Osorio et al. 1994; DiMartini et al. 1995; Pageaux et al. 1995a; Stefanini et al. 1997; Pereira and Williams 1997; Fabrega et al. 1998) for their cohorts of alcoholic cirrhotics. A relapse rate of 21% was reported in one study that included some longer follow-up times (18 to 46 months) (Tringali et al. 1996). By contrast, in alcohol research it is understood that the definition of "relapse" is complex and does not fit well with attempts to define it as a dichotomous phenomenon. Depending on the focus and definition, very different pictures of outcome are obtained. For example, in the general alcoholic population, using a dichotomous (either abstinence or relapse) outcome can result in very low success rates (Miller and Sanchez-Craig 1996). In one US study of 38 patients diagnosed with DSM-IIIR alcohol dependence, followed 6 to 63 months (mean 36 months) after OLTX, relapse was defined as *any* alcohol exposure (Campbell et al. 1993). Another study defined "harmful drinking as more than one drinking *episode* and moderate drinking as a single *episode* during follow-up" (Berlakovich et al. 1994), though episode was not defined. The risk of alcoholic relapse by these criteria after 1, 2, and 3 years was 15%, 27%, and 31%, respectively (Berlakovich et al. 1994). Another study included post-OLTX follow-up times from 12 to 48 months in 25 patients given transplants for alcoholic cirrhosis and found the "frequency of exposure to alcohol" increased to 30% at 2 to 4 year follow-up. However, they believed that the rate of return to pathologic drinking, defined as drinking that results in withdrawal symptoms or in physical or social injury, remained at about 10% (Beresford 1994b). Another study concluded that, over the long term, the majority (69%) of alcohol-dependent recipients abstain completely, whereas an additional minority (18%), experience brief relapses that do not result in liver graft injury or require hospitalization. A small minority (13%) return to pathologic drinking leading to hospitalization and infrequently death (Campbell et al. 1993). Some studies report a return to drinking mostly occurring within the first year post-OLTX, with an average of nine months post-transplantation sobriety before relapsing (Lucey et al. 1992; Tringali et al. 1996). Other studies suggest high abstinence rates during that first year (up to 90%), with recidivism rates increasing during the second to third years post-OLTX (Campbell et al. 1993; Beresford 1994b; Berlakovich et al. 1994), suggesting the need for intensive long-term follow-up. Nonetheless, in another study, 10 of 12 patients who admitted to relapsing post-OLTX returned to regular drinking, supporting the contention that a return to "social" levels of controlled drinking is not possible (Tringali et al. 1996).

Monitoring post-OLTX alcohol use for alcoholic cirrhotics

To identify individuals and percentages of those who use alcohol post-OLTX, many transplant centers have used medical or surgical clinic interviews (Starzl et al. 1988; Kumar et al. 1990; Tringali et al. 1996), alcohol use documentation in the medical chart, telephone interviews (Kumar et al. 1990; Tringali et al. 1996), or laboratory evidence suggestive of a return to drinking (Bird et al. 1990; Berlakovich et al. 1994). Some centers randomly check urine or blood alcohol levels (Tringali et al. 1996). Some studies presumed alcohol use on the basis of liver biopsy results (Bird et al. 1990; Berlakovich et al. 1994) or liver enzyme profiles (Bird et al. 1990) even when patients denied using alcohol. Many studies do not report psychiatric diagnosis or employing psychiatric/psychologic interviews post-OLTX (Starzl et al. 1988; Kumar et al. 1990; Bird et al. 1990; Osorio et al. 1994; Pageaux et al. 1995a). Some centers report using collateral sources (reports from transplant coordinators and family members) to help to identify post-OLTX alcohol use (Howard et al. 1994; Tringali et al. 1996). One study found using interviewers not associated with the transplant team can increase the yield of post-OLTX alcohol consumption reporting (Howard et al. 1994). In one study, standardized questionnaires were used at one time post-OLTX in addition to clinical interviews to identify post-OLTX alcohol use and alcohol behaviors (Howard et al. 1994).

In addition to clinical follow-up interviews, some transplant centers use liver enzymes as biochemical markers to monitor post-OLTX alcohol consumption, with an elevated γ-glutamyl-transferase (GGTP) indicating possible alcohol use. However, elevated GGTP has much lower specificity rates for the detection of alcohol consumption in patients with liver disease (Mihas and Tavassoli 1992), which may confound its interpretation during post-OLTX follow-up. In the general medical population, statistical constructions of groups of other clinical laboratory variables (including direct and total bilirubin, aspartate aminotransferase, alanine aminotransferase and mean corpuscular volume), are not clinically useful in screening for the presence of covert alcoholism (Beresford et al. 1990a). In one study of actively relapsing patients post-OLTX, a specific pattern of liver function tests related to abnormal alcohol abuse could not be determined. However, at the end of the relapse, liver function tests returned to preevent values (Berlakovich et al. 1994). Diagnosis of drinking was made by patient admission, suggestive laboratory values or in some cases by liver biopsy (Berlakovich et al. 1994). These methods alone may underestimate (as in chart review or uncorroborated self-report) or overestimate (as in abnormal laboratory data) the true frequency of alcohol use.

It has been established that the production of a deglycosylated form of the hepatically synthesized protein transferrin occurs during heavy alcohol consumption. Levels of carbohydrate-deficient transferrin (CDT), a biochemical marker of heavy drinking, may provide a more specific marker of post-OLTX drinking than GGTP, which is a nonspecific marker of liver tissue damage. CDT may be a useful adjunct to other commonly sampled biochemical markers such as GGTP, but will need to be tested in liver transplant recipients. In a pilot study in post-OLTX patients, CDT was found to have 80% sensitivity and 90% specificity when correlated with the assessment of a trained psychologist (Berlakovich 1996). Though CDT can identify only those who are drinking heavily (60 g ethanol/day for one week), data suggest that post-transplantation alcohol consumption can be regular and heavy (Tringali et al. 1996). During alcohol abstinence, the values normalize with a mean half-life of 14 to 17 days (Pharmacia 1994). In one study of alcohol abusers who had not had transplants, and controls, a comparison between CDT and GGTP demonstrated that the sensitivity of GGTP in detecting alcohol abusers was 65% in males and 44% in females. Using data from several studies, they found at specificities of $> 90\%$ the sensitivity of CDT was 79% and 44%, respectively (Anton and Moak 1994). However, because CDT and GGTP levels are independent markers of alcohol consumption, their combined measurement should increase the sensitivity of detection of heavy alcohol use. When both tests were used simultaneously, the sensitivity for the detection of alcohol abuse increased to 95% for males and 72% for females (Anton and Moak 1994). However, because CDT levels can be falsely positive in severe hepatic insufficiency (Stibler and Borg 1988; Heinemann et al. 1998), its usefulness in post-OLTX patients needs further investigation. In fact, in one study the use of CDT in a pre-liver transplant clinic was abandoned due to an unacceptable specificity rate (as low as 20% to 40%) resulting in a high rate of false positives (Heinemann et al. 1998). Newer biochemical markers, such as fatty acid ethyl esters, may offer better clinical indicators of acute and chronic alcohol use (Laposata 1997), but will need to be developed in liver disease and transplant patients.

Predictors of post-OLTX alcohol use

Despite over a decade of transplant experience with alcoholic cirrhotics, research on post-OLTX outcome, particularly post-OLTX alcohol consumption, is still limited. Studies have examined medical and surgical outcomes and basic drinking outcomes (usually defined dichotomously as "yes" drinking or "no" not drinking) but many have not dealt with the behavioral distinctions of alcoholism. Studies have frequently suffered from small cohort size (usually from a single transplant program cohort), lack of standarized measures or diagnoses, or short time of follow-up. Large cohort studies are needed that use standardized behavioral diagnoses and standardized outcome or follow-up measures. Studies on post-OLTX alcohol use have used a traditional alcohol research paradigm, i.e., assessing patients at pre-OLTX intake and then at several points post-OLTX. This method typically overestimates the impact of social background and drinking history on outcome (Marlatt and Gordon 1980; Moos, Finney and Cronkite 1990). Some studies have combined results from multiple studies in a descriptive analysis (De Maria, Colantoni, and Van Thiel 1998) or used the combined data to evaluate the predictive utility of specific variables (Foster et al. 1997). Opportunities now exist for large longitudinal studies using pre- and post-transplantation variables to model predictors of outcome (DiMartini and Beresford, 1999). The work to date suggests two main areas for further research: (a) clarification and standardization of definitions of alcoholism, alcohol-related liver disease, and alcohol relapse; and (b) development of prognostic models to predict post-transplantation alcohol use and outcome (DiMartini and Beresford 1999).

Preliminary investigations suggest pre-OLTX variables such as short duration of pre-OLTX sobriety (commonly defined as < 6 months), available social support, and previous rehabilitation experience individually do not reliably predict post-OLTX relapse. Though studies report higher recidivism rates (between 43% and 100%) for patients whose pretransplantation sobriety was less than six months (Bird et al. 1990; Kumar et al. 1990; Osorio et al. 1994) not all studies concurred. In fact one study, combining data from six published studies, found that while the presence of six months pre-OLTX sobriety was very predictive of post-OLTX abstinence, the absence of six months pre-OLTX sobriety was a relatively poor predictor of post-OLTX abstinence (sensitivity 50%, predictive value positive 61%) (Foster et al. 1997). The inability of short length of sobriety to predict post-OLTX outcome is not surprising, given evidence in alcohol research that outcome classifications from the first six months have been found to be unrelated to long-term outcome status (Miller et al. 1992). From multidecade studies of alcoholism in the USA (not necessarily cirhosis), it is known that sustained sobriety is measured in years, not months, and abstinences of six months duration reveal little about long-term relapse outcome (Vaillant 1988).

Many studies of post-OLTX alcohol use did not investigate the contribution of other variables such as other psychiatric diagnoses (Starzl et al. 1988; Kumar et al. 1990; Bird et al. 1990; Berlakovich et al. 1994; Howard et al. 1994; Osorio et al. 1994; Pageaux et al. 1995a; Tringali et al. 1996), nor did any study investigate the influence of post-OLTX psychological factors (e.g. stress or coping) on alcohol use. One study found that patients with polydrug use (i.e. at least one other drug besides alcohol) had a significantly higher rate of relapse post-OLTX than others without a substance abuse history ($p = 0.003$) (Foster et al. 1997). Another study, however, found that patients with a past history of comorbid substance abuse were not more likely to relapse (Coffman et al. 1997), perhaps because these patients were many years remitted from their substance abuse before transplantation. Character pathology is often explored as a risk factor for relapse. In one study of patients with alcohol-related liver disease awaiting transplantation, subjects with severe personality disorders had higher rates of divorce, comorbid drug abuse or dependence, and higher scores on indicators of emotional impairment (Yates, LaBrecque, and Pfab 1998). However, three patients with severe personality disorders who received transplants did not relapse or become noncompliant in the early postoperative phase (Yates et al. 1998). Another study reporting a relapse rate of 13% found that four of the five most significant relapses occurred in patients with personality or affective disorders (Tripp et al. 1996). In one study modeling of pre-OLTX variables was attempted and found that neither the length of preoperative abstinence nor a scale that quantified the prognostic factors at baseline (Beresford's Alcohol Prognostic Scale) reliably predicted subsequent alcohol use (Campbell et al. 1993). Indeed, investigations to date have not found any pre-OLTX variable that could reliably predict post-OLTX relapse (Osorio et al. 1994). One study reported higher odds for women and the unemployed to relapse (Tringali et al. 1996), though age, marital status, durations of pretransplantation sobriety and heavy drinking, and previous rehabilitation did not predict relapse. In another study 6 of 29 patients (21%) relapsed post-OLTX and 4 of these 6 relapsers had a comorbid axis II personality disorder (Gish et al. 1993).

In the field of addictions, research on relapse tends to follow patients after treatment to investigate post-treatment variables that place them at risk or precipitate relapse. In the existing transplant literature on patients with alcoholic liver disease, efforts have been directed primarily at identifying pretransplantation variables rather than post-transplantation factors that predict who will relapse. Studies of liver transplant recipients have focused primarily on pre-OLTX variables because so far these are the only measures that have been routinely collected. In addition, the identification of pre-OLTX variables that predict post-OLTX relapse, would be especially useful in the pre-OLTX evaluation and selection phase. However, the natural history of addictions is complex and most likely, in these patients, is influenced by post-OLTX factors and events. To date, attempting to predict post-OLTX outcome solely from pre-OLTX characteristics has not been successful and most likely will not be. For alcoholics in general, pretreatment drinking predictors may not predict post-treatment relapse due to the fact that treatment may have suppressed some of the tendency to repeat past patterns (Stout, Longabaugh, and Rubin 1996). This process may be accentuated by undergoing liver transplantation, which is felt by some to be the ultimate sobering experience (Kumar et al. 1990).

Post-transplant alcohol-related morbidity and mortality

Definitions of alcohol relapse correlating alcohol consumption with medically related consequences, such as elevated liver enzymes, graft injury, or graft failure, are needed to investigate alcohol-related morbidity and mortality in liver transplant recipients. Nevertheless, the overall survival of this group is comparable with that of patients receiving transplants for other types of liver disease. Furthermore, the cumulative probability of surviving without retransplantation 5 years after liver transplantation is 0.66 for all adults and 0.80 for alcoholic cirrhotics (Belle et al. 1996). In a comparative analysis of the literature, Foster et al. (1997) found death caused by alcohol-induced noncompliance or toxic alcohol intake ranged from 2% to 5% of those patients given a transplant because of alcoholic cirrhosis.

While the prevalence of post-OLTX drinking is an important variable, whether post-OLTX drinking results in increased morbidity and mortality is also a question needing further research. As a hepatotoxin, alcohol can damage the engrafted liver as well as the native organ. Post-OLTX drinking may cause alcohol-related sequelae, such as fatty changes seen on liver biopsy, but its contribution to increased post-OLTX morbidity or mortality is less clear. In a retrospective study of actively relapsing alcoholic cirrhotic transplant recipients, the 1-year survival rate and retransplantation rate did not differ from abstainers (Lucey et al. 1997), and liver biopsy revealed that the major histologic abnormality for both groups was non-alcoholic hepatitis (Lucey et al. 1997). Another study looked at the influence of alcohol recidivism on clinical outcome following liver transplantation for alcoholic cirrhosis (Pageaux et al. 1995b). They studied 44 patients given transplants for alcoholic cirrhosis who survived more than three months post-OLTX and found that 27% had some alcohol use (mean intake of 69 g ethanol/day). In the group of patients who were drinking, one died from lymphoma but another died from a cerebral hematoma related to alcohol use. Another patient had immuosuppression noncompliance due to drinking that resulted in several episodes of acute rejection. However alcohol consumption did not impact on survival rates at 1, 2, and 3 years post-OLTX (100%, 80%, 80% versus 89%, 72%, 66%, respectively, for drinkers versus non-drinkers, nonsignificant). In this study, liver biopsies showed steatosis of $> 50\%$ in 8 of the 10 drinkers. Nevertheless, they concluded that alcohol use did not seem to influence post-OLTX outcome (Pageaux et al. 1995b).

There is additional, surprising evidence that alcoholics who use alcohol post-OLTX had significantly *fewer* episodes of acute or chronic rejection than those who were continuously abstinent (2.24 episodes of acute cellular rejection/alcohol-abstinent patient compared with 0.75 episodes/alcohol using patient, $p < 0.01$) (Van Thiel et al. 1995). Some have suggested an immunological benefit of alcohol consumption after liver transplantation (Cotton 1994; Van Thiel et al. 1995), perhaps accounting for fewer episodes of rejection. One study of the histologic pathology seen on liver biopsies post-OLTX for alcoholic cirrhotics reported that some of the patient biopsies showed evidence of steatosis, a pattern typically considered to be associated with alcohol-induced changes (Baddour et al. 1992). Despite the authors of the study cautioning about the overlap of biopsy findings consistent with alcoholic hepatitis versus viral hepatitis, graft rejection, or graft preservation/reperfusion injury, these data have been cited as demonstrating evidence of alcoholic hepatitis and cirrhosis in post-OLTX relapsing alcoholics (Cotton 1994; Sherlock 1995), which could be a misinterpretation of biopsy findings. Such liver biopsy data need to be matched with information about post-OLTX alcohol consumption, including quantity, frequency, and timing of alcohol use compared to when the biopsy is sampled. It is possible that the liver was donated from someone who was actively drinking alcohol (Hassanein et al. 1991) and it may have had pre-engraftment alcoholic damage or steatosis. This underscores the problems of data clarity, interpretation of existing data, and the need to investigate these issues in a rigorous scientific manner.

Heart transplantation

Data about alcohol use in heart transplant recipients are limited. Even in studies where post-transplantation alcohol use is noted, a pre transplantation diagnosis of alcoholic cardiomyopathy is not specified. In one of the earliest studies of psychiatric outcomes in heart transplantation, nearly 19% of recipients were found to have excessive alcohol use post-transplantation (Freeman et al. 1988). In another study, post-transplantation alcohol abuse that met diagnostic criteria, was reported at a rate of 2% per 100 person-years (Dew et al. 1996; Paris et al. 1994). This study of 53 patients post-cardiac transplantation showed that patients with pretransplantation DSM-III-R diagnoses of alcohol abuse ($n = 8$) and illicit drug abuse ($n = 3$) were more likely to develop post-transplantation depressive or anxious disorders, or to be noncompliant with medical regimens (Paris et al. 1994). Three of the four patients with less than six months pretransplantation abstinence from drugs or alcohol relapsed within the first post-transplantation year (Paris et al. 1994). Another study found that 63% of patients with a pretransplantation history of alcohol abuse resumed alcohol use post-transplantation (Bell and Van Triget 1991). A study of medical compliance in heart transplantation found persistent heavy drinking in 9% post-transplantation, though a pre-transplantation diagnosis of alcoholic cardiomyopathy was not reported (Dew et al. 1996). Specific predictors of relapse other than a prior history of alcohol use have not yet been studied. Clearly, more research on patients with alcoholic cardiomyopathy and on alcohol use in the total population of cardiac transplant recipients is needed.

Heart transplant alcohol-related morbidity and mortality

In contrast to OLTX, there is clearer evidence in the heart literature that post-transplantation alcohol or substance use is deleterious, though not directly related to its cardiotoxic effect. Alcohol use can cause noncompliance with medical regimens, thereby increasing morbidity and mortality. After organ transplantation, noncompliance with postoperative medical therapy is a major cause of late morbidity and mortality (Addonizio et al. 1990; Paris et al. 1994; Dew et al. 1996). One study determined that a substance abuse history (past or current) is a powerful predictor of noncompliance (relative risk 3.75, $p = 0.047$) in cardiac post-transplantation patients (Shapiro et al. 1996), though a delineation between alcohol and other substance abuse was not made. Though in one study no death could be attributed to post-transplantation psychosocial factors such as substance abuse (Paris et al. 1994), another study suggests that mortality risk would not become evident until years 2 to 5 post-transplantation (Hanrahan et al. 1991). In addition, in this second study 48% of patients with a pretransplantation history of substance abuse (drug and alcohol) returned to active substance abuse post-cardiac transplantation and deaths related to noncompliance in this group were statistically higher ($p < 0.01$) (Hanrahan et al. 1991). One study of heart transplantation showed no difference in survival or numbers of infection episodes between heart transplant recipients with or without a history of alcohol use prior to transplantation (alcohol use defined as any prior alcohol use – occasional, regular, or severe) (Skotzko et al. 1996). However, compared to the non-alcoholic recipients of heart transplants, the alcohol-using patients were demographically different with respect to age, marital status, race and had significantly more rehospitalizations and a trend towards increased rejection rates, though these differences were not directly related to alcoholism (Skotzko et al. 1996). This study did not report whether patients had a diagnosis of alcoholic cardiomyopathy, nor was the rate of post-transplantation relapse identified for outcome comparison.

Summary

There are limited data addressing issues of transplanting alcoholics, especially for alcoholic cardiomyopathy and heart transplantation. Much research still needs to be done. Standarized selection criteria and research methods need to be employed. Definitions of alcohol relapse need to be clarified, standardized alcohol measures/instruments need to be used, and correlations to medical outcomes needs to be investigated. If relapse does not portend a worse outcome, assumed risks for relapse (i.e., short duration of sobriety, poor social supports, no alcohol rehabilitation) may not be good measures of transplantation candidacy. Longer-term studies investigating multiple pre dictors of outcome, not just relapse, may be underway, but have not yet provided the information necessary for clinical decision making. Nevertheless, our current selection methods are consistently choosing good candidates who achieve outcomes and survival similar to patients with other diagnoses and have low relapse rates compared to the general alcoholic population in the USA. Until new evidence emerges, we must guard against individual prejudices and anecdotal cases that can create strong and lasting opinions about patients with alcoholism.

References

Addonizio, L. J., Hsu, D. T., Smith, C. R. et al. (1990). Late complications in pediatric cardiac transplant recipients. *Circulation* **82** (5 Supplement IV), 295–301.
Anton, R. F. and Moak, D. H. (1994). Carbohydrate-deficient transferrin and gamma-

glutamyltransferase as markers of heavy alcohol consumption: gender differences. *Alcoholism Clin Exp Res*, **18**, 747–54.

Arria, A. M., Tarter, R. E., and Van Thiel, D. H. (1991). Vulnerability to alcoholic liver disease. *Rec Dev Alcohol*, **9**, 185–204.

Arthur M. J. P., Lee, A., and Wright, R. (1984). Sex differences in the metabolism of ethanol and acetaldehyde in normal subjects. *Clin Sci*, **67**, 397–401.

Atterbury, C. E. (1986). The alcoholic in the lifeboat: should drinkers be candidates for liver transplantation? *J Clin Gastroenterol*, **8**, 1–4.

Baddour, N., Demetris, A. J., Shah, G. et al. (1992). The prevalence, rate of onset, and spectrum of histologic liver disease in alcohol abusing liver allograft recipients. *Gastroenterology*, **102**, A777.

Bell, M. and Van Triget (1991) Addictive behavior patterns in cardiac transplant patients [abstract]. *J Heart Lung Transplant*, **10**, 158.

Belle, S. H. and Detre, K. M. (1997). Liver transplantation for alcoholic liver disease in the U. S. 1988–1995. *Liver Transplant Surg*, **3**, 212–19.

Belle S. H., Berringer K. C., and Detre K. M. (1996). Recent findings concerning liver transplantation in the United States. In *Clinical Transplants*, ed. J. M. Cecke and P. I. Terasaki, pp. 15–29. UCLA Tissue Typing Laboratory: Los Angeles, CA.

Beresford, T. P. (1992). Alcoholism prognosis scale for major organ transplant candidates. In *Psychiatric Aspects of Organ Transplant*, ed. J. Craven and G. M. Rodin, pp. 31–2. Oxford University Press: Oxford.

Beresford, T. (1994a). Liver transplantation and alcoholism rehabilitation. *Alcohol Health Res World*, **18**, 310–12.

Beresford, T. P. (1994b). Psychiatric follow-up care of alcohol-dependent liver graft recepients. In *Liver Transplantation & the Alcoholic Patient*, ed. M. R. Lucey, R. Merion and T. P. Beresford pp. 96–112. Cambridge: Cambridge University Press.

Beresford, T. P., Blow, F. C., Hill, E., Singer, K., and Lucey, M. R. (1990a). Clinical practice comparison of CAGE questionnaire and computer-assisted laboratory profiles in screening for covert alcoholism. *Lancet*, **336**, 482–5.

Beresford, T. P. and Lucey, M. R. (1994). "Does alcoholic liver disease indicate alcohol dependence?" Paper presented at the Academy of Psychosomatic Medicine Annual Meeting 18 November.

Beresford, T. P. and Lucey, M. R. (1995). "Duration of abstinence prior to liver transplant: can we justify the 6 month rule? Paper presented at the Academy of Psychosomatic Medicine Annual Meeting, 11 November.

Beresford, T. P., Turcotte, J. G., Merion, R. et al. (1990b). A rational approach to liver transplantation for the alcoholic patient. *Psychosomatics*, **31**, 241–54.

Berlakovich, G. A. (1996). Detection of alcohol relapse in patients following liver transplantation for alcoholic cirrhosis. Poster abstract at the Liver Transplantation for Alcoholic Liver Disease Conference, 6–7 December.

Berlakovich, G. A., Steininger, R.,Herbst, F., Barlan, M., Mittlbock, M., and Muhlbacher, F. (1994). Efficacy of liver transplantation for alcoholic cirrhosis with respect to recidivism and compliance. *Transplantation*, **58**, 560–5.

Bernstein, M. J. (1983). Consensus conference: liver transplantation. *JAMA*, **250**, 2961–4.

Bird, L. A. G., O'Grady, J. G., Harvey, F. A. H., Calne, R. Y., and Williams, R. (1990). Liver transplantation in patients with alcoholic cirrhosis: selection criteria and rates of survival and relapse. *British Medical Journal,* **301**, 15–17.

Blume, S. B. (1986). Women and alcohol. A review. *JAMA,* **256**, 1467–70.

Campbell, D. S., Beresford, T. P., Merion, R. N. et al. (1993). Alcohol use relapse following liver transplantation for alcoholic cirrhosis: long-term follow-up. Abstract, *Proceedings of the American Society of Transplant Surgeons.* Houston, TX, 20–22 May, p. 131.

Caplan, A. L. (1989). Problems in the policies and criteria used to allocate organs for transplantation in the United States. *Transplant Proc,* **21**, 3381–7.

Caplan, A. L. (1994). Ethics of casting the first stone: personal responsibility, rationing, and transplants, *Alcohol Clin Exp Res,* **18**, 219–21.

Coffman, K. L., Hoffman, A., Sher, L., Rojter, S., Vierling, J., and Makowka, L. (1997). Treatment of the postoperative alcoholic liver transplant recipient with other addictions. *Liver Transplant Surg,* **3**, 322–7.

Cohen, C. and Benjamin, M. (1991). Alcoholics and liver transplantation. The Ethics and Social Impact Committee of the Transplant and Health Policy Center, Ann Arbor, Michigan. Alcoholics and liver transplantation. *JAMA,* **265**, 1299–1301.

Cotton, P. (1994) Alcohol's threat to liver transplant recipients may be overstated. *JAMA,* **271**, 1815.

Cuervas-Mons, V., Millan, I., Gavaler, J. S., and Starzl, T. S. (1986). Prognostic value of preoperatively obtained clinical and laboratory data in predicting survival following orthotopic liver transplantation. *Hepatology,* **6**, 922–7.

Currie, K., Jones, D., and Piedmont, M. (1994). Chemically dependent vs. non-chemically dependent: a survival study with liver transplant candidates. Paper presented at the Third Biennial International Transplant Psychiatry Meeting at the Medical College of Virginia, 6–8 October.

Demakis, J. G., Proskey, A., Rahimtoola, S. H. et al. (1974). Natural course of alcoholic cardiomyopathy. *Ann Intern Med,* **80**, 293–7.

De Maria, N., Colantoni, A., and Van Thiel, D. V. (1998). Liver transplantation for alcoholic liver disease. *Hepato-Gastroenterol,* **45**, 1364–8.

Dew, M. A., Roth, L. H., Thompson, M. E., Kormos, R. L., and Griffith, B. P. (1996). Medical compliance and its predictors in the first year after heart transplantataion. *J Heart Lung Transplant,* **15**, 631–45.

Diehl, A. M. (1997). Alcoholic liver disease: natural history. *Liver Transplant Surg.* **3**, 206–11.

DiMartini, A. and Beresford, T. (1999). Alcoholism and liver transplantation. *Curr Opin Organ Transplant,* **4**, 177–81.

DiMartini, A., Fitzgerald, M.G., Magill, J., and Irish, W. (1996). Evaluation and listing of alcoholic cirrhotics for liver transplantation. Poster presentation at the Liver Transplantation for Alcoholic Liver Disease Conference, 6–7 December.

DiMartini, A. F., Jain, A., Fung, J. J. et al. (1995). Liver transplantation in alcohol and non-alcoholic cirrhosis: survival according to UNOS status, sobriety and rehabilitation. *Liver Transplant Surg,* **6**, 446.

DiMartini, A. F., Khera, G., Yates, W., Irish, W., Magill, J., and Fitzgerald, M. G. (1997). Use of a high risk alcohol relapse scale in evaluating liver transplant candidates. Presentation at the Academy of Psychosomatic Medicine Annual Meeting, 21 November.

Evans, R. W., Mannine, D. L., and Dong, F. B. (1991). *The National Cooperative*

Transplantation Study: Final Report. Battelle-Seattle Research Center: Seattle, WA.

Fabrega, E., Crespo, J., Casafont, F., De las Heras, G., de la Pena, J., and Pons-Romero, F. (1998). Alcoholic recidivism after liver transplantation for alcoholic cirrhosis. *J Clin Gastroenterol*, **26**, 204–6.

Fabrizio, L. and Regan, T. J. (1994). Alcoholic cardiomyopathy. *Cardiovasc Drugs ther*, **8**, 89–94.

Flavin, D. K., Niven, R. G., and Kelsey, J. E. (1988). Commentary: alcoholism and orthotopic liver transplantation. *JAMA*, **259**, 1546–7.

Foster, P., Fabrega, F., Karademir, S., Sankary, H. N., Mital, D., and Williams, J. W. (1997). Prediction of abstinence from ethanol in alcoholic recipients following liver transplantataion. *Hepatology*, **25**, 1469–77.

Freeman, A. M., Folks, D. G., Sokol, R. S., and Fahs, J. J. (1988). Cardiac transplantation: clinical correlates of psychiatric outcome. *Psychosomatics*, **29**, 47–54.

Frierson, R. L. and Lippmann, S. B. (1987). Heart transplant candidates rejected on psychiatric indications. *Psychosomatics*, **28**, 347–55.

Gish, R. G., Lee, A. H., Keefe, E. B., Rome, H., Concepcion, W., and Esquivel, C. (1993). Liver transplantation for patients with alcoholism and end-stage liver disease. *Am J Gastroenterol*, **88**, 1337–42.

Glannon, W. (1998). Responsibility, alcoholism and liver transplantation. *J Med Philos*, **23**, 31–49.

Grant, B. F. (1994). Alcohol consumption, alcohol abuse and alcohol dependence. The United States as an example. *Addictions*, **89**, 1357–65.

Grant B. F., DeBakey S., and Zobeck T. S. (1991). Liver cirrhosis mortality in the United States 1973–1988. In *U.S. Alcohol Epidemiologic Data Reference Manual*, Alcohol Epidemiologic Data System. Rockville, MD: US Department of Health and Human Services, Public Health Service, Drug Abuse and Mental Health Administration, National Institute on Alcohol Abuse and Alcoholism.

Hanrahan, J. S., Taylor, D. O., Eberly, C. et al. (1991). Cardiac allograft survival in "reformed" substance abusers. *J Heart Lung Transplant*, **10**, 158.

Hassanein, T. I., Gavaler, J., Fishkin, D. et al. (1991). Does the presence of a measurable blood alcohol level in a potential organ donor affect the outcome of liver transplantation? *Alcohol Clin Exp Res*, **15**, 300–3.

Heinemann, A., Sterneck, M., Kuhlencordt, R. et al. (1998). Carbohydrate-deficient transferrin: diagnostic efficiency among patients with end-stage liver disease before and after liver transplantation. *Alcohol Clin Exp Res*, **22**, 1806–12.

Hosenspud, J. D. (1994). The cardiomyopathies. In *Congestive Heart Failure*, ed. J. D. Hosenspud and B. H. Greenberg, pp. 196–222. New York: Springer-Verlag.

Hosenspud, J. D., Novick, R. J., Breen, T. J., Keck, B., and Daily, P. (1995). The Registry of the International Society for Heart and Lung Transplantation: Twelfth official report – 1995. *J Heart Lung Transplant*, **14**, 805–15.

Howard, L., Fahy, T., Wong, P., Sherman, D., Gane, E., and Williams, R. (1994). Psychiatric outcome in alcoholic liver transplant patients. *Q. J. Med*, **87**, 731–6.

Jensen, K. and Gluud, C. (1994). The Mallory body: morphological, clinical, and experimental studies (part 1 of a literature survey). *Hepatology*, **20**, 1061–77.

Keeffe, E. (1997). Milestones in liver transplantation for alcoholic liver disease. *Liver Transplant Surg*, **3**, 197–8.

Knechtle, S. J., Fleming, M. F., Barry, K. L. et al. (1993). Liver transplantation in alcoholics: assessment of psychological health and work activity. *Transplant Proc,* **25**, 1916–18.

Krom, R. (1994). Liver transplantation and alcohol: who should get transplants? *Hepatology,* S28–S32.

Kuhn, W. F., Myers, B., Brennan, A. F. et al. (1988). Psychopathology in heart transplant candidates. *J Heart Transplant,* **7**, 223–6.

Kumar, S., Stauber, R. E., Gavaler, J. S. et al. (1990). Orthotopic liver transplantation for alcoholic liver disease. *Hepatology,* **11**, 159–64.

Laposata, M. (1997). Fatty acid ethyl esters: short-term and long-term serum markers of ethanol intake. *Clin Chem,* **43**, 1547–54.

Lefkowitch, J. H. and Fenoglio J. J. Jr. (1983). Liver disease in alcoholic cardiomyopathy: evidence against cirrhosis. *Hum Pathol,* **14**, 457–63.

Lelbach, W. K. (1975). Cirrhosis in the alcoholic and its relation to the volume of alcohol abuse. *Ann NY Acad Sci,* **252**, 85–105.

Levenson, J. L. and Olbrish, M. E. (1993). Psychosocial evaluation of organ transplant candidates: a comparitive survey of process, criteria, and outcomes in heart, liver and kidney transplantation. *Psychosomatics,* **34**, 314–23.

Lucey, M. R., Carr, K., Beresford, T. P. et al. (1997). Alcohol use after liver transplantation in alcoholics: a clinical cohort follow-up study. *Hepatology,* **25**, 1223–7.

Lucey, M. R., Merion, R. M., Henley, K. S. et al. (1992). Selection for and outcome of liver transplantation in alcoholic liver disease. *Gastroenterology,* **102**, 1736–41.

Maricle, R. A., Hosenspud, J. D., Norman, D. J. et al. (1989). Depression in patients being evaluated for heart transplantation. *Gen Hosp Psychiatry,* **11**, 418–24.

Marlatt, G. A., Baer, J. S., Donovan, D. M., and Kivlahan, D. R. (1988). Addictive behaviors: etiology and treatment. *Ann Rev Psychol,* **39**, 223–52.

Marlatt, G. A. and Gordon, J. R. (1980). Determinants of relapse: implications for the maintenance of behavior change. In *Behavioral Medicine: Changing Health Lifestyles,* ed. P. O. Davidson and S. M. Davidson, pp. 410–52. Brunner/Mazel: New York.

Marshall, A. W., Kingstone, D., Boss, M. et al. (1983). Ethanol elimination in males and females: relationship to menstrual cycle and body composition. *Hepatology* **3**, 701–6.

McCurry, K. R., Baliga, P., Merion, R. M. et al. (1992). Resource utilization and outcome of liver transplantation for alcoholic cirrhosis. *Arch Surg,* **127**, 772–7.

Mihas, A. A. and Tavassoli, M. (1992). Laboratory markers of ethanol intake and abuse: a critical appraisal. *Am J Med Sci,* **303**, 415–28.

Miller, W. R., Leckman, A. L., Delaney, H. D., and Tinkcom, M. (1992). Long-term follow-up of behavioral self-control training. *J Studies Alcohol,* **53**, 249–61.

Miller, W. R. and Sanchez-Craig, M. (1996). How to have a high success rate in treatment: advice for evaluators of alcoholism programs. *Addiction,* **91**, 779–85.

Moos, R. H., Finney, J. W., and Cronkite, R. C. (1990). *Alcoholism Treatment: Context, Process and Outcome.* New York: Oxford University Press.

Moss, A. H. and Siegler, M. (1991). Should alcoholics compete equally for liver transplantation? *JAMA,* **265**, 1295–8.

Neuberger, J. and Tang, H. (1997). Relapse after transplantation: European studies. *Liver Tranplant Surg,* **3**, 275–9.

Olbrisch, M. E., Levenson, J. L., and Hamer, R. (1989). The PACT: a rating scale for the study of clinical decision-making in psychosocial screening or organ transplant candidates. *Clinical Transplant*, **3**, 164–9.

Osorio, R. W., Ascher, N. L., Avery, M., Bacchetti, P., Roberts, J. P., and Lake, J. R. (1994). Predicting recidivism after orthotopic liver transplantation for alcoholic liver disease. *Hepatology*, **20**, 105–10.

Pageaux, G. P., Fabre, J. M., Perrigault, P. F. et al. (1995a). Liver transplantation for alcoholic cirrhosis: a monocentric experience about 44 patients with control group over a five-year period. *Liver Transplant Surg*, **1**, 446.

Pageaux, G. P., Fabre, J. M., Perrigault, P. F. et al. (1995b). Alcoholism recurrence does not influence clinical outcome of patients transplanted for alcoholic cirrhosis. *Liver Transplant Surg*, **1**, 446.

Paris, W., Muchmore, J., Pribil, A., Zuhdi, N., and Cooper, D. K. C. (1994). Study of the relative incidences of psychosocial factors before and after heart transplantation and the influence of posttransplant psychosocial factors on heart transplantation outcome. *J Heart Lung Transplant*, **13**, 424–32.

Parrish, K. M., Higuchi, S., and Dufour, M. C. (1991). Alcohol consumption and the risk of developing liver cirrhosis: implications for future research. *J Substance Abuse*, **3**, 325–35.

Pereira, S. P. and Williams, R. (1997). Liver transplantation for alcoholic liver disease at King's Hospital: survival and quality of life. *Liver Transplant Surg*, **3**, 245–50.

Pharmacia (1994). *CD test for detection of carbohydrate-deficient transferrin, Directions for Use*. Uppsala: Pharmacia AB.

Piazza, N. J., Vrbka, J. L., and Yeager, R. D. (1989). Telescoping of alcoholism in women alcoholics. *Int J Addict*, **24**, 19–28.

Presberg, B. A., Levenson, J. L., Olbrisch, M. E., and Best, A. M. (1995). Rating scales for the psychosocial evaluation of organ transplant candidates: comparison of the PACT and TERS with bone marrow transplant patients. *Psychosomatics*, **36**, 458–61.

Rubin, E. and Urbano-Marquez, A. (1994). Alcoholic cardiomyopathy. *Alcohol Clin Exp Res*, **18**, 111–14.

Scharschmidt, B. F. (1984). Human liver transplantation: analysis of data on 540 patients from four centers. *Hepatology*, **4**, S95–S101.

Schenker, S. (1984). Medical treatment vs. transplantation in liver disorders. *Hepatology*, **4**, S102–S106.

Schenker, S., Perkins, H. S., and Sorrell, M. F. (1990). Editorial: Should patients with end-stage alcoholic liver disease have a new liver? *Hepatology*, **11**, 314–19.

Schroeder, J. S. and Hunt, S. (1987). Cardiac transplantation: update 1987. *JAMA*, **258**, 3142–5.

Schwartz, F., Mall, G., Zebe, H. et al. (1984). Determinants of survival in patients with congestive cardiomyopathy: quantitative morphologic findings and left ventricular hemodynamics. *Circulation*, **70**, 923–8.

Shapiro, P. A., Williams, D. L., Foray, A. T. et al. (1996). Psychosocial variables and outcomes of heart transplantation. *Psychosomatics*, **37**, 197.

Shelton, W. and Balint, J. A. (1997). Fair treatment of alcoholic patients in the context of liver transplantation. *Alcohol Clin Exp Res*, **21**, 93–100.

Sherlock, S. (1995). Alcoholic liver disease. *Lancet*, **345**, 227–9.

Sherman, D. and Williams, R. (1995). Commentary: liver transplantation and the alcoholic patient. *Alcohol Alcoholism*, **30**, 141–3.

Shugoll, G. I., Bowen, P. J., Moore J. P. et al. (1972). Follow-up observations and prognosis in primary myocardial disease. *Arch Intern Med*, **129**, 67–71.

Simko, V. (1983). Patterns of alcohol abuse and the role of diet in alcoholic liver disease. *Comp Ther*, **9**, 37–44.

Skotzko, C. E., Miotto, K., Wheeler, J. G., and Rudis, R. (1996). Alcohol use and outcome following cardiac transplantation. *Psychosomatics*, **37**, 195.

Snyder, S. L., Drooker, M., and Strain, J. (1996). A survey estimate of academic liver transplant teams' selection practices for alcohol-dependent applicants. *Psychosomatics*, **37**, 432–7.

Starzl, T. E., Van Thiel, D., Tzakis, A. G. et al. (1988). Orthotopic liver transplantation for alcoholic cirrhosis. *JAMA*, **260**, 2542–4.

Stefanini, G. F., Biselli, M., Grazi, G. L. et al. (1997). Orthotopic liver transplantation for alcoholic liver disease: rates of survival, complications, and relapse. *Hepato-Gastroenterol*, **44**, 1356–9.

Stibler, H. and Borg, S. (1988). The value of carbohydrate-deficient transferrin as a marker of high alcohol consumption. In *Biomedical and Social Aspects of Alcohol and Alcoholism*, ed. K. Kuriyama, A. Takada and H. Ishil, pp. 503–6. Elsevier Science Publishers: Amsterdam.

Stout, R. L., Longabaugh, R., and Rubin, A. (1996). Predictive validity of Marlatt's relapse taxonomy versus a more general relapse code. *Addiction*, **91**, S99 S110.

Tringali, R. A., Trzepacz, P. T., DiMartini, A., and Dew, M. A. (1996). Assessment and follow-up of alcohol-dependent liver transplantation patients. *Gen Hosp Psychiatry*, **18**, S70–S77.

Tripp, L., Clemons, J. R., Goldstein, R. R., and Stewart, L. M. (1996). Drinking patterns in liver transplant recipients. *Psychosomatics*, **37**, 249–53.

Twillman, R. K., Manetto, C., Wellisch, D. L., and Wolcott, D. L. (1993). The transplant evaluation rating scale: a revision of the psychosocial levels system for evaluating organ transplant candidates. *Psychosomatics*, **34**, 144–53.

Urbano-Marquez, A., Estruch, R., Fernandez-Sola, J., Nicholas, J. M., Pare, J. C., and Rubin, E. (1995). The greater risk of alcoholic cardiomyopathy and myopathy in women compared with men. *JAMA*, **274**, 149–54.

Vaillant, G. E. (1983). *The Natural History of Alcoholism*. Havard University Press: Cambridge, MA.

Vaillant, G. E. (1988). What can long-term follow up teach us about relapse and prevention of relapse? *Addiction*, **83**, 1147–57.

Van Thiel, D. H., Bonet, H., Gavaler, J. et al. (1995). Effect of alcohol use on allograft rejection rates after liver transplantation for alcoholic liver disease. *Alcohol Clin Exp Res*, **19**, 1151–55.

Van Thiel, D. H., Schade, R. R., Gavaler, J. S., Shaw, B. W., Iwatsuki, S., and Starzl, T. (1984). Medical aspects of liver transplantation. *Hepatology*, **4**, S79–S83.

Wall, W. J. (1998). Trends in liver transplantation: hepatocellular cancer and alcoholic liver disease. *Transplant Proc*, **30**, 1822–5.

Yates, W. (1996). The validity of the six months of abstinence criteria for liver transplantation. Paper presented at the Fourth Biennial Psychiatric, Psychosocial, and Ethical Issues in Organ Transplantation Conference, 13 November.

Yates, W. R., Booth, B. M., Brown, K., and Masterson, B. (1992). A model to estimate alcoholism relapse risk: implications for liver transplantation candidates. Paper presented at the Annual Academy of Psychosomatic Medicine Meeting, 31 October.

Yates, W. R., Booth, B. M., Reed, D. A., Brown, K., and Masterson, B. J. (1993). Descriptive and predictive validity of a high-risk alcoholism relapse model. *J Studies Alcohol*, **54**, 645–51.

Yates, W. M., LaBrecque, D. R., and Pfab, D. (1998). Personality disorder as a contraindication for liver transplantation in alcoholic cirrhosis. *Psychosomatics*, **39**, 501–11.

9

Ethics and images in organ transplantation

Grant Gillett D.Phil.

Introduction

The ethical issues associated with organ transplantation encompass some of the most basic features of our moral belief systems about human beings as embodied individuals. Here we find a deeply challenging mixture of images and arguments that concern life, death, and what is essential to being an intact human being. On the face of it, the issues seem clear, one person donating tissue or an organ that they are willing to give or can no longer benefit from to another person who needs that organ to live. But this is only the beginning of the discussion because of the inevitable mixed feelings that arise in relation to body parts from one person being used in another. Consider, for example, the problem of a heart transplant from a beating heart donor: if the heart is still beating and the donor is still breathing, then in what sense is the donor dead? This question has provoked one commentator to argue "that the heartbeat 'counts for life'" (Evans 1990). It has also led some to a vigorous contemporary debate on strategies for obtaining organs for transplantation (Price 1996). The exact nature of human death and what defines life are among a number of questions that must be addressed in discussing these issues. These questions include:

1. Are there individuals who should be treated as freely accessible sources for organs and tissues for transplantation, such as fetuses and anencephalic infants?
2. If you are alive and could give a kidney to save somebody else's life, then could you also decide to donate your heart to your child?
3. Should we ever accept donations from relatives even when the organs or tissues can be given safely?
4. Should we allow people to donate organs for money?
5. If kidneys are needed in greater quantities those in which than they are available from voluntary donations, should we be able to take kidneys except when the person had specified otherwise?
6. Should a person's wishes about the use of his or her organs following

death be over-ridden by the wishes of relatives?

7. Is it discriminatory to bar organ donations from people with human immunodeficiency virus (HIV) or acquired immune deficiency syndrome (AIDS)?

These questions indicate the range of current ethical debates surrounding organ and tissue transplantation. In addition they introduce the key role of mental images or symbols in our ethical thinking.

The justification for transplantation

In general, most would agree that there is something right about improving the life of other persons by transplanting organs for which one person, unfortunately and for whatever tragic reasons, has no further use. So why do we have reservations about the donation and transplantation of organs? In part, these reservations seem to stem from lingering mysticism about death and respect for the dead. Other concerns center around the idea, expressed by the English journalist Malcolm Muggeridge, that it is unnatural for people to have "spare parts" that have been derived from other people. Some of these feelings are very deep and probably primeval, having descended from our prehistoric forebears. However, ethical debate is sometimes broadly based and sensitive to our basic emotive and value commitments, and is not restricted narrowly to a "purely rational" analysis. Ethical concerns can therefore plunge us into mythical and imagistic territory to which we shall return.

The most accessible ethical justification for organ transplantation is utilitarian and the reasoning is as follows:

1. The recipient wants a future life with certain benefits.
2. That future life depends on the recipient receiving a certain organ.
3. An organ of the requisite type is available without disvalue to the donor or to other persons.
4. Therefore the organ should be transplanted.

We ought to be cautious about a too ready acceptance of this utilitarian argument because "the trolley problem" (Thomson 1986) suggests that a utilitarian argument can be used to prove too much. In the trolley problem we are asked whether it would be correct for the driver of an out of control trolley to divert it onto a spur of track where it will kill one person if that is the only way of avoiding the death of five people on the main track. The utilitarian answer is "Yes". The problem is that if five patients could be saved by transplanting organs into each by killing one healthy person, should we do it? Most people say "No," although the utilitarian answer seems to be "Yes".

To resist the "Yes" conclusion is difficult if we are confined to utilitarian arguments, which suggests that there are important moral considerations missing from this theoretical view. Notice that we accept the position outlined in points 1 to 4 above, but the trolley problem shows us that this is not purely for reasons grounded in utilitarian theory. This implies that something is wrong with the utilitarian argument.

The crucial premise in the utilitarian argument is point 3 above, which is widely disputed by those who feel that it is always a wrong to the donor to take an organ from him or her. It is also argued that any society in which transplantation occurs has a moral disvalue because of this practice. However, using dead donors does not seem to justify this concern about wronging a human being by removing organs. Considering that ordinary human death is the end of embodied life as a biological organism (irrespective of our views about events after death), it would seem that the taking of an organ does not harm the dead person. In fact, removing an organ seems less destructive than burning a body or leaving it out for vultures to eat, both of which are acceptable practices in some cultures. However, religious or social concerns about mutilating the dead may fuel an argument based on the harm to society; I examine these later.

A larger ethical concern is that organ donation creates an incentive for death itself, particularly in fit, young, incompetent or vulnerable patients. Some argue that widespread organ transplantation may encourage either less than optimal medical treatment or premature pronouncements of death to obtain donor organs (Arnold and Younger 1993). Thus, we need to examine the ethical issues surrounding the determination of death in contemporary medical settings in order to see whether such abuse is likely or even possible.

Is the donor really dead?

In the Monty Python movie *The Meaning of Life*, collectors come to the house of a woman who has signed a donor card to collect her liver. The fact that she is not dead does not deter them. Is there a similar attitude creeping into contemporary transplant practice (Arnold and Younger 1993)?

The criteria for brain death were originally formulated in the late 1960s (Beecher 1968). The philosophical basis for decisions about brain death were widely discussed in the USA and UK subsequent to the adoption of these criteria (Jennett 1977; Pallis 1982). Pallis (1982) argued that the decision was based on "irreversible loss of the capacity for consciousness combined with irreversible loss of the capacity to breathe". When defining consciousness, Pallis based his argument largely on "the centrality we instinctively allocate to persisting brain stem function". In fact, on one hand, the irreversible loss of breathing function seems particularly irrelevant because there are a number of patients who have been kept alive and conscious for years on ventilators. On the other hand, the capacity for consciousness is critically important (Cranford 1986; Gillett 1990). Most argue that the characteristic features that "make me the person I am, my life a life that is worth living, and my actions more than primitive reflexes" are crucial in the moral value of the life of a person. These are all lost in persistent vegetative state (PVS). To some, this suggests that PVS is a kind of death – the death of a person. Therefore we seem to lack a good reason why we should distinguish PVS from brain death, except that PVS patients are obviously alive (Gillett 1986). However, even if PVS is ethically troubling, few have difficulties with the idea that loss of cortical function means death of unique personhood. Using this basis, the diagnosis of brain death would appropriately signal an opportunity to gift vital organs to a living person.

What if the availability of organ transplantation means that we are less concerned about saving the lives of potential donors than if they were our only focus of care? This is theoretically problematic in an environment where medical care market-driven policy places greater incentives on good outcome, hi-tech, transplant surgery than on poor outcome, expensive, resuscitative care for victims of severe multitrauma. This possibility is counterbalanced in part by the dedication of doctors in intensive care units to high standards of excellence in critical care medicine. Nonetheless, these issues highlight the need for clear standards in a health care system where incentives may conflict with the welfare of individual patients.

The medical profession has, in fact, developed strict provisions regarding the determination of death, in particular brain death, and these can safeguard the potential donor against undesirable pressures. Clear ethical guidelines for intensive and terminal care are more difficult to develop when health care systems are increasingly evolving to emphasize the marketability and profile of a given service unit and to rely on concepts such as effectiveness and efficiency in determining which health care procedures ought to be delivered and how. The medical profession must stand behind the principle that defends the right of every patient to expect care directed primarily at his or her own benefit as far as justice permits. Only when this is firmly entrenched as the standard of care for any patient do we have adequate safeguards against medical decisions tainted by economic pressures.

Donors whose life is not-life

In addition to the PVS patient, another group whose lives are ethically ambiguous comprises anencephalic infants. In both cases the cerebral functions needed to support the mental life of an adequately functioning person are absent (Gillett 1990) or irreversibly lost and not just temporarily lacking.

PVS patients were previously conscious with a distinct identity and conscious life of thought and action, whereas anencephalic infants will never attain that capacity. Yet, in both cases there is something that is both human and alive. One theologian refers to a being of this type as a "completely depersonalized biological larva, where nothing remains – nothing can be revived – except the minimal operations of the lower nervous system and the rudimentary bodily functions" (Thielicke 1970). For this reason it seems futile to offer any life-sustaining treatment to such patients. But, should we take the further step of regarding such individuals as suitable sources for donated organs?

In both the PVS and anencephalic situations, a minor amendment to our definition of brain death would allow us to set limits and avoid possible misuse or descend the slippery slope of extending the argument to patients with brain injuries of lesser severity. These criteria would be:

1. Loss of all the higher brain functions required for an integrated and recognizably human thought life
2. Absence of the capacity ever to develop such a mental life.

Clearly these conditions do not obtain for a patient who has a lesser degree of brain injury and they definitely do not hold with fetuses or other at risk neonates (such as those with Down's syndrome). However, the issues surrounding anencephaly are still widely debated. Some argue that there is no moral difference between anencephaly and brain death due to absence of integrated brain function, while others argue that the anencephalic is a person, is not dead but rather dying, and that the use of their organs involves using people (what is more, vulnerable people) as means to serve the interests of others (Capron 1987).

This is an area where rational considerations point in one direction and our traditional intuitions point in another. In one sense, the young patient in PVS is an ideal source for donor organs: the organs are undamaged, they have shown that they are healthy and viable, they can be removed at any time without harm to a patient because nothing can constitute harm or benefit in the state under consideration, and it is a way of salvaging something from a tragedy. However, the human being concerned is going to grimace and perhaps even shed tears based on the intact reflexes and responses of the lower brain. This means that, to assist the organ retrieval surgery, some kind of anesthetic will be given. Now, whereas we might not mind the prospect of a person who has already been pronounced dead not waking up from a terminal anesthetic, to give a terminal anesthetic knowing that doing so would effectively end the life of that person is a different kind of act. Even if, in purely rational terms, using organs from anencephalic children and PVS patients is permissible, there are, therefore, some deep and intuitive misgivings about it.

Another ethical delemma is raised by the possibility of fetal tissue trans-plantation. The status of the human embryo or fetus is complex and different from that of either anencephalic or PVS patients because it typically has the potential to grow into a fully functioning human being (Poplawski and Gillett 1991). Experimental work is ongoing for the use of fetal tissue grafts in patients who have a variety of degenerative diseases of the brain including Parkinson's disease and Alzheimer's disease. Jones (1991) has classified the arguments into abortion-dependent and abortion-independent varieties. Some regard fetal tissue transplants as inseparable, ethically, from the abor-tion that provides the fetus as a source of brain tissue. Others argue that the cause of a person's death is morally separable from the transplantations that might ensue. Imagine, for instance, that one were offered kidneys from a young man who had been brutally murdered as part of a vendetta against his family or a young woman killed by a drunken driver. It is ludicrous to suggest that the transplant doctor colluded with the murderers in the first case or should take any of the blame due to the drunken driver in the second. However, this argument succeeds only if the fetal tissue transplant and the abortion are truly morally separable. Thus, for instance, were a couple to conceive a child merely to provide tissue for transplantation into the brain of their favorite uncle the issues would be inseparable and the ethics of the situation thereby complicated. For those who maintain that killing a fetus with the potential to become a normal human being is wrong, the abortion and transplant would be wrong in the case of deliberate conception to provide tissue in a way that it is not when the intention is to save the life of the mother. In the deliberate conception and use situation, the wrongness would arise from:

1. The avoidance of harm or danger being less clear-cut in the fetal tissue transplant case, in fact amounting to little more than an unproven attempt to benefit another.
2. The cynical attitude to fetal life that it expresses.

It seems, therefore, that we feel some ethical unease about a couple conceiv-ing specifically to harvest tissue for transplantation from their to-be-aborted fetus. Thus, the abortion-independence condition needs to be satisfied before the two sets of arguments can be disentangled. However, in real-world terms our worry is probably unfounded, given that many women who have, for what were considered good reasons, had a fetus aborted feel a sense of loss, arguing against the idea that women might take the cynical attitude required to conceive a child solely to provide tissue. Recent legal moves that have attempted to make abortion separation a requirement for fetal tissue research and use have been criticized on the basis of invasion of a woman's privacy and the unlikelihood of the cynical stance being taken by any woman

(Kearney, Vawter, and Gervais 1991). Indeed Gillam (1998) has suggested that, although the practice is vindicated if the fetal tissue transplant and the abortion are truly morally separable, the argument about more abortions is not conclusive even if there is a connection. She claims that the more-abortions argument has two forms: a weak form that concentrates on social attitudes and a strong directly causal form (the possibility of fetal transplants causes more abortions). When she examines both forms she concludes that there is no conclusive objection on the basis of abortions. However, even where there is a clear separation between the abortion decision and the transplant decision, there are still two major positions possible based on other features of fetal tissue transplants.

The first position is that fetal tissue transplants should be pursued as part of the advancement of medical science, given that they have a small but as yet unproven therapeutic potential. Against this, some argue that the innovators are performing major brain operations on a vulnerable and often desperate group of patients without good enough results to support this procedure. The latter ignores the common difficulties in evaluating any new medical technique's efficacy (Jennett 1986: Bailey 1990). Thus, what Jones (1991) calls "scientific pragmatism" argues both for and against fetal tissue grafts. We should note that these arguments, along with real concerns about the abuse of parental trust and the discounting of animal rights, were in the forefront of debates about Baby Fae, an infant who was used as an experimental xenograft recipient of a baboon heart (Pence 1990).

Living healthy donors

Living healthy donors bring up issues about altruism and payment. Most believe that there should not be an "organ market" (Murray 1987), although this is hotly debated for renal and some other types of transplantation. Heart transplants are excluded from the debate because of the one-to-one correspondence between functioning hearts and living human beings. However, there could be a situation when one person wants to give his or her life to save another.

The issues raised by kidney donation from living donors center on the coercion that a potential living donor might feel because of either financial inducements or family relationships. Both types of coercion are problematic.

The problem of donor relatives is especially difficult. There is emotional coercion on any family with a severely ill member, though it is not clear that there should not be or that it is wrong for an individual to respond to such pressure. There is a fine line of distinction between, on the one hand, a sacrifice made out of commitments to people dear to oneself and, on the other, coercion that exploits an individual without regard for that individual's real wishes. One would give a great deal to help a loved one, especially if one's gift were the only means to save his or her life. It would be hard to claim that there was any demeaning of a person by complying with that person's request to help a person they dearly loved and one might even view the donation as an exemplary moral act. However, emotional coercion might occur via an expectation that traps the donor into compliance. Counseling and support for individuals in such a situation need to be sensitive to the psychodynamics and family system issues that may, from behind the scenes, be distorting the decisions that a potential donor is making.

Arguments similar to those that apply in adults apply to living related child donors (Ross 1994). A child may be considered to risk losing a great deal if a dearly loved sibling dies or is incurably and lingeringly ill. Therefore, it would be wrong to adopt prohibition against organ or tissue donation by children for the reason that donation may be made because the child genuinely wants, more than anything else, to help the sibling or relative. We might, however, want to insist that such motivations, while acceptable in the case of a child who can make an authentic or autonomous choice in accordance with their own values and commitments, can never be assumed in a child who is too young to understand. This would imply also that parental consent alone would never suffice and that such transplants are out of the question in children too young to give meaningful consent. However, this is also an arguable position. Imagine the following case:

Hetty is now sixteen. She recalls, and has often talked about, her older sister Jacquie who would now be twenty but who died when Hetty was six. One evening she asks what her sister died of and finds that Jacquie died of leukemia. She remarks that she has just learned about the disease at school and heard that people can be saved by chemotherapy and bone marrow transplantation. The parents agree and after some further questioning by Hetty it emerges that she could have been used as a transplant donor but the ethics committee of her hospital thought that a girl of six was too young to be involved and refused to allow the procedure. Hetty is mortified and protests that it should have been allowed because she now feels that the sacrifice asked of her in undergoing the procedure is one she would willingly have made for the possible joy of still having Jacquie as a sister.

It seems obvious that Hetty has a point. Her justification is similar to that used by Redman (1986) in arguing that children might later be glad of having contributed to medical research. Indeed, in such a situation there is some merit in crediting a child, otherwise too young to give valid informed consent, with a very real interest in donating tissue to a sibling. If that is so, then it is not justified to issue a blanket ethical prohibition in the use of incompetent minors for transplant procedures. However, one might want to insist on certain safeguards to prevent abuse, such as:

1. The minor should not be exposed to too great a risk of personal harm.
2. The parents should be in agreement.
3. An independent advisor, such as an ethics committee ought to be assured that the donation is one the child might reasonably be pleased to have made when he or she reaches an age to understand the issues.

Provided these conditions are met, it seems reasonable to allow tissue donation from minors particularly where it would be natural for them to appreciate the ongoing presence of the person to whom the donation was made.

A related set of issues is posed by the possibility of total self-sacrifice for the purpose of saving another. Imagine, for instance, that I were a modern day Dickensian Sydney Carton without that character's drinking problem but with a relatively insignificant role in life by my own estimation. I have become aware that the person I most admire, my gentle and brilliant cousin, a good husband and father to a family I dearly love, is dying of a severely damaged heart caused by a viral inflammation and subsequent progressive degeneration. My cousin needs a heart transplant and I happen to know I am a close tissue type match from previous matching for blood transfusion purposes. I volunteer to give my heart to my cousin just as Sydney Carton volunteered to give his life for Charles Darnay. Why should I not be regarded as heroic just as Sydney Carton was? I have made a competent rational decision and decided that my cousin's life and the happiness of his children is worth more than my life. In the current literature, the main argument against this is an analogy with John Stuart Mill's condemnation of selling oneself into slavery (Brecher 1994). However, if, in another situation, I had given my life for his, I would be honored, so why is it that, here, I am prevented from helping him? It is not easy to say in rational terms why that should be so. The outcome of the surgery is inherently more uncertain but so might an heroic rescue attempt in which I lose my life. The image here is one of the uniqueness of each life. I have life and my own history to trace and my cousin has his. The possibility of medicine colluding in such a radical and ghoulish sacrifice therefore horrifies our sense of human life, death, and destiny.

The organ market

Financial inducements to organ donation tend to be rejected on the basis that it is wrong, without qualification, to trade in human bodies. Some link this to fundamental human rights; Justice Manohar remarked "profiteering by procuring organs and inducing the poor and needy to violate their bodily integrity are violations of these rights" (Manohar 1990). However, consider a poor family with four children living in severe deprivation. If one or two of them took the (comparatively minor) risk of being organ donors, should they not be allowed to make that choice? The proponents of this argument claim that it is only those of us who have the resources to indulge our refined moral sensibilities who oppose this option. They point to the fact that we are quite willing to let other relatively disadvantaged people do other life-threatening things, such as work in coal mines and clean the windows of skyscrapers for financial inducements.

On the other hand, it could be argued that the existence of systems in which such oppression can occur is, in itself, an evil and that we cannot condone an action as ethically right simply because it is inescapable as a result of other evil acts (Brecher 1994). An analogy is the concentration camp guard who executes inmates because he has no choice given the circumstances. His lack of real choice does not make his action right, although it does spread the burden of evil beyond him as an individual. Nonetheless, there are significant differences between the concentration camp guard and the family making a choice to obtain money from an exploitative system. The guard may be under extreme inducements, perhaps even to the extent of forcing him to choose between doing his duty and exposing his own family to persecution. But because he is doing some intrinsically evil things, such as torture and maybe even mass murder, these actions are almost impossible to condone, whatever the inducements. Such crimes morally separate him from the actions of family members who give organs as the only means of providing for their other family members. Their actions not only do not harm others but, in fact, benefit the recipients of the organs. There is admittedly a fine line between a considered choice made by a family in response to difficult circumstances, and a situation where they are coerced into making decisions by direct and oppressive exploitation at the hands of an organ-procuring organization. The problem reminds us that we need to be aware both of the difficulties faced by disadvantaged groups for whom the whole of life can be a series of life-and-death choices and of the need for health care ethics to embrace some concern for social justice.

Another concern is the idea of a market for human organs, perhaps obtained in ways that may not meet our ethical criteria for organ donation. The harvesting of organs for money does begin to make us look at the human body as a collection of commodities (Campbell 1992), which violates our respect for the human body and, therefore, our respect for human life. The sensitivities of relatives and loved ones of deceased persons may be callously overridden in the interest of a thriving trade. The practices of obtaining donors might neglect some of the important safeguards about death and terminal care. Our concerns about transplant organ availability should not blind us to the dignity and importance of each human being. It is a large step, but not conceptually impossible, from the view that each of us is a collection of valuable resources to the idea of individuals being sacrificed in the pursuit of the transplant enterprise.

Social justice and organ transplantation

Even if we were to have unlimited health care finance the problem of scarce resources would be raised by the scarcity of transplantable organs. In this case our ability to act for the benefit of any given individual must be tempered by the requirements of justice. If there is one kidney and more than one possible recipient, some basis has to be found to make the choice between recipients. It is tempting to believe that there must be some ethical way of regulating such choices.

The obvious way is to accept the principle of first-come first-served. To some this seems just too haphazard; surely people can be ranked in terms of some measure of ethical entitlement just as medical triage can tell us which patients are most likely to benefit from a given intervention. This idea has special appeal when we consider a case such as that of the heart patient who is also a pedophile and whose angina has prevented him from molesting children. It is hard to believe that this person should take a turn equitable to others on the cardiac waiting list. However attractive this concept may seem, it is incredibly difficult to formulate in useful terms. If we try to defend the idea that some individuals are more worthy or more deserving than others, we end up making value judgments about human lives which inevitably reflect a kind of elitism based in a narrow idea of the ideal society. For most of us this is invisible because we naturally assume that people like ourselves are deserving but who is to say whether we should attempt to rank an out-of-work newly graduated arts major above or below a prosperous businessman. We are, therefore, cast back on the utilitarian maxim that "Every individual should count for one and nobody for more than one." This is, for practical purposes, the waiting list, modified only by purely medical indications of the likely success of a transplant in the potential recipient. The more one debates the issue, the more it seems the only fair way to determine how to distribute scarce resources.

Dangerous donors

There are certain restrictions that should be applied on the other side of the donor–recipient relation. The basic justification for transplantation is that, despite all its conflicting ethical features and the associated difficulties, there is a great benefit to the recipient. But when there is reason to believe a donor will transmit a life-threatening disease to the recipient we do not accept donations from that person. Patients with cancer might transmit live cancer cells to the recipient, thus turning a gift of life into a gift of death. Similar considerations apply to an HIV positive donor. The issue is not decided in terms of the rights of the donor, but rather in terms of the action's underlying crucial value, which is an attempt to help the recipient. The "first do no harm" maxim demands that we do not expose the recipient to a gratuitous and lethal risk in an attempt to help. This maxim mitigates against accepting donors with certain conditions and, therefore, cannot be considered discriminatory.

Xenotransplantation

The transplantation of animal organs and tissues into human beings has raised "Fundamental questions of ethics technology and social policy" (Fox and McHale, 1998). In fact the practice has been with us in the form of transplantable porcine heart valves for some time but the recent moves have been provoked by the shortfall in availability of human organs and expanded indications to take in solid organ transplantation. The arguments focus on animal rights, scientific uncertainty, and some intuitions about human nature and integrity. The first group of arguments focus on the fact that the donor animals have rights and interests not served by any policy of animal organ procurement. It is given particular force by the fact that the animals most suitable for transplantation are those closest to us in biology (and therefore have the attributes which ground the value we attach to human life). Given the widespread acceptance of the destruction of animals such as pigs and sheep to feed human beings it is a bit hypocritical to deny their use in the transplantation context for the reason of animal rights alone.

The issues of scientific uncertainty (concerning "immunology, anatomy, physiology, and potential risks of infection", Fox and McHale, 1998, p. 52) are difficult for any new technology. Decisions have to be made in the light of partial knowledge and some of these will turn out to be unfortunate in the long run. That is an intrinsic problem of innovation and has to do with the fact that foresight is inherently limited but hindsight is 20/20. We do not know what the long-term results of persuading immune systems to accept xenografts might be and we do not know what viral and microbial adaptations such practices might potentiate but to fail to move because of imperfect knowledge of a new area is to stagnate in terms of medical advances.

The third set of issues revolves around our intuitions about the integrity of human beings as a unique class of inhabitants of the biosphere. Perhaps these intuitions will be eroded if we accept that more and more bits of us are replaceable by bits of other creatures. This has much in common with the spare-parts image that has already been alluded to and carries us into the debate about imagery and ethical reasoning.

Images and ethical problems

The concept of transplantation is subject to a number of widely shared sentiments and stereotypes, heart transplantation perhaps being surrounded by more misconceptions than most. It is said that the ancient Britons had a custom of eating the hearts of their newly dead forebears, so partaking of the prowess and wisdom that the dead person had shown. The contrast between imagistic thoughts of the ancient British custom and of our contemporary mores is profound. In the ancient setting, the act is regarded as loving and respectful because of its symbolic links of belonging and continuity, and the reverence paid to one's ancestors. In our world it is considered revolting, treating the human body as meat and desecrating the memory of the person who has died. Depending on which imagery one associates with the act of eating the heart of an ancestor, one will see the act take on one of two sharply contrasting moral characters. Despite these differences, there is a certain core of the old beliefs about the heart that persist in contemporary society: even now we give the heart a central place in our thoughts about the nature and identity of the person whose heart it is. Imagine, for example, that it were proposed to use donated hearts from condemned death row prisoners. If the hearts were associated with the antisocial behaviors of the their donors, heart transplantation would intensify the concerns that surround organ donation and transplant surgery in general.

Symbolic concerns, unlike scientific issues, are deeply imagistic and in a very real way important to the modes of moral identification that define a society (Lamb 1992). The idea of having a part of someone living inside another person seems to import into the debate images of identity and the persisting life of the dead person. These images and the role of the donor become particularly strong when we consider donation to humans from other animals in xenotransplantation (Nelson 1992). Such a symbolically potent gift may need to be cleared of the association with the donor and his or her character. Although the Western mind regards this type of thinking as mystical and perhaps irrational, it would be very meaningful particularly to many indigenous cultures who regard the taking of an animal life as an occasion for spiritual release of the associated significance in terms of life and spirit. The altruistic giving of a gift seems, in some way, to serve as a sanctification of the gift. The PVS patient could perhaps be seen as such a giver in the same spirit as such a human being can be seen as not wanting to be left hopelessly alive in such a state. In the cases of the anencephalic infant and the fetus the image is much harder to ground. The acceptability of loving or altruistic gifts may well be for reasons that have to do with the sacrificial gift tradition. It is in that tradition that I believe we will find the fundamental ethical image that endorses organ transplants.

The idea of a gift

Many of us intuitively share semi-mythical fears about the grafting into one person a part of another's body. This goes beyond concerns about AIDS or any other rational considerations and embraces the deep, indeed symbolic, associations that underlie many of our value commitments. The thought that, when transplantation occurs, a person both literally and symbolically takes into him or herself aspects of the donor person is understandable to us at one level even though it seems irrational at another. When such symbolic associations are operative, stongly countervailing images are needed to resolve these worries in a satisfying way. One key countervailing concept, as has already been suggested, is the concept of a gift. Tom Murray (1987) has argued that this concept is an underpinning for many of the aspects of collective human life that we most value. He has also argued that it is fundamentally different from other types of social transaction.

The most powerful image associated with such giving of self is expressed in the words, familiar to many Christian Westerners, "Take, eat, this is my body which is broken for you". Similar to this eucharistic image, organ donation can focus on the gift-giving when one person is enabled to give life where there otherwise was no hope of life. This so closely parallels the highest ideals of most moralities, be they religious or secular, that it is a fitting image to apply to transplant issues both in abstracto (in ethical discussion) and in concreto (at the bedside of the newly dead person). A dignified recognition that one human life has ended and the sensitive suggestion that this person may have wanted to give a gift of life to someone else has shades of meaning that are on a moral level different from that of the ideas central to the paid procurement of organs.

Cardiac transplantation, as we have noted, is burdened with imagery and associations that have deep roots in our fundamental feelings about ourselves and other human beings. When our thoughts and responses are engaged in this deeper way, an ethical problem is not susceptible to purely rational resolution because those deeper aspects of our being need to be recognized and respected. I have suggested that the concept of a gift, particularly as exemplified in the Christian eucharist, is eminently suited to inform our ethics in this area. The eucharistic image that symbolizes (among other things) a sacrificial giving of self to give life to another is so central to our highest moral ideals that it can serve outside of the particular faith and doctrine that specifically celebrates it. The idea that a donated heart is a precious gift given by a fellow human being who has died does exactly what is needed to restore to a situation of moral and emotional unease a feeling of "rightness".

Thus, we can conclude that transplantation is a realm in which rational arguments seem unerringly to lead toward certain conclusions, but meet, at certain points, almost immovable intuitive barriers. These barriers are resistant to argument and deserve deep respect because of their place in our sense of what is right and wrong in human life. The reservations we feel about transplantation can be countered by images that direct our intuitive associations toward the graciousness of giving and the supreme value of the gift of life. For each ethical issue we need to scrutinize it using both reasoned arguments based on a commitment to human life and a set of images and symbols that allow us to see things in a different light from the one that immediately comes to mind. The combination of both kinds of reflection is our best protection against unprincipled responses on the one hand or coldly rational and often superficial arguments on the other. This eclectic path allows us to be true to those deeper moral intuitions central in good ethical judgment and yet also to address issues when evolving technology demands novel ethical thought.

References

Arnold, R. M. and Younger, S. J. (1993). The dead donor rule: should we stretch it, bend it, or abandon it? *Kennedy Inst Ethics J*, **3**, 263–78.

Bailey, L. L. (1990). Organ transplantation: a paradigm of medical progress. *Hastings Center Rep*, **20**(1), 24–7.

Beecher, H. K. (1968). A definition of irreversible coma: report of the ad hoc Committee of the Harvard Medical School to examine the definition of brain death. *J Am Med Assoc*, **205**, 337–40.

Brecher, B. (1994). Organs for transplant: donation or payment. In *Principles of Health Care Ethics*, ed. R. Gillon, pp. 993–1002. Wiley & Sons: Chichester.

Campbell, C. (1992). Body, self and the property paradigm. *Hastings Center Rep*, **22**(5), 34–42.

Capron, A. M. (1987). Anencephalic donors: separate the dead from the dying. *Hastings Center Rep*, **17**(1), 5–9.

Cranford, R. N. (1986). Patients with permanent loss of consciousness. In *By No Extraordinary Means: The Choice to Forego Life Sustaining Food and Water*, ed. J. Lynn, pp. 186–94. Indiana University Press: Indianapolis.

Evans, M. (1990). A plea for the heart. *Bioethics*, **4**, 227–31.

Fox, M. and McHale, J. (1998). Xenotransplantation: the ethical and legal ramifications. *Med Law Rev*, **6**, 42–61.

Gillam, L. (1998). The more-abortions objection to fetal tissue transplantation. *J Med*

Phil, **23**, 411–27.

Gillett, G. (1986). Why let people die? *J Med Ethics,* **12**, 83–6.

Gillett, G. (1990). Consciousness, the brain, and what matters. *Bioethics,* **4**, 181–98.

Jennett, B. (1977). The diagnosis of brain death. *J Med Ethics,* **4**, 5–7.

Jennett, B. (1986). *High Technology Medicine.* Oxford University Press: Oxford.

Jennett, B. and Plum, F. (1977). Persistent vegetative state after brain damage. *Lancet,* **i**, 734.

Jones, D. G. (1991). Fetal neural transplantation: placing the ethical debate within the context of society's use of human material. *Bioethics,* **3**, 23–43.

Kearney, W., Vawter, D. E., and Gervais, K. G. (1991). Fetal tissue research and the misread compromise. *Hastings Center Rep,* **21**(5), 7–12.

Lamb, D. (1992). Organ transplants and anencephalic infants. In *Philosophy and Health Care,* ed. E. Matthews and M. Menlowe, pp. 124–34. Avebury Press: Aldershot.

Manohar, S. V. (1990). Medicolegal issues of the 1990s: an Indian perspective. In *Papers of the 9th Commonwealth Law Conference,* pp. 453–6. Commerce Clearing House: Auckland.

Murray, T. (1987). Gifts of the body and the needs of strangers. *Hastings Center Rep,* **17**(2), 30–8.

Nelson, J. L. (1992). Transplantation through a glass darkly. *Hastings Center Rep,* **225**, 6–8.

Pallis, C. (1982). ABC of brain stem death. *Br Med J,* **285**, 1409–12.

Pence, G. E. (1990). *Classic Cases in Medical Ethics.* McGraw-Hill: New York.

Poplawski, N. and Gillet, G. (1991). Ethics and embryos. *J Med Ethics,* **17**, 62–9.

Price, D. P. T. (1996). Contemporary transplantation initiatives:
where's the harm in them? *J Law Med Ethics,* **24**, 139–49.

Redman, R. B. (1986). How children can be respected as ends yet still be used as subjects in non-therapeutic research. *J Med Ethics,* **12**, 77–82.

Ross, L. F. (1994). Justice for children: the child as organ donor. *Bioethics,* **8**, 105–26.

Thielicke, H. (1970). *The Doctor as Judge of Who Shall Live and Who Shall Die,* Fortress: Philadelphia.

Thomson, J. J. (1986). Killing, letting die, and the trolley problem. In *Rights, Restitution, and Risk: Essays in Moral Theory,* by J. J. Thomson, ed. W. Parent, pp. 85–6. Harvard University Press: Cambridge, MA.

10

Psychoneuroimmunology and organ transplantation: theory and practice

Richard Kradin M.D. and Owen Surman M.D.

Introduction

Psychoneuroimmunology (PNI) is the science of nervous, endocrine, and immune interactions in health and disease. Unfortunately, the field of PNI has been largely neglected by transplant biologists, who traditionally have been inclined to view the immune system as an autonomous network of host defense. However, the last decade has witnessed considerable progress in our understanding of the structural and functional pathways of neuroimmune interaction. In light of these advances, the role of PNI in organ transplantation warrants increased attention.

Transplantation is a viable clinical option for patients with a variety of end stage organ disorders. However, despite its overall success, this approach poses a variety of clinical challenges. Patients come to organ transplantation after a protracted illness, in which at least one vital organ has failed. As a rule they have previously been subjected to prolonged polypharmaceutical interventions. Anxiety and mood disorders are common, often reflecting either failed coping mechanisms including immunosuppresant mediator or the complications of metabolic encephalopathy. Frequent hospitalizations and invasive procedures also predispose these patients to developing phobias, panic disorder, and post-traumatic stress disorder (PTSD) (Surman 1989).

Successful integration of the transplanted organ is a psychosomatic challenge. From a psychodynamic perspective, the graft can be viewed as a liminal object, one that is foreign, yet also part of self. Castelnuovo-Tedesco (1981) has suggested that the graft is not psychologically inert and that mental factors can affect graft outcome. However, the successful psychological integration of "graft-as-self" is impeded by the interminable requirements of immunosuppression and clinical monitoring.

No systematic study has addressed whether psychological factors can influence the immune response to the allograft. Viederman has presented case reports, in which he attributed allograft rejection primarily to psychological conflicts (Viederman 1974, 1975; Castelnuovo-Tedesco 1981). Surman (1989) has suggested that unresolved conflicts between the recipient and donor can lead to poor compliance with immunosuppressant medication regimens. For example, he attended to a man in his early twenties with chronic renal failure who had harbored longstanding anger toward his father. When his father subsequently became the patient's living kidney donor, the patient grew noncompliant with his immunosuppressive regimen and a serious episode of acute allograft rejection ensued. A psychiatric hospital admission was required, in order to address the impact of his intrapsychic conflicts and major depression. As these conditions improved, stable allograft function was also achieved.

Immunity and the mind

Both Sigmund Freud and Élie Metchnikoff adopted metaphors of defense in their respective models of mind and immunity (Kradin et al. 1997). The appropriateness of this common "military" metaphor is founded in the remarkable strategic similarities shared by the nervous and immune systems. For example, both systems have developed processes for the reception, processing, storage, and recall of information. Whereas transplant immunologists traditionally adhere to the position that the immune system represents a functionally autonomous unit, there are good reasons to reconsider this limited perspective and begin to address how immune and neuroendocrine activities are integrated in the host response to the allograft antigens. Progress towards this goal has been substantially fostered by recent findings that immune, nerve, and endocrine cells communicate with each other via networks of nerves and soluble "information factors."

The discrimination of "self" from "nonself" is the aim of many neuronal and immune responses. In this regard, Kradin has proposed that Edelman's model of learning and remembering in the central nervous system (CNS) has important parallels in the immune system (Kradin 1995). Common strategies that yield specific "recall" in these systems include: (a) isomorphic recognition of informational stimuli, (b) categorization of stimuli, and (c) the attribution of "value" to the stimulus with respect to self.

In the immune system, specific isomorphic responses to antigen are mediated by T and B cells. These cells express receptors with invariate antigen-combining sites (Jerne 1971), so that during a recall, or "memory," response, isomorphic accuracy is assured by the clonal expansion of antigen-specific T lymphocytes and by the secretion of specific antibodies by B cells. Categorization is generated by subsystems of lymphokines that display pleiotropic biological activities during an encounter with antigen. Physicochemical features of the antigen, as well as factors produced by non-major histocompatability complex (MHC) restricted antigen-presenting cells (Janeway and Bottomly 1994), determine the types of cytokines

Table 10.1. Summary of type 1 (T helper-1) and type 2 (T helper-2) cytokines

	Type 1	Type 2
Characteristic cytokines	IL-2, IFN-γ, TNF-α	IL-4, IL-5, IL-6, IL-10, IL-13
Major immune functions	DTH (delayed type hypersensitivity), cytotoxicity	B cell help, eosinophil and mast cell stimulation
Responses	Proinflammatory, graft rejection, endogenous pyrogen release	Graft tolerance, hypothalamic release of ACTH

IL interleukin; IFN, interferon; TNF, tumor necrosis factor; ACTH, adrenocorticotropic hormone.

produced by antigen-specific T-cells.

At least two major categories of lymphokines (Table 10.1) exist (Mossman and Coffman 1994), and immune responses may be considered as either "balanced" or "polarized" with respect to these types of cytokines provided. Type 1, or T helper (H) 1, lymphokines, including interleukin (IL)-2, interferon (IFN)-γ, and tumor necrosis factor (TNF)-α (Carter and Dutton 1996), mediate proinflammatory responses with features of delayed type-hypersensitivity (DTH) and lymphocyte-mediated cytotoxicity. These responses play critical roles in effecting cell-mediated allograft rejection. Type 1 cytokines also are active within the CNS, where they promote pyrogenic responses at the level of the hypothalamus and the release of adrenocorticotropic hormone (ACTH) by anterior pituicytes (Weigent and Blalock 1994).

A complementary subset of type 2 (TH-2) lymphokines includes IL-4, IL-5, IL-6, IL-10, and IL-13. These cytokines antagonize the production and activities of type 1 cytokines (Mossman and Coffman 1994), so that a "yin–yang" of immune homeostasis exists. Polarized type 2 responses are associated with atopy and immune tolerance to antigens in the allografts (Gianello, Fishbein, and Sachs 1993).

Bidirectional transfer and processing of information may occur between the nervous and immune systems. For example, sensory afferent neuropeptide-immunoreactive nerves, which are distributed within the mucosal linings of gut and lung, have been demonstrated to project to thalamic and hypothalamic nuclei in the rat brain. These areas in turn show rich associative input from the limbic system, and project to nuclei of the autonomic nervous system (C. Saper, personal communication). As these are areas that also participate in the generation of affect and mood, it is possible that input from mucosal immune responses may influence psychological states. Conversely, neuronal projections from higher cortical centers in the CNS may influence autonomic nervous and endocrine system output to peripheral immune tissues and potentially contribute to the modulation of immune responses.

The immune system, by virtue of its ability to recognize and respond to antigen with "memory," develops its own unique history (Blalock 1984). And like neuronal memory, anamnesis by the immune system appears to represent a "reconstruction" of immune events (Edelman 1989), and one that is potentially subject to inaccuracies, or "false immune memories." The total set of possible anamnestic immune responses constitutes an "immune self," that is, in turn, a subset of the larger psychosomatic "self" (Tauber 1995). In this regard, organ transplantation represents a major event in the history of the immune system and in the psychology of self.

The mechanisms of recognition, learning, and response in the immune system are obviously different from those in the nervous system; however, strategic similarities are evident. For example, in the nervous system, exteroceptive stimuli are first detected by sensory afferent nerves distributed along mucosal and cutaneous surfaces. Information from these encounters is rapidly transmitted centrally to the neuraxis, where it is further processed.

A similar strategy has been adopted by the immune system, in which afferent cells capable of recognizing antigen are strategically located at sites where nonself is likely to be encountered (Blalock 1984). During an antigen-specific immune response, this initial recognition of nonself antigen is mediated by dendritic cells (DC), highly specialized antigen-presenting cells that express high levels of "self" major histocompatibility antigens, (Xia, Pinto and Kradin 1995). The DC at mucosal surfaces generate a network of interdigitating processes that closely resembles a neuronal network. (Figure 10.1) The DC are also located in immediate proximity to substance P-immunoreactive nerve fibers within the mucous of lung (Kradin et al. 1997) and gut, and in skin. In addition, DC respond functionally to neuropeptides, suggesting that neuroimmune interactions may modulate the early response to antigen.

Following this initial encounter, antigen is "processed" by DC in tissues and transported by DC to lymph nodes, where it is presented directly to B and T lymphocytes. In the lymph node, critical decisions are made concerning whether a "productive" or "tolerant" response will be generated. In cases where a secondary exposure to antigen yields immune inflammation, there is evidence to suggest that peripheral autonomic nerves participate in the localization of circulating immune cells to sites of antigen deposition (Kradin 1995; Kradin et al. 1997).

Psychoneuroimmune communication

The status of PNI has been fostered by evidence that a network of communication (Figure 10.2) exists between neuroendocrine and immune cells. This

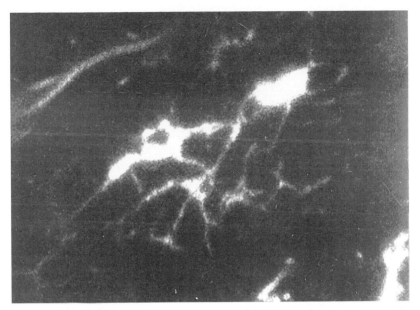

Figure 10.1. Network of dendritic antigen-presenting cells in the tracheal mucosa. Note the pattern of interconnecting dendritic processes mimicking neuronal networks. Cells were stained for class II major histocompatibility (Ia) antigens and examined by confocal microscopy ($\times$ 400).

bidirectional cross-talk promotes integration of neuroimmune responses and significantly enhances the complexity and diversity of immune responses.

While the functional anatomy of neuroimmune interactions is still being elucidated, it is generally accepted that two major output pathways of signaling from the central nervous system (CNS) to immune cells exist: (a) the neuroendocrine hypothalamic pituitary adrenal axis (HPA) (Figure 10.3) and (b) peripheral nerve fibers derived from nuclei of the autonomic nervous system.

Much of the evidence supporting the ability of the CNS to modulate the immune response is based on lesioning of the brain (Felten et al. 1991). Ablation of selected cortical regions and subcortical nuclei alters immune reactivities, and areas of the brain that are concerned primarily with the generation and regulation of affect, e.g. the limbic system, appear to be critical in influencing immunity. For example, lesioning the preoptic/anterior hypothalamic nuclei yields suppression of both cell-mediated and humoral responses. These effects are mediated primarily by the HPA axis and are abrogated by hypophysectomy.

The influence of brain hemispheres on immunity is asymmetric; lesions of right versus left brain yield enhancement or suppression of T cell immune responses, respectively (Renoux and Bizzierre 1991). These observations raise important questions concerning the impact of hemispheric dominance,

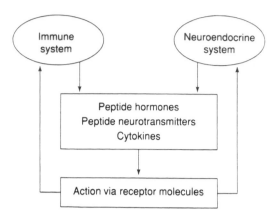

Figure 10.2. Molecular communication between neuroendocrine and immune systems. (From Blalock 1994.)

handedness, and imaginal versus linguistic informational processing on immunity.

Pituitary cells, hypothalamic and sensory neurons, and glial-support cells synthesize and secrete certain regulatory cytokines that are identical at both the gene and protein levels to those produced by immune leukocytes (Blalock 1994). In addition, lymphocytes secrete a variety of neuropeptides and traditional endocrine hormones (Table 10.2), including ACTH, endorphins, thyroid-stimulating hormone, growth hormone, and prolactin (Mitrova and Mayer 1976; Smith and Blalock 1981; Cross and Roszman 1989; Blalock 1994; Weigent and Blalock 1994). Lymphoid cells possess functional receptors for many of the endocrine factors produced along the HPA axis, whereas neuronal and endocrine cells express receptors for a variety of cytokines, e.g., IL-1, IL-2, IL-3, and IL-6, that are released by immune cells.

Certain proinflammatory cytokines, including IL-1, IL-2, IL-6 and TNF-α, bind to nerve cells in the CNS and modulate the homeostasis of vegetative functions, including body temperature, appetitive drives, and sleep. Cytokines also participate in the somatic response to stress, by binding to cells along the HPA axis and increasing adrenergic tone.

Direct neuronal influences on immunity are well documented. Both central and peripheral lymphoid tissues are richly innervated by postganglionic sympathetic nerve fibers (Felten et al. 1985). These axons terminate in immediate proximity to lymphocytes and macrophages, yielding effector junctions that are physiologically capable of transmitting signals to lymphoid cells. As lymphocytes are motile cells that circulate from lymphoid tissues via the peripheral blood to extralymphoid tissues, direct neuronal influences are probably short lived. However, the vasculature and certain "fixed" stromal cells within lymphoid tissues may represent targets of neuronal modulation.

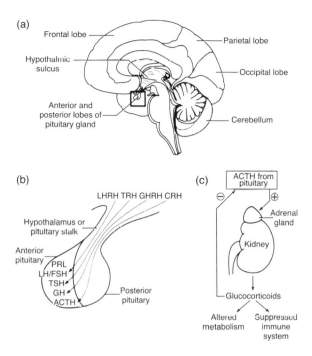

Figure 10.3. The hypothalamic–pituitary–adrenal axis. (a) Medial surface of brain showing cortical and subcortical relationships; (b) effects of hypothalamic releasing hormones in pituitary hormone release; effects of ACTH and adrenal cortical release of glucocorticoids.

PRL, prolactin-releasing hormone; LHFSH, luteinizing hormone/follicle-stimulating hormone; TSH, thyroid-stimulating hormone; GH, growth hormone, ACTH, adrenocortico-tropic hormone; LHRH, luteinizing hormone-releasing hormone; TRH, thyrotropin-releasing hormone; GHRH, growth hormone-releasing hormone; CRH, corticotropin-releasing hormone. (From Blalock 1994.)

Sympathetic innervation has a positive trophic effect on lymphoid tissue, and pharmacological ablation of postganglionic adrenergic neurons leads to lymphoid atrophy in vivo (Madden, Felten, and Felten 1994). Unlike, the sympathetic nervous system, the effects of parasympathetic innervation on lymphoid tissues have not been well established. However, epithelium-lined organs are rich in parasympathetic nerves, and it is likely that the cholinergic system affects mucosal immunity. This hypothesis is supported by the fact that many cholinergic nerves also produce neuropeptides (see below).

A third set of nonadrenergic and noncholinergic (NANC) nerves synthe-size and release neuropeptides (Weigent and Blalock 1994) and participate in immune responses. Substance P (SP), neurokinins A/B, vasoactive intestinal peptide (VIP), calcitonin gene-related peptide (CGRP) and others, released

Table 10.2. Cellular sources of peptide hormones and neurotransmitters in the immune system

Source	Peptides or proteins
T lymphocytes	ACTH, endorphins, TSH, chorionic gonadotropin, GH, PRL, [Met]enkephalin, parathyroid hormone-related protein, IGF-I
B lymphocytes	ACTH, endorphins, GH, IGF-I
Macrophages	ACTH, endorphins, GH, substance P, IGF-I, atrial naturetic peptide
Splenocytes	LH, FSH, CRH
Thymocytes	CRH, LHRH, AVP, OT
Mast cells and PMN cells	VIP, somatostatin
Megakaryocytes	Neuropeptide Y

ACTH, adrenocorticotropic hormone (corticotropin); AVP, arginine-vasopressin; GRH, corticotropin-releasing hormone; FSH, follicle-stimulating hormone; GH, growth hormone; IGF-I, insulin-like growth factor I; LH, luteinizing hormone; LHRH, luteinizing hormone-releasing hormone; OT, oxytocin; PMN, polymorphonuclear; PRL, prolactin; TSH, thyroid-stimulating hormone; VIP, vasoactive intestinal peptide.
From Blaloch 1994.

by NANC sensory afferent nerves and by a subset of cholinergic nerves in lung, gut and skin, can diffuse locally to bind to peptide receptors expressed by regional immune cells. Recent findings indicate that a constitutive isoform of nitric oxide synthase (B-NOS) that catalyzes the production of nitric oxide (NO) from arginine is co-localized in NANC nerve endings (Fischer and Hoffman 1996). NO, a short-lived radical with pleiotropic biological activities, is a potent vasodilator and an inhibitor of T lymphocyte activities (Bilyk and Holt 1995).

The importance of peripheral nerves in inflammation is evidenced by the failure of certain immune disorders, including mast cell-mediated urticaria and autoimmune arthritis (Felten et al. 1992), to develop in denervated limbs. Both capsaicin, a toxin of the Cayenne pepper that damages small unmyelinated nerves containing neuropeptides, and pharmacological inhibitors of tachykinins (SP and neurokinins) can potently suppress the development of pulmonary delayed-type hypersensitivity responses in rats (Kradin et al. 1997; Kaltreider et al. 1997). This finding raises the possibility that tissue denervation, an invariable complication of organ extirpation and implantation during transplantation, may influence the local immune response to the allograft.

Behavioral aspects of psychoimmune interaction

Attempts have been made to link immunological function to behavioral changes. In a now classic study of behavioral conditioning in the immune system, Ader and Cohen developed a taste-aversion conditioning paradigm to generate immunosuppression using cyclophosphamide as an unconditioned stimulus (Ader and Cohen 1985; Ader 1987). Mice stimulated in this protocol were eventually able to produce immunosuppressive responses to a stimulus in their drinking water in the absence of cyclophosphamide, the "active" immunomodulating drug. A similar model has been successfully adapted to suppress autoimmune reactivity in NZB-mice and to suppress graft-versus-host responses (Borbjerg, Ader, and Cohen 1982; Ader et al 1991).

Investigations in clinical psychobiology suggest that immune and neuronal responses are genetically codetermined. For example, while examining the psychologic and physiologic differences between "shy" and "bold" children, Kagan and colleagues noted that the shy and behaviorally inhibited children, who are at increased risk of developing panic disorder and social phobia as adults, displayed evidence of sustained sympathetic tone and an increased prevalence of atopic allergies (Arcus 1994).

Differences in immune reactivity have also been associated with personality differences. Heisel et al. (1986) studied scores on the Minnesota Multiphasic Personality Inventory (MMPI) in 114 college students. Their scores on the "ego strength scale" were correlated positively with natural killer (NK) cell activity, whereas evidence of "ego fragility" and psychopathology on other psychometric scales was associated with diminished NK cell activity.

Stress and immunity

Since antiquity, there has been a widespread belief among the lay public that stress is deleterious to health. The association between stress and susceptibility to infection in humans was elegantly characterized in Dubos' account of how the destruction of the Irish potato crop in the mid-nineteenth century contributed to the epidemic spread of pulmonary tuberculosis (Dubos 1959). Social stress related to love loss was correlated with increased morbidity from pulmonary tuberculosis by Kissen (1958), who was working with subjects in the slums of Glasgow. More recently, Keicolt-Glaser et al. found decreased cellular immune function in the spouses of dementia patients (Keicolt-Glaser, Dura, and Spreicher 1991). In those studies, subjects with the most severe immunologic deficits proved to have the least social support.

A relationship between stress and immunity has been demonstrated in laboratory animals. At a National Institutes of Health (NIH) conference in

Table 10.3. Catecholamines and immune function

Anatomic findings	Sympathetic fibers innervate primary and secondary lymphoid tissues Chemical denervation by 6-hydroxydopamine leads to lymph node atrophy Lymphoid cells express adrenergic receptors
Effects of T cell migration	Adrenaline decreases circulating CD4$^+$ T cells in vivo Decreased CD4$^+$ lymphocytes in spleen and increased CD4$^+$ lymphocytes in lung following parenteral injection of adrenaline Adrenaline yields a specific compartmental shift of CD4$^+$CD45RO$^+$ lymphocytes from spleen to lung Increased T cell motility in vitro
Functional responses to adrenaline	Minimal changes in proliferation and IL-2 production to mitogens in vitro Augments response to HEL antigen in genetically low responder mice (B6) but decreases response to HEL in high responder Balb/c

IL, interleukin; HEL, hen-eggs lysozyme.

1992, Sternberg and coworkers stressed that activation or suppression of the HPA axis "is not simply an epiphenomenon, but has physiologic relevance for the severity of susceptibility to inflammation..." (Sternberg et al. 1992). Take for example the diverse and complex effects of catecholamines on immunologic function (Table 10.3).

As noted above, Felten and coworkers demonstrated that central and peripheral lymphatic tissues are innervated by fibers of the sympathetic autonomic nervous system, and that chemical denervation by 6-hydroxydopamine leads to lymph node cell depletion (Felten et al. 1985). Crary et al. (1982) showed that physiologic levels of adrenaline in humans decreased the number of circulating CD4$^+$ lymphocytes. Kradin and coworkers demonstrated that parenteral injection of adrenaline yielded a rapid decrease in labeled murine splenic CD4$^+$ lymphocytes with a concomitant increase of these cells in the lung (Rodberg, Surman, and Kradin, 1999). This finding was accounted for by a specific compartmental shift in CD4$^+$CD45RO$^+$ "memory" cells in the lung and was blocked in vivo by propranolol.

An "unmasking" effect on T cell immunity has also been observed in response to adrenaline (Rodberg and Kradin 1998). B6 strain mice, which normally respond weakly to ovine antigen, hen-egg lysozyme (HEL), developed normal responses to HEL after receiving daily injections of adrenaline during the phase of antigen sensitization. Interestingly, when treated comparably, a high responder strain of mice (A/J) displayed decreased reactivity to HEL, suggesting that the genetic background, or state of the responding mice, can influence whether immune activities are augmented or decreased by adrenaline. The immune-enhancing effects of adrenaline in the B6 strain were specifically abrogated by the elimination of CD8$^+$ lymphocytes *in vivo*, indicating that these cells play a critical role in mediating the response.

Activation of the HPA axis leads to release of glucocorticoids, which have a wide variety of effects on the immune response (Barnes 1996). Glucocorticoids suppress the secretion of IL-1b, IL-2, TNF-α, granulocyte–macrophage colony-stimulating factor, IL-3, IL-4, IL-5, and IL-6, and block the synthesis of chemokines, including IL-8 and monocyte chemoattractant protein (MCP)-1. Synthetic inhibition reflects the ability of glucocorticoids to bind AP-1, a nuclear factor that normally complexes with NF-AT, in order to initiate cytokine gene transcription. Steroids also antagonize the synthesis of inducible nitric oxide synthase (iNOS) and the expression of endothelial cell adhesion molecules, including intercellular adhesion molecule (ICAM)-1, vascular adhesion molecule (VCAM)-1, and endothelial cell (E)-selectin. The effects of HPA activation and glucocorticoid release on lymphocyte circulation and endothelial adhesion have been reviewed elsewhere by Ottaway and Husband (1994).

Steroids regulate a variety of receptor molecules critical to immune homeostasis. The expression of neurokinin-1 receptors, which mediate the response to SP, are reduced, whereas β-adrenergic receptors are increased by steroids. Finally, glucocorticoids promote lymphocyte cytolysis by signaling pathways of apoptosis (Penninger and Kroemer 1998).

Psychiatric disorders and immunity

Depressive disorders became a popular focus of immunologic investigation after diminished lymphocyte responses to mitogen were noted in bereaved individuals. While the mechanisms of this finding are uncertain, major depression probably diminishes immune function in part by yielding elevated plasma cortisol levels (Levy et al. 1991). Unfortunately, the effects of depression on immunity have often appeared contradictory. In a review of the psychoimmunology literature, Stein, Miller, and Trestman (1991) noted that variables including age, sleep patterns, activity level, diet, substance abuse, degree and type of depression, medications, and immunologic methodology were often uncontrolled. Despite these confounding variables, a recent meta-analysis by Herbert and Cohen (1993) clearly supports the conclusion that cellular immunity is reduced in major depression.

The effects of anxiety disorders on immune function have also been investigated. Patients with untreated panic disorder have shown immune abnormalities in some studies. Whereas a study of mitogen-induced lymphocyte proliferation in 36 panic patients showed no diminution in immunologic function, Ramesh et al. (1991) examined 59 panic disorder patients and found significantly lower lymphocyte levels and higher levels of serum IgA. Perini and coworkers recently noted a decreased number of $CD3^+$ lymphocytes in the blood of patients with panic disorder (Perini et al. 1995).

Kradin and coworkers detected a significant increase in naive $CD45RA^+$ lymphocytes and increased expression of the CD62L (L-selectin) lymph node homing receptor in 30 untreated patients with panic disorder. This was associated with "high-normal" plasma levels of cortisol and decreased ex vivo IL-2 production by blood lymphocytes (Manfro et al., 1999). Levels of lymphocyte CD62L correlated positively with Hamilton-Anxiety (HAM-A) and Hamilton-Depression (HAM-D) scores, as well as with the severity of panic. CD62L expression also correlated with cortisol levels in panic disorder. Parallel ex vivo experiments showed that CD62L expression is normally downregulated by IL-2 following mitogen stimulation, but remained elevated when lymphocytes were activated in the presence of dexamethasone, suggesting that elevated glucocorticoid levels might be responsible for the diminished conversion of $CD62L^+$ naive to $CD62L^-$ memory lymphocytes in panic disorder.

The immunological changes in anxiety disorders are apparently heterogeneous. In a study from the same laboratory, van der Kolk and co-workers (Wilson et al. 1999) examined 10 never-treated sexually traumatized patients who met DSM-IV criteria for post-traumatic stress disorder (PTSD). A trend towards increased immune memory $CD45RO^+$ lymphocytes in the peripheral blood of patients was detected and a significantly increased ratio $CD45RO^+/CD45RA^+$ lymphocytes in the peripheral blood was observed, consistent with increased immune activation in vivo. Unlike in panic disorder, basal cortisol levels were "low-normal" in patients with PTSD, a finding that is consistent with previously noted abnormalities in HPA axis activation in PTSD and chronic stress.

Endocrine regulators of immunity

Whereas the role of sex hormones in regulation of immune function is poorly understood, their importance may be evidenced by the increased female to male incidence of autoimmune disorders, including systemic lupus erythematosus (SLE) (9 : 1) and rheumatoid arthritis (4 : 1). Vidaller et al.

(1986) cited evidence of increased prolactin in some men with SLE and suggested a role for prolactin in suppressor cell responses during pregnancy.

Kincade et al. (1994) have reviewed the effects of estrogen and progesterone on B cell lymphopoiesis in pregnancy and in non-gravid women. In addition to its effects at the level of marrow stromal cell estrogen receptors, estrogen may influence B cell formation by inhibiting insulin growth-factor binding proteins, cellular adhesion molecules, and other mediators. Clarke and Kendall (1994) have reviewed the neuronal, immune, and endocrine effects on thymic involution in pregnancy, a time-limited state during which immune tolerance is required to protect the developing allogeneic fetus.

The immune enhancing effects of prolactin are antagonized by cyclosporine A, which competitively binds to a site on the T cell prolactin receptor (Heistand et al. 1986). Bernton postulated that prolactin might act as a counterregulatory hormone and that its suppression of glucocorticoid activity could play a role in both stress and aging (Bernton 1989; Bernton, Bryant, and Holaday 1991).

Neuropharmacology and allograft rejection

In view of the current understanding of neuronal transmission and receptor expression by immune and other cells in allografts, the effects of neuropharmacologic interventions on graft activity and survival are pertinent. Pierpaoli and Maestroni (1978) used a combination of drugs with neuroimmunologic activity in mice undergoing skin grafting. By combining dopamine, 5-hydroxytryptamine, phentolamine, and haloperidol, they were able to achieve a mean graft prolongation of 21 days.

Unfortunately, the results of psychoimmunologic animal studies are often in apparent conflict. In the Pierpaoli and Maestroni study, this effect was reversed by 5-hydroxytryptamine (HT). Surprisingly, ketanserine, an antihypertensive serotonin type-2 receptor antagonist, was shown to inhibit delayed-type hypersensitivity, and this effect was reversed by a HT 2R agonist (Ameisan, Meade, and Askenase 1989). These contradictory results may reflect differences in the functional activities mediated by serotonin receptor subtypes.

Bromocriptine, a dopamine agonist that produces hypoprolactinemia, has been reported to mediate immunosuppressive effects in animal studies and has also been used successfully to promote graft viability in experimental heart–lung transplantation (DiStefano et al. 1990). In contrast, Vidaller et al. (1986) reported that decreased cellular immune function in four patients with prolactin-secreting tumors was reversed by bromocriptine.

Clinical effects of psychotropic medications in the transplant patient population

Surman (1993) has reviewed the immunologic effects of standard psychotropic medications. Aside from the direct effect of these agents, we have observed that when clinical anxiety and depression in the post-transplantation period are recognized and effectively treated there can be a significant favorable effect on patient compliance with the demanding immunosuppressive drug regimens. The putative effects of the major subclasses of psychotropic medications on the immune response are reviewed briefly below.

Neuroleptic agents

Neuroleptic agents, including haloperidol, α-butyrophenone, and the phenothiazines, trifluoperazine and metaclopromide, are frequently used in the transplant population to control psychotic symptoms, nausea, and symptoms of diabetic neuropathy. These agents increase prolactin levels and may theoretically stimulate immune function via this pathway. However, Mitrova and Mayer (1976) found that neuroleptic agents suppressed cellular and humoral immune function in experimental tick-borne encephalitis. Neuroleptics also have cytoprotective effects and they can potentially suppress immune function via α-adrenergic blockade.

Benzodiazepines

Anxiolytic agents, such as alprazolam, lorazepam, and oxazepam, are often used perioperatively in the transplant population. Among these agents, alprazolam is known to inhibit thromboxane-2 and platelet-activation factor. A benzodiazepine inverse agonist, FG 7142, decreases cytotoxic T cell and NK cell activity (Arora, Hanna, and Skolnick 1991).

Antidepressants

The successful treatment of major depression with antidepressants may reverse the immunosuppressive effects thought to be associated with this disease. Several of the tricyclic antidepressants (TCAs), including doxepin, amitriptyline, and clomipramine, and all of the selective serotonin reuptake inhibitors (SSRIs), i.e., fluoxetine, sertraline, paroxetine, and fluvoxamine, can increase central and possibly peripheral nervous system levels of serotonin. The widespread prescription and startling success of the SSRIs in the treatment of a variety of psychiatric disorders raises important questions concerning the role of serotonin and the effects of these drugs on the immune response.

Serotonin has activities within and outside of the CNS. Whereas a number of studies have implicated a role for serotonin in immunity, little is known concerning the immunological effects of the SSRIs. Schwartz et al. (1977) demonstrated that serotonin leads to inhibition of delayed-type hypersensitivity in mice. Calogero et al. (1990) reported induction of the HPA axis in the rat by 5-HT 1A agonist activity.

Other drugs used in the treatment of depression, notably methylphenidate, bupropion, and sertraline have dopamine-agonist properties. Miller and Lackner (1989) found a reduction in NK cell activity in depressed patients treated with the TCA desipramine. However, the effect required blood levels in excess of 625 ng/ml, which exceeds the accepted therapeutic range.

Lithium carbonate

Among psychotropic agents, lithium carbonate is perhaps most intriguing with respect to its potential immunologic properties. In the nervous system, lithium acts as a mood stabilizer, ameliorating both depressive and manic forms of psychopathology. Baraban et al. suggested that lithium decreases synaptic activity in overactive systems by inhibiting inositol phosphatase and blocking the activation of G-proteins (Baraban, Worley, and Snyder 1989).

Lithium has long been recognized to reduce neutropenia in patients undergoing cancer chemotherapy (Lyman, Williams, and Preston 1980). However, it also has effects on antigen-specific immune cells. For example, lithium modulates T cell signal transduction (Conroy et al. 1995; Deckert et al. 1995); Gelfand et al. (1979) found that it blocked cyclic AMP suppression of T cell function in patients with agammaglobulinemia. In addition, lithium may have antiviral effects, as it has been shown to limit the reactivation of herpetic infection (Lieb 1979; Amsterdam, Maislin, and Winokur 1989). In view of the recognized deleterious effects of T cell immune activation and DNA virus infections on allograft survival, a possible role for lithium in the immunological management of the allograft merits further consideration.

Summary

The study of PNI in organ transplantation is in its infancy. The nervous system and the immune system share a variety of strategies that are critical in discriminating self from nonself, making the transplantation arena an ideal site to explore neuroimmune interactions. There is currently irrefutable evidence to support neuroimmune interactions in the response to antigens, and it is likely that mind–body communication may be able to modify not only the general well-being of the organ recipient, but also the fate of the allograft. Psychotropic medications used to manage the psychiatric complications of end-organ failure and transplantation-related stress can modulate immunity, either indirectly via their effects on the nervous system, or by direct effects on immune cells. Focusing on the role of PNI in organ transplantation will substantially increase our understanding of psychosomatic interactions and contribute to the therapeutic management of this unique patient population.

References

Ader, R. (1987). Conditioned immune responses: adrenocorticol influences. *Prog Brain Res*, **72**, 79–90.

Ader, R. and Cohen, N. (1985). CNS-immune interactions: conditioning phenomena. *Behav Brain Sci*, **8**, 379–94.

Ader, R., Grota, L., Moynihan, J., and Cohen, N. (1991). Behavioral adaptations in autoimmune disease-susceptible mice. In *Psychoneuroimmunology*, 2nd edn, ed. R. Ader, N. Cohen, and D. Felten, pp. 685–708. Academic Press: New York.

Ameisan, J., Meade, R., and Askenase, P. (1989). A new interpretation of the involvement of serotonin in delayed type hypersensitivity: serotonin-2 receptor antagonists inhibit contact sensitivity by an effect on T-cells. *J Immunol*, **142**, 3171–9.

Amsterdam, J., Maislin, G., and Winokur, A. (1989). Lithium prophylaxis and recurrent labial herpes infection. (Abstract). In *28th Annual Meeting of the American College of Neuropharmacology*, Maui, Hawaii.

Arcus, D. (1994). Biological mechanisms and personality: evidence from shy children. *Advances*, **4**, 40–50.

Arora, P., Hanna, E., and Skolnick, P. (1991). Suppression of cytotoxic T-lymphocyte (CTL) activity by FG 7142, a benzodiazepine receptor "inverse agonist." *Immunopharmacology*, **21**, 91–7.

Barbaran, J., Worley, P., and Snyder, S. (1989). Second messenger system and psychoactive drug action: focus on the phosphoinositide system and lithium. *Am J Psychiatry*, **146**, 1251–60.

Barnes, P. (1996). Mechanisms of action of glucocorticoids in asthma. *Am J Resp Crit Care Med*, **154**, 521–7.

Bernton, E. (1989). Prolactin and immunity. *Prog Neuroendocr-Immunol*, **2**, 21–8.

Bernton, E., Bryant, H., and Holaday, J. (1991). Prolactin and immune function. In *Psychoneuroimmunology*, 2nd edn, ed. R. Ader, N. Cohen, and D. Felten, pp. 403–28. Academic Press: New York.

Bilyk, N. and Holt, P. (1995). Cytokine modulation of the immunosuppressive phenotype of pulmonary alveolar macrophage populations. *Immunology*, **86**, 231–7.

Blalock, J. (1984). The immune system as a sensory organ. *J Immunol*, **132**, 1067–70.

Blalock, J. (1994). The syntax of immune–neuroendocrine communication. *Immunol Today*, **15**, 504–11.

Borbjerg, D., Ader, R., and Cohen, N. (1982). Behaviorally conditioned suppression of a graft-versus-host response. *Proc Natl Acad Sci USA*, **79**, 583–5.

Calogero, A., Bagdy, G., Szemeredi, K, Tartaglia, M., Gold, P., and Chrousos, G. (1990). Mechanisms of serotonin agonist-induced activation of the hypothalmic–pituitary–adrenal axis in the rat. *Endocrinology*, **126**, 1888–94.

Carter, L. and Dutton, R. (1996). Type 1 and type 2: a fundamental dichotomy for all T-cell subsets. *Curr Opin Immunol*, **8**, 336–42.

Castelnuovo-Tedesco, P. (1981). Transplantation: psychological implications of change in body image. In *Psychonephrology I: Psychological Factors in Hemodialysis and Transplantation*, ed. N. Levy, pp. 218–25. Plenum: New York.

Clark, A. and Kendall, M. (1994). The thymus in pregnancy: the interplay of neural, endocrine and immune influences. *Immunol Today*, **15**, 545–51.

Conroy, L., Jenkinson, E., Owen, J., and Michell, R. (1995). Phosphatidylinositol 4,5-bisphosphage hydrolysis accompanies T-cell receptor-induced apoptosis of murine thymocytes within the thymus. *Eur J Immunol*, **25**, 1828–35.

Crary, B., Hauser, S., Borysenko, M. et al. (1982). Epinephrine induced changes in the distribution of lymphocyte subsets in peripheral blood of humans. *J Immunol*, **131**, 1178–81.

Cross, R. and Roszman, T. (1989). Neuroendocrine modulation of immune function: The role of prolactin. *Prog Neuroendocr Immunol*, **2**, 17–29.

Deckert, M., Ticchioni, M., Mari, B., Mary, D., and Bernard, A. (1995). The glycosyl-phosphatidylinositol-anchored CD59 protein stimulates both at cell receptor delta/ZAP-70 dependent and independent signaling pathways in T-cells. *Eur J Immunol*, **25**, 1815–22.

DiStefano, R., Carmellini, M., Carobbi, F. et al. (1990). Bromocriptine plus suboptimal cyclosporine treatment abrogates acute rejection of rat cardiac allografts. *Transplant Proc*, **22**, 2015–16.

Dubos, R. (1959). *Mirage of Health: Utopias, Progress and Biological Change*. Harper and Row: New York.

Edelman, G. (1989). *The Remembered Present*. Basic Books: New York.

Felten, D., Cohen, N., Ader, R. et al. (1991). Central neural circuits involved in neural–immune interactions. In *Psychoneuroimmunology*, 2nd edn, ed. R. Ader, N. Cohen, and D. Felten, pp. 3–25. Academic Press: New York.

Felten, D., Felten, S., Bellinger, D. et al. (1992). Noradrenergic and peptidergic innervation of secondary lymphoid organs: role in experimental arthritis. *Eur J Clin Invest*, **22**, 37–41.

Felten, D., Felten, S., Carlson, S., Olschowka, J., and Livnat, S. (1985). Noradrenergic and peptidergic innervation of lymphoid tissue. *J Immunol*, **135**, 755S–765S.

Fischer, A. and Hoffman, B. (1996). Nitric oxide synthase in neurons and nerve fibers of lower airways and in vagal sensory ganglia in man. *Am J Respir Crit Care Med*, **154**, 209–16.

Gelfand, E., Dosch, H., Hastings, B., and Shore, A. (1979). Lithium: a modulator of cyclic AMP-dependent events in lymphocytes? *Science*, **203**, 365–7.

Gianello, P. Fishbein, J., and Sachs, D. (1993). Tolerance to primarily vascularized allografts in miniature swine. *Immunol Rev,* **133,** 19–33.

Heisel, J., Locke, S., Kraus, L., and Williams, R. (1986). Natural killer cell activity and MMPI scores of a cohort of college students. *Am J Psychiatry,* **143,** 1382–6.

Heistand, P., Mekler, P., Nordmann, R. et al. (1986). Prolactin as a modulator of lymphocyte responsiveness provides a possible mechanism of action for cyclosporine. *Proc Natl Acad Sci USA,* **83,** 2599–603.

Herbert, T. and Cohen, S. (1993). Depression and immunity: a meta-analytic review. *Psychol Bull,* **113,** 472–86.

Janeway, C. and Bottomly, K. (1994). Signals and signs for lymphocyte responses. *Cell,* **76,** 275–85.

Jerne, N. (1971). The somatic generation of immune recognition. *Eur J Immunol,* **1,** 1–9.

Kaltreider, H., Ichikawa, S., Byrd, P. et al. (1997). Upregulation of neuropeptides and neuropeptide receptors in a murine model of immune inflammation in lung parenchyma. *Am J Resp Cell Mol Biol,* **16,** 133–44.

Keicolt-Glaser, J., Dura J., and Spreicher, C. (1991). Spousal caregivers of dementia victims: longitudinal changes in immunity and health. *Psychosom Med,* **53,** 345–62.

Kincade, P., Medina, L, Smithson, G., and Scott., D. (1994). Pregnancy: a clue to normal regulation of B lymphopoiesis. *Immunol Today,* **15,** 539–44.

Kissen, D. (1958). *Emotional Factors in Pulmonary Tuberculosis.* London: Tavistock.

Kradin, R. (1995). The immune self. *Perspect Biol Med,* **38,** 605–82.

Kradin, R., MacLean, J., Duckett, D. et al. (1997). Pulmonary response to inhaled antigen: I. Neuroimmune interactions promote the recruitment of dendritic cells and the cellular immune response to antigen. *Am J Pathol,* **150,** 1735–43.

Levy, E., Borrelli, D., Mirin, S. et al. (1991). Biological measures and cellular immunological function in depressed psychiatric inpatients. *Psychiatric Res,* **36,** 157–67.

Lieb, J. (1979). Remission of recurrent herpes infection during therapy with lithium (letter). *N Engl J Med,* **301,** 942.

Lyman, G., Williams, C., and Preston, D., (1980). The use of lithium carbonate to reduce infections and leukopenia during systemic chemotherapy. *N Engl J Med,* **302,** 257–60.

Madden, K., Felten, S., and Felten, D. (1994). Sympathetic nervous system modulation of the immune system. II. Evaluation of lymphocyte proliferation and migration in vivo by chemical sympathectomy. *J Neuroimmunol,* **49,** 67–75.

Manfro, G., Pollack, M., Otto, M., Scott, E., Rosenbaum, J., and Kradin., R. (1999). Altered immune function in patients with panic disorder. *Anxiety,* in press.

Miller, A. and Lackner, C. (1989). Tricyclic antidepressants and immunity. In *Progress in Psychiatry 16,* ed. A. Miller, pp. 85–103. American Psychiatric Press: Washington, DC.

Mitrova, E. and Mayer, V. (1976). Phenothiazine induced alterations of immune response in experimental tick-borne ecephalitis: morphological models of analysis of events. *Acta Virol (Praha),* **20,** 479–85.

Mossman, T. and Coffman, R. (1994). Different patterns of lymphokine secretion lead to different functional properties. *A Rev Immunol,* **7,** 145–73.

Ottaway, C. and Husband, A. (1994). The influence of neuroendocrine pathways on lymphocyte migration. *Immunol Today,* **511,** 511–17.

Penninger, J. and Kroemer, G. (1998). Molecular and cellular mechanisms of T lymphocyte apoptosis. *Adv Immunol*, **68**, 51–144.

Perini, G., Zara, M., Carraro, C. et al. (1995). Psychoimmunoendocrine aspects of panic disorder. *Human Psychopharmacol*, **10**, 461–5.

Pierpaoli, W. and Maestroni, G. (1978). Pharmacologic control of the hormonally modulated immune response. III. Prolongation of allogeneic skin graft rejection and prevention of runt disease by a combination of drugs acting on neuroendocrine function. *J Immunol*, **120**, 1600–13.

Ramesh, C., Yeragani, V., Balon, R., and Pohl, R. (1991). A comparative study of immune status in panic disorder patients and controls. *Acta Psychiatry Scand*, **84**, 396–7.

Renoux, G. and Bizzierre, K. (1991). Neocortex lateralization of immune function and of the activities of immuthiol, a T-cell specific immunopotentiator. In *Psychoneuroimmunology*, 2nd edn, ed. R. Ader, N. Cohen, and D. Felter, pp. 127–48. Academic Press: New York.

Rodberg, G., Surman, O., and Kradin, R. (1999). Epinephrine augments T-cell responses to antigen in low responder mice. *Pathobiology*, in press.

Rodberg, G. and Kradin, R. (1998). Epinephrine augments specific T-cell responses to antigen in C57BL/6 (H-26) weak-responder mice by a CD8⁺ lymphocyte-dependent mechanism. *Pathobiology*, **66**, 84–9.

Schwartz, A., Askenase, P., and Gershon, R. (1977). The effect of locally injected vasoactive amines on the elicitation of delayed type hypersensitivity. *J Immunol*, **118**, 159–65.

Smith, E. and Blalock, J. (1981). Human lymphocyte production of corticotropin and endorphine-like substances: Association with leukocyte interferon. *Proc Natl Acad Sci USA*, **78**, 7530–4.

Stein, M., Miller, A., and Trestman, R. (1991). Depression, the immune system and health and illness: findings in search of meaning. *Arch Gen Psychiatry*, **48**, 171–7.

Sternberg, E., Chrousos, G., Wilder, R., and Gold, P. (1992). The stress response and the regulation of inflammatory disease. *Ann Intern Med*, **117**, 854–66.

Surman, O. (1989). Psychiatric aspects of organ transplantation. *Am J Psychiatry*, **146**, 972–82.

Surman, O. (1993). Possible immunological effects of psychotropic medication. *Psychosomatics*, **34**, 139–43.

Tauber, A. (1995). *The Immune Self: Theory or Metaphor*. Cambridge University Press: New York.

Vidaller, A., Llorencte, L., Larrea F., Mendez, J., Alcocer-Varela, J., and Alarcon-Segovia, D. (1986). T-cell dysregulation in patients with hyperprolactinemia: effect of bromocriptine treatment. *Clin Immunol Immunopathol*, **38**, 337–43.

Viederman, M. (1974). The search for meaning in renal transplantation. *Psychiatry*, **37**, 283–90.

Viederman, M. (1975). Psychogenic factors in kidney transplant rejection: a case study. *Am J Psychiatry*, **132**, 957–9.

Weigent, D. and Blalock, J. (1994). Role of neuropeptides in the bidirectional communication between the immune and neuroendocrine systems. In *Neuropeptides and Immunoregulation*, ed. B. Scharrer, E. Smith, and G. Stefano, pp. 14–27. Springer-Verlag: Berlin.

Wilson, S., Kradin, R., Burbridge, J., Fisler, R., and van der Kolk, B. (1999). Immunologic activation in post traumatic stress disorder. *Psychosomatics*, in press.

Xia, W., Pinto, C., and Kradin R. (1995). The antigen-presenting activities of Ia+ dendritic cells shift dynamically from lung to lymph node after an airway challenge with soluble antigen. *J Exp Med*, **181**, 1275–83.

11

Pediatric transplantation

Robert D. Canning Ph.D. and Margaret L. Stuber M.D.

Introduction

Pediatric recipients of organ transplants and their families present a variety of psychological and ethical challenges to transplant teams and the psychologists and psychiatrists who work with them. Some of these are relatively similar to those of adult patients, but others differ in significant ways. For example, a primary difference between adult and pediatric transplants is that the majority of organ transplantation done in children is for congenital disorders such as biliary atresia or cardiac malformations (Fox and Swazey 1992). This means that the recipients are often very young, and require an adult, usually a parent, to act as the decision maker. Congenital illnesses also mean that the child has been chronically ill, often without an experience of normal development, and sometimes with quite delayed development. A third implication of a congenital illness is that it is not acquired by the patient, and thus is not subject to the recrimination about causation or concern for recurrence frequently raised by organ damage secondary to alcohol use, cigarette smoking, or diet, and often seen in the adult population (Craven and Rodin 1992).

These areas of difference between adult and pediatric organ transplantation will be the focus of the first part of this chapter: the unique epidemiology, role of the family, issues of development, and responses of staff for pediatric organ transplant recipients. The second part of the chapter will then discuss the usual psychological assessment and follow-up of pediatric organ transplant recipients, given these considerations.

Epidemiology

Pediatric patients accounted for 8.2% (1577) of all organ transplants in the USA in 1995 (UNOS 1997). From 1988 to 1995 only 6.6% (5160) of kidney transplantation performed in the U.S. were done on pediatric patients (UNOS 1997). In the same period, 10.7% (1802) of heart transplants, 17.3% (85) of heart–lung transplants, and 6.4% (230) of lung transplants in the USA were performed on pediatric patients (UNOS 1997). Almost 4000 liver transplants (16.7%) were performed on patients of less than 18 years of age,

Therefore, the meaning of the illness and treatment will change with the context, such as whether post-transplant medications are greater or smaller in number than those taken before (Stuber 1993). Previous functional level will also play a prominent role in the ability of the child to adapt following transplantation. Children with transplanted organs may not have attended school and, although cognitively intact, may be at a disadvantage when compared to their peers who have never missed substantial time from school (Stewart et al. 1991).

Although understanding ceases to be a limitation in the teen years, other developmental considerations become important (Stuber 1992). Adolescents are often quite capable of making their own decisions and should be involved in most medical decision making. It is also highly appropriate for adolescents to be responsible for their own medication. However, adolescents' usual suspicion of adults and their need to feel independent may lead to noncompliance. Developmental tasks of individuation must be considered in the assessment and follow-up of adolescent transplant patients (Stuber and Nader 1995).

Responses of staff

Children are generally viewed both as innocent victims of disease and as capable of behavioral change. These assumptions become important in the attitude of transplant teams toward selection of transplant candidates. Though there is no fixed set of psychosocial criteria for acceptance to the candidate list for adults (Olbrisch and Levenson 1996), there is somewhat more clarity than there is for children. Since the child is not the decision maker, was not responsible for the damage to the organ, and is not the primary agent for compliance, many of the usual concerns are not applicable. An argument could be made that the same issues apply to children as to adults, but instead must be applied to the assessment of the parents or guardian. Though this appears reasonable, it may lead to a child being disqualified for transplantation owing to a parent's problem, which is an uncomfortable situation for many clinicians.

Adolescents also raise emotional and controversial responses from the team. Some clinicians have gone so far as to say that the prevalence of noncompliance is high enough that adolescence should be considered at least a relative contraindication for organ transplantation (Stuber 1992). Those who view adolescents as people in transition argue that past or present behaviors are not adequate predictors of the future for these patients, and they must be given assistance and the benefit of the doubt. Others see adolescents as inherently high risk patients, who must be carefully screened and followed.

Clinical applications

Given the differences discussed above, how is the role of the psychiatrist or psychologist different when dealing with pediatric rather than adult transplant patients? The remainder of this chapter examines the tasks within the major phases of the transplantation: the pretransplantation evaluation, the waiting period, the transplantation hospitalization, and the post-transplantation follow-up.

Pretransplantation evaluation

Several review articles on pediatric transplantation have suggested outlines to be used in the initial transplant evaluation (Sexson and Rubenow 1992; Stuber 1993; Slater 1994). However, there are no formal pediatric screening instruments, at present, as exist for adults (Olbrisch, Levenson, and Hammer 1989; Levenson and Olbrisch 1993; Twillman et al. 1993). The following five basic areas of evaluation are common to most assessment batteries (Stuber and Canning, 1998):

1. Does the patient and family (however that is defined) understand the reasons for the transplantation, and have a realistic understanding of what will be required of them post-transplantation?
2. Are the patient and at least one significant adult committed to having this transplant?
3. Do the patient and family have the basic support and skills to provide the necessary medical care after the transplantation (e.g., telephone, transportation to the hospital or clinic, ability to administer a complex set of medications multiple times per day, judgment to perceive and respond to a medical emergency)?
4. Has the patient and responsible adult demonstrated an ability to adhere to medical instructions (e.g., compliance with medications, attendance at medical appointments)?
5. Are there any major psychiatric disturbances in this candidate or responsible adult?

The importance of the family changes the focus of the pretransplantation assessment for pediatric candidates, and complicates the teams' decision. Transplant teams are reluctant to disqualify a child for any reason, and are particularly unlikely to refuse to carry out a transplantation on a child because a parent has a psychiatric disorder. Added to this is the absence of any standardized assessment tools that might predict those who would have difficulties. Nonetheless, clinical experience is clear that, for children, the level of family chaos and parental psychopathology are important predictors of problems. Though it is possible that almost any child can be brought through a transplantation with sufficient interventions, cost is becoming a consideration that cannot be ignored (Stuber 1993; Slater 1994).

An intriguing recent study of adult transplant recipients found that axis I psychopathology was predictive of distress, both acutely and over time (Chacko et al. 1996). However, it was specifically character psychopathology that predicted noncompliance (Chacko et al. 1996). Clinical experience also suggests that it is axis II psychopathology in the parents that is most problematic for pediatric transplantations, predicting the amount of staff and psychosocial time the family will demand. Adolescents, who cannot have personality disorders by definition, also can present a history of behavior that signals a warning to the team. An obvious example is the teen presenting for liver transplantation after a suicide attempt with an overdose of acetaminophen. As noted in Olbrisch and Levenson's (1996) excellent article, there is a great deal of variability in the attitude of transplant teams to such scenarios. Those who hesitate to "waste" an organ that could save another life are very cautious about those who are seen as poor risks. Other teams are most concerned that they do not judge the relative value of lives, and neglect to save someone who could live. Often the question comes down to whether sufficient resources can be mobilized to help a child and family get through the transplantation and the subsequent treatment until the anti-rejection regimen can be stabilized and the child is functioning again.

Waiting

The period of time after the child has been placed on the candidate list, but before a match has been found, is extremely trying, full of excitement as well as fear. For those who plan a living related donor transplant, the uncertainty is greatly reduced, as is the time of waiting. However, the knowledge that the odds are good, but not perfect, remains to haunt all.

The waiting period is an ideal time to establish a therapeutic relationship, and provide the child and family with coping strategies to use during and after the transplant hospitalization. However, since families often live at some distance from the transplant center, such interventions are rarely done in any systematic way unless the family remains hospitalized or comes for outpatient follow-up. Relaxation techniques can be used to help the child and family to prepare for, or deal with, anticipatory anxiety or pain (Fanning 1988; Ross and Ross 1988). Practical help regarding discipline, school, and peer interactions can be useful for children who are still functioning in these normal arenas of childhood. Marital counseling is often necessary, as each spouse deals with the stress in his or her own way, and financial and parental worries can overwhelm the couple. Families may need to be made aware of the distress of the siblings, and the extra attention they will require (Stewart et al. 1993).

For younger children and families who are unfamiliar with the hospital, a tour can be extremely helpful in decreasing pretransplantation anxiety and allowing the family to prepare. Introductions to some of the staff and explanations of the types of machinery and tubes, especially in the intensive care unit and recovery room, are often provided by child development or child life workers. Explanations must be geared at a developmentally appropriate level, so that the child's questions are answered without being overwhelming.

The meaning of replacing an organ, or of receiving a donated organ, is an ongoing issue, but it is best to begin addressing this during the time before the transplantation. For some families, the type of organ has significance (such as the common attributions to the heart), while for others it is the source of the organ that has meaning. The living related donor's role can be complicated. Though it is important to acknowledge the sacrifice that is being made, family and staff must be careful not to create a situation in which the donor feels responsibility for the success or failure of the transplant. This is particularly true for siblings and parents who serve as donors.

Children who require extended pretransplantation hospitalizations present special challenges to their families and staff. The psychiatric consultant may have to assist the family and staff to understand the coping approaches each employs to avoid conflict and blame in this inherently stressful situation. Parents who are perceived by the staff as "abandoning" their children in reality may have conflicting demands, such as other young children, or may have difficulty tolerating the sense of helplessness they experience in watching their children's deterioration (Stutzer 1989; Stuber et al. 1995). Staff may take on nursing tasks that are perceived by the parents as intrusions on the parental role. At times, the boundaries may be blurred, and parents may take on tasks that are inappropriate, such as adjusting ventilator settings. Such extreme situations usually can be prevented by earlier interventions, particularly in cases in which there is overt evidence of parental psychopathology.

Transplantation hospitalization

The initial transplantation hospitalization raises fewer psychiatric concerns for solid organ transplant recipients, whose primary issues are pain control and adjustment of medication, than for bone marrow transplants. Bone marrow transplantation has quite a different type of hospital course. The prolonged period of protective isolation, while the new marrow is engrafting and while the recipient is immunocompromised, can be a crisis for the family (Stuber et al. 1996). The probability of death, both acutely and long term, is also higher for bone marrow transplantation than for solid organ transplantation.

Delirium is a less frequent consultation issue for pediatric transplant patients than for adults, though it is not clear whether this represents a difference in incidence or detection (Smith, Breitbart, and Platt 1995). Management is similar to that used for adults, with careful titration of intravenous droperidol or haloperidol being the most frequently successful approaches (Trzepacz, DiMartini, and Tringali 1993a,b).

Although depressed mood is common among post-transplant patients, it is rare for a pediatric patient to require antidepressant medication. If medication is used, dosages must be carefully titrated, as young children are more sensitive to the cardiovascular side effects, in addition to the usual issues of compromised metabolism or excretion in people with end-stage organ failure (Shaffer 1992). Often psychosocial interventions, such as the involvement of a child development specialist, can help the child to find some distractions, and improve their mood. At times, the depression reflects an inappropriate hopelessness, based on misinterpretations of events or comments. These can be investigated and clarified, in a developmentally sensitive manner. Staff often forget that young children may be able to repeat far more than they can understand, and they often hear much more than is intended. The concrete interpretations appropriate to the cognitive developmental stage of school-age children can also lead to confusion. A little investigation and discussion can accomplish a great deal for children who are misinterpreting events or who overheard conversations to mean that the transplant is failing or that they will never get any better.

Post-transplant follow-up

Once out of the hospital, the adjustment to post-transplant life must be made. For some, this is a liberation, with parents and children having to learn to tolerate new independence for children who were never before able to attend school or play with peers. For others, such as victims of acute viral cardiomyopathy, the limitations are new, as are the frequent doctor visits and medications. All must deal with the fear of rejection and keep constant vigilance for its subtle indicators. Side effects of medications are also common and are particularly difficult for children and adolescents who are sensitive to anything that makes them different from their peers.

Failure to take the medications as prescribed is common and dangerous. Recipients have many reasons for failing to comply, including the belief that the grafted organ is now a part of them and should no longer be seen as "foreign" (Didlake et al. 1988). Adolescents are particularly likely to wish to stop actions that set them apart or serve as reminders of the ways in which they differ from other teens. Anxiety may be triggered by reminders, and thus medications or medical visits may be avoided, in an effort to forget. The post-transplant vulnerability can also be used for manipulation. Unaware of the danger they were courting, adolescent recipients have stopped taking their medications in attempts to resolve custody disputes or fights with their parents. Unfortunately, the obvious symptoms of rejection are rather late, and do not provide an immediate disincentive for noncompliance with immunosuppressive drugs.

Transplantation is now common enough that schools have generally had some experience with recipients. However, schools with no prior experience may be very anxious, and require assistance in accepting students into their programs, and even into physical education programs. Classroom presentations also can be given to help the other students in the class to understand what has happened and to accept and support their classmate.

The long-term prognosis for pediatric transplant recipients is quite good. Studies of liver, kidney, and heart transplant recipients have found normal growth, return to school, and an absence of significant complications (Simmons, Klein, and Simmons 1977: Gersony 1990; Stewart et al. 1991). However, families who hope to return to "normal" may be quite upset with the number of medications and clinic visits that are required, especially in the first post-transplant year. The complications and monitoring make it difficult for both parents to return to full-time employment. The child's appearance is generally improved over the immediate pretransplantation time, but may not resemble the pre-morbid state, due to steroid-related weight gain or the hirsutism and gum hyperplasia associated with cyclosporine A. Similarly, although it appears that children do better cognitively after transplantation than before, there still may be deficits, particularly in children who had cyanotic heart disease (Hobbs and Sexson 1993; Stewart et al. 1994).

Some recent studies of children and adults have found evidence that medical life threat can be sufficient to precipitate post-traumatic stress symptoms, that can persist for years in both survivors and their parents (Alter et al. 1996; Pelcovitz et al. 1996; Kazak et al. 1997). Parents report more symptoms than children, and appear to influence the perceptions of life threat of their children (Kazak et al. 1998). This line of research has been fruitfully pursued with bone marrow transplantation (Pot-Mees 1989; Stuber et al. 1991; Stuber and Nader 1995), but only preliminary data are available to suggest that pediatric organ recipients (in particular adolescents) also suffer negative long-term psychological effects of medical trauma (M. L. Stuber, personal communication).

Psychopathology in the child or parents will be most problematic long term. These are the children who are difficult to get back to school, who have frequent unexplained incidents of rejection, or who simply drive the staff to distraction with their frequent telephone calls. Most worrisome are the parents with personality disorders, as they can cause splitting in the team in addition to the other types of problem. Psychiatric consultation can assist the team in setting clear expectations and limits, with equally clear and immediate consequences. In extreme circumstances, foster placement may be necessary to remove the child from a potentially dangerous family setting.

Summary

The role of a psychiatrist or psychologist in pediatric transplantation differs from adult work largely in the emphasis on family, developmental issues, and the response of the staff. The option of living related liver donors for young children raises additional ethical and psychological issues. Though transplant teams are reluctant to disqualify children as candidates for transplantation, there are clinical issues that can signal a need for significant intervention if rejection or other complications are to be avoided. Society has not yet decided how much we are willing to finance the psychosocial support that is necessary to pull some families through the transplant experience. Further research is needed to clarify the predictors, the types of intervention that appear to work, and the costs associated with these interventions. The role of the pediatric transplant psychiatrist or psychologist of the future may be to predict the needs and supply specific, targeted interventions for organ recipients and their families.

References

Alter, C. L., Pelcovitz, D., Axelrod, A. et al. (1996). Identification of PTSD in cancer survivors. *Psychosomatics*, **37**, 137–43.

Caplan, A. (1993). Must I be my brother's keeper? Ethical issues in the use of living donors as sources of liver and other solid organs. *Transplant Proc*, **25**, 1997–2000.

Chacko, R.C., Harper, R.G., Kunik, M., and Young, J. (1996). Relationship of psychiatric morbidity and psychosocial factors in organ transplant candidates. *Psychosomatics*, **37**, 100–7.

Chang, I. (1991). Baby girl's bone marrow transplanted into sister. *Los Angeles Times*, 5 June, p. 1.

Craven, J. and Rodin, G. M. (1992). *Psychiatric Aspects of Organ Transplantation*. Oxford: Oxford University Press.

Didlake, R.H., Dreyfus, K., Kerman, R.H., Van Buren, C.T., and Kahan, B.D. (1988). Patient noncompliance: a major cause of late graft failure in cyclosporin-treated renal patients. *Transplant Proc*, **20**, 63–9.

Fanning, P. (1988). *Visualization for Change*. Oakland, CA: New Habinger Publications.

Fox, R. C. and Swazey, J. P. (1992). *Spare Parts: Organ Replacement in American Society*. New York: Oxford University Press.

Gersony, W. M. (1990). Cardiac transplantation in infants and children. *J Pediatr*, **116**, 266–8.

Goldman, L. S. (1993). Liver transplantation using living donors: preliminary donor psychiatric outcomes. *Psychosomatics*, **34**, 235–40.

Hobbs, S. A. and Sexson, S. (1993). Cognitive development and learning in the pediatric organ transplant recipient. *J Learning Disabilities*, **26**, 104–13.

Kazak, A. E., Barakat, L. P., Meeske, K. et al. (1997). Posttraumatic stress, family functioning, and social support in survivors of childhood leukemia and their mothers and fathers. *J Clin Consult Psychol*, **65**, 120–9.

Kazak, A. E., Stuber, M. L., Barakat, L. P., Meeske, K., Guthrie, D. and Meadows, A. T. (1998). Predicting posttraumatic stress symptoms in mothers and fathers of survivors of childhood cancers. *J Am Acad Child Adolescent Psychiatry*, **37**, 823–31.

Kinrade, L. C. (1987). Preparation of sibling donor for bone marrow transplant harvest procedure. *Cancer Nur*, **10**(2), 77–81.

Kocoshis, S. A., Tzakis, A. G., Todo, S., Reyes, J., and Nour, B. (1993). Pediatric liver transplantation: history, recent innovations, and outlook for the future. *Clin Pediatr*, **32**, 386–92.

Levenson, J. and Olbrisch, M. (1993). Psychosocial evaluation of organ transplant candidates: a comparative study. *Psychosomatics*, **34**, 314–23.

Olbrisch, M. E. and Levenson, J. H. (1996). Psychological assessment of organ transplant candidates. *Psychosomatics*, **36**, 236–43.

Olbrisch, M. E., Levenson, J. H., and Hammer, R. (1989). The PACT: a rating scale for the study of clinical decision-making in psychosocial screening of organ transplant candidates. *Clin Transplant*, **3**, 164–9.

Pelcovitz, D., Goldenberg, B., Kaplan, S. et al. (1996). Post-traumatic stress disorder in mothers of pediatric cancer survivors. *Psychosomatics*, **37**, 116–26.

Pot-Mees, C. (1989). *The Psychosocial Effects of Bone Marrow Transplantation in Children*. Eubron Publishers: Delft.

Ross, D. M. and Ross, S. A. (1988). *Childhood Pain, Current Issues, Research, and Management*. Urban and Schwarzenberg: Baltimore, MD.

Sexson, S. and Rubenow, J. (1992). Transplants in children and adolescents. In *Psychiatric Aspects of Organ Transplantation*, ed. J. Craven and G. M. Rodin, pp. 33–49. Oxford: Oxford University Press.

Shaffer, D. (1992). Pediatric psychopharmacology. *Psychiatric Clin North Am*, **15**, 1–28.

Simmons, R. G., Klein, S. D., and Simmons, R. L. (1977). *Gift of Life: The Psychological and Social Impact of Organ Transplantation*. New York: John Wiley & Sons.

Singer, P. A., Siegler, M., Whittington, P. F. et al. (1989). Ethics of liver transplantation with living donors. *N Engl J Med*, **321**, 620–2.

Slater, J. A. (1994). Psychiatric aspects of organ transplantation in children and adolescents. *Child Adolescent Psychiatric Clin North Am*, **3**, 557–98.

Smith, M. J., Breitbart, W., and Platt, M. (1995). A critique of instruments and methods to detect, diagnose and rate delirium. *J Pain Symptom Management*, **10**, 35–77.

Stewart, S. M., Hiltebeitel, C., Nici, J., Waller, D. A., Uauy, R., and Andrews, W. S. (1991). Neuropsychological outcome of pediatric liver transplantation. *Pediatrics* **87**, 367–76.

Stewart, S. M., Kennard, B. D., De Bolt, A., Petrik, K., Waller, D. A., and Andrews, W. S. (1993). Adaptation of siblings of children awaiting transplantation. *Children's Health Care*, **22**, 205–15.

Stewart, S. M., Kennard, B. D., Waller, D. A., and Fixler, D. (1994). Cognitive function in children who receive organ transplantation. *Health Psychol*, **13**, 3–13.

Stuber, M. L. (1992). Psychologic care of adolescents undergoing transplantation. In *Textbook of Adolescent Medicine*, ed. E. R. McNarney, R. E. Kreipe, D. P. Orr, and G. D. Comerci, pp. 1138–42. Philadelphia, PA: W. B. Saunders Company.

Stuber, M. L. (1993). Psychiatric aspects of organ transplantation in children and adolescents. *Psychosomatics*, **34**, 379–87.

Stuber, M. L. and Canning, R. D. (1998). Organ transplantation. In *Handbook of Pediatric Psychology and Psychiatry*, vol. II, ed. R. T. Ammerman and J. V. Campo, pp. 369–82. Allyn & Bacon: Boston, MA.

Stuber, M. L., Caswell, D., Cipkala-Gaffin, J., and Billett, B. (1995). Nursing concerns regarding liver transplantation: a case for more nursing involvement. *Nurs Management*, **26**, 62–70.

Stuber, M. L. and Nader, K. (1995). Psychiatric sequelae in adolescent bone marrow transplant survivors: implications for psychotherapy. *J Psychother Prac Res*, **4**, 30–42.

Stuber, M. L., Nader, K. O., Houskamp, B. M., and Pynoos, R.S. (1996). Appraisal of life threat and acute responses in pediatric bone marrow transplant patients. *J Traumatic Stress*, **9**, 673–85.

Stuber, M. L., Nader, K., Yasuda, P., Pynoos, R. S., and Cohen, S. (1991). Stress responses after pediatric bone marrow transplantation: preliminary results of a prospective, longitudinal study. *J Am Acad Child Adolescent Psychiatry*, **30**, 952–7.

Stutzer, C. A. (1989). Work-related stresses of pediatric bone marrow transplant nurses. *J Pediatric Oncol Nurs*, **3**, 70–8.

Twillman, R. K., Manetto, C., Wellisch, D. K. et al. (1993). The transplant evaluation rating scale: a revision of the psychosocial levels system for evaluating organ transplant candidates. *Psychosomatics*, **34**, 133–54.

Trzepacz, P. T., DiMartini, A., and Tringali, R. (1993a). Psychopharmacologic issues in organ transplantation. Part I: Pharmacokinetics in organ failure and psychiatric aspects of immunosuppressant and anti-infectious agents. *Psychosomatics*, **34**, 199–207.

Trzepacz, P. T., DiMartini, A., and Tringali, R. (1993b). Psychopharmacologic issues in organ transplantation. Part II: Psychopharmacologic medications. *Psychosomatics*, **34**, 290–8.

UNOS (United Network of Organ Sharing) (1997). Database.

12

Current trends and new developments in transplantation

Maureen Martin M.D., F.R.C.S. (C)

Introduction

In less than 40 years organ transplantation has advanced from the experimental laboratory to clinical reality. As such, transplantation is now viewed as the treatment of choice for most forms of organ failure. The critical shortage of organ donors has resulted in the development of innovative surgical techniques, including reduced size organ partitioning, and a greater emphasis on living donation. Likewise, the public and legislators are being asked to consider novel approaches to organ donation such as Presumed Consent and financial incentives to organ donor families. The 1990s and the century beyond hold even greater promise for significant advances in our scientific knowledge and management of allograft rejection, immune tolerance, and cross-species transplantation. This chapter focuses on recent major advances in organ transplantation in the last decade and a better understanding of immunology introduced in clinical settings with new immunosuppressant agents that now challenge conventional protocols.

In addition, the concept of chimerism has invited new and exciting approaches to tolerance induction using bone marrow and stem cell-derived factors, combined with solid organ transplantation. Cell and intestinal transplants have also been initiated and will soon be included in routine clinical practice. Finally, the previously impossible feat of xenotransplantation has now been successfully carried out by the pivotal experiments in baboon to human liver transplants.

Special recognition for the exciting field of organ transplantation was recently awarded to Drs. Joseph Murray and E. Donnall Thomas, who received the 1990 Nobel Prize in Medicine for their visionary contributions to the fields of renal and bone marrow transplantation, respectively. The introduction of cyclosporine in the early 1980s, together with improvements in surgical technique and perioperative care, have resulted in unprecedented patient and graft survival. In addition, the last decade has seen an explosion of new immunosuppressive agents and innovative approaches to tolerance induction and more refined allograft survival.

Despite rapid proliferation in the number of transplant programs and, consequently, the number of candidates awaiting transplantation worldwide, the number of organ donors has remained relatively stable. This has seriously hampered the potential impact of many recent advances in immunosuppression and technology. Between 31 December 1988, and 31 December 1991, the number of American patients awaiting transplantation grew by 54% (from 16 026 to 24 719), while the number of organ donors increased by only 15.5%. Of concern were the number of deaths on the 1991 waiting list, which constituted a 59% increase over 1988 (UNOS 1991). In addition to the many challenges facing the transplant community, the most pressing one has been the dilemma of how to expand the organ donor pool. The problem does not appear to be simply a lack of organ donors, but rather a failure to identify suitable donors, obtain consent, and ultimately procure these scarce organs (Nathan et al. 1991).

Possible solutions to improving organ donation

Expansion of the pool of potential organ donors can be made possible by a number of novel approaches as noted below.

Increased public awareness

Many initiatives have been introduced to educate the public about organ donation, including publicity campaigns, media coverage of transplant events, and the widespread availability of organ donor cards. Aggressive organ procurement organization (OPO) efforts have resulted in the establishment of hospital-based organ donor protocols, reimbursement of organ procurement costs, and important educational programs for hospital personnel and others. Although these factors may help to increase donor availability, they have been insufficient to dramatically increase actual donor supply and many patients continue to die while awaiting organs. In the USA, organ donor retrieval rates were approximately 16 per million of the population in 1988 and 1989. In 1992, cadaveric donors in European countries were not much better, with a wide variation between countries, ranging from 9.1 per million in Greece to 21.7 per million in Spain (Cohen and Wight 1993).

Support and involvement of health care professionals is critical to the success of organ donation. The entire process begins with identification of suitable candidates, declaration of brain death, and, most importantly, approach of family members for permission to use the organs. In a survey of medical and surgical residents, 92% considered organ donation to be very important and 89% stated that they would donate their own organs after death (Spital and Kittur 1990). Only 45% of these "health care givers," however, knew how to recognize an organ donor or whom to contact to initiate the process. Another survey involving 100 nonphysician health care professionals noted that, while 90% of respondents had no moral objection to organ donation, only 45% indicated a willingness to donate their own organs and 50% would donate organs of their family members (Gaber et al. 1990b). This study underscored the importance of professional education. In fact, respondents who attended in-service training on organ donation and transplantation were significantly more aware of the need for organ procurement and were more likely to donate their organs or those of their relatives. Failure to ask or obtain consent from relatives, permission being withheld by the coroner, and failure to test all potential donors for brain death appear to be the most frequent causes for loss of potential organ donors. Of critical importance was reluctance of primary physicians, anesthesiologists, and nurses to initiate any intervention in a patient if its specific intention was to provide donor organs.

Use of minority requesters for donor recruitment

It has been estimated that of over 300 organ procurement coordinators working in 72 organizations only 14 were African-American. This is a particular problem in the USA, because there is a higher percentage of African-American than white patients awaiting renal transplantation (Kusserow 1991). The introduction of a minority education program in 1989, which focused on schools, churches, and employers, resulted in an increase in consent rates from black families from 12% in 1989 to 31% in 1994. This report also emphasized the importance of using minority requesters when dealing with minority organ donor families in an attempt to overcome the distrust or misconceptions of health care delivery systems or any cultural and/or religious differences.

Widening organ donor criteria

Another means of increasing potential donors would be to initiate donation from what in the past have been considered "marginal" organ donors. These would include elderly, diabetic, or hypertensive patients and hemodynamically labile patients who are being maintained on excessive doses of vasopressors (Alexander and Vaughan 1991).

Use of nonheart beating donors

Advances in organ preservation techniques offer greater viability of organs in a nonheart beating donor until consent can be obtained. Until recently, donors without cardiovascular function at the time of organ procurement were not considered suitable for solid organ transplantation. The transplant community, however, believes that these unique donors may be an important source of transplantable organs, in particular, victims of trauma or those who die of cardiac arrest soon after arrival to the hospital. This could potentially increase numbers of available organ donors by five- to tenfold. The chief problem with implementing the use of nonheart beating donors has been difficulty in obtaining consent for organ recovery before vital organs are irreparably damaged by lack of blood supply, so called "warm ischemia.". It may now be possible to reduce this damage by preserving organs in situ using minimally invasive techniques. At this point, search for organ donor consent can be obtained by the health care professionals treating the patient. Recent reports from experienced centers have now documented the feasibility of transplanting kidneys and other lifesaving organs from nonheart beating donors (Varty et al. 1993).

The use of non-related living donors

Although living donors have been utilized in renal transplantation since its inception, unrelated living donor renal transplantation has been recognized as a successful means of treating end stage renal disease. Excellent results have been reported both with and without the use of donor-specific blood trans-fusions (Squifflet et al. 1990). Most centers, however, have insisted that these donors be emotionally related to the recipient, i.e., spouse, step-parent, or step-child.

Presumed consent

In the mid-1980s, Required Request legislation was introduced in the USA in an attempt to relieve the organ shortage (Gaber, Hall, and Britt 1990a). However, this legislation has not fulfilled its promise because most forms of request law mandate that hospital administrators be responsible for ensuring that next of kin be asked to donate organs or tissues of the deceased when death occurs in a hospital setting. An alternative would be to initiate Pre-sumed Consent legislation, as has been practiced in European countries (Austria, Belgium, France) so that organs can be harvested without explicit consent. In those countries, cadaveric organ procurement is significantly higher than in countries with a Next of Kin consent system. In one study, cadaveric kidney procurement increased 86% and extra-renal procurement 183% after Presumed Consent law was approved in Belgium in 1986 (Roels et al. 1990). Despite Presumed Consent laws, however, most physicians in these countries have been unwilling to remove organs without first consulting family members. The one exception has been Austria, which has a long history of autopsy without consent. In this regard, there is also a more favorable attitude toward Presumed Consent within the Austrian medical community than exists in other European countries.

Currently in the USA, a person is not considered an organ donor unless he/she or the family gives permission. On the other hand, Presumed Consent indicates that the person is willing to have his/her organs harvested upon death unless the family objects. In recent years serious consideration of Presumed Consent has been put forth by a number of states. Unfortunately, surveys of the general public have suggested that this actually may have a negative impact on organ procurement.

Financial incentives to potential organ donor families

Various types of financial inducement to enhance organ donation have been proposed. Some of these ideas include the concept of a death benefit paid directly to organ donor families and/or possible reductions in state or local income taxes, payment of some or all of the costs associated with burial of the donor, or payment of some portion of the hospital costs incurred by the donor family (Financial Incentives, 1991). This issue remains highly controversial and there are concerns that payment for cadaver organs would result in a loss of altruistic values while inviting a sense of free enterprise (Peters 1991).

Xenotransplantation

The use of xenografts (cross-species transplantation) not only serves as a possible solution to the critical shortage of donor organs, but also would allow access to a less limited supply of pristine organs to permit elective timing of transplantation before patients became critically ill. However, limitations include the xenograft response, which involves both cellular and antibody-mediated arms of the immune response, and can result in an intense host reaction to the alien graft. The term "discordant" applies to cross-species combinations where preformed antibodies destroy grafts quickly within minutes or hours (hyperacute rejection) and "concordant" for more favorable combinations lacking preformed antibodies in which rejection is more indolent (Calne 1970).

Although Keith Reemtsma carried out the first clinical study of concordant xenotransplantation in the 1960s (Reemtsma et al. 1964), attempts to substitute organs between other species and humans have taken place only sporadically in the last 25 years. Without exception, each xenotransplantation performed during this time has failed, usually very rapidly. In the vast majority of cases failure was due to vigorous immune responses mounted by the host against the alien graft. In other cases, though the xenograft functioned, the intense and dangerously high levels of immunosuppression required to control rejection resulted in fatal infectious complications. Thus, immunological differences between species may limit the use of xenografts.

Recently, xenotransplantation has been revived by the performance in 1992 of the first three animal-to-human transplants since 1984. Two patients at the University of Pittsburgh received baboon-to-human liver transplants in the face of actively replicating hepatitis B (Starzl et al. 1993). Hepatitis B is considered by many transplant centers as an absolute contraindication to liver transplantation due to rapid reinfection of the human allograft by this virus. Though both patients died at 70 and 25 days post-transplantation respectively, currently available immunosuppressant agents attenuated the immune response to these concordant xenografts. The success of xenotransplantation may ultimately depend upon the ability to induce long-term tolerance to foreign tissue antigens. Without further improvement in this technology, it is likely that xenotransplantation may serve only as a temporary "bridge" until a suitable human donor organ becomes available.

Later in 1993 at Cedars-Sinai Medical Center in Los Angeles, a young woman in desperate need of a liver received a porcine xenograft intended to function as a "bridge" until a human liver could be located (Makowka et al. 1993). In spite of excellent surgical results and prompt graft function, the patient died of brain edema less than one day later while doctors were preparing to transplant a human liver.

Physiological and immunological barriers to the use of animal organs are not the only factors to be considered. A number of important ethical issues have been raised by the performance of xenotransplants.

New immunosuppressive agents

In the next decade a number of new, potent, immunosuppressive agents will be introduced for treatment of transplant recipients and patients with autoimmune diseases. Many of these agents will be used as primary immunosuppressive therapy (e.g., FK506). Others may be used in combination (e.g., mycophenolate) to permit dose reductions and avoid synergistic toxicities, while maximizing immunosuppressive potential.

The expansion of the immunosuppressant drug armamentarium will offer more flexibility and potency in clinical management, hopefully with reduced side effects. The introduction of newer cyclosporine analogues will improve absorption and lower dosing requirements of this drug. FK506 (tacrolimus) will probably emerge as a rescue agent in addition to a primary therapy following liver transplantation. Though recent clinical trials conducted in the USA and Europe have shown that FK506 is quite similar to cyclosporine, its unique properties make it an attractive alternative for the rescue of failing grafts or prevention of rejection in liver transplant recipients. Azathioprine may be challenged by RS-61443 (mycophenolate mofetil) or brequinar sodium as part of triple therapy regimens. Immunosuppressive protocols combining rapamycin or brequinar sodium with cyclosporine will allow for reductions in cyclosporine dosing and a potential lowering of its nephrotoxicity profile. The availability of these agents will challenge the dominant role of steroids in transplantation and result in either a "sparing" use or their total elimination. Finally, emerging monoclonal antibody technology may allow for more specific targeting of the immune response and preserve the ability of transplant recipients to fight infection and cancer.

The following are descriptions of newer immunosuppressant agents.

FK506

The US Food and Drug Administration (FDA) recently approved FK506 (tacrolimus) for preventing allograft rejection in liver transplant recipients. FK506, a member of the macrolide antibiotic family, is metabolized in the liver with peak serum concentrations seen one to four hours after oral administration. Although structurally unrelated, its action is similar to that of cyclosporine (Johansson and Moller 1990). Both agents bind to immunophilin and interfere with signal transduction pathways in T lymphocytes (Thomson 1990). FK506 inhibits T cell proliferation and the production of interleukins 2, 3, and 4. Milligram for milligram, FK506 is 10 to 100 times more potent than cyclosporine. Experimentally, FK506 prolongs allograft survival in skin, cornea, heart, liver, kidney, and small bowel transplants (Murase et al. 1990, 1991a).

Clinical experience with FK506 has now extended to liver, kidney, heart, and heart–lung allograft recipients. FK506 is also highly effective in conjunction with low dose steroids as primary antirejection therapy in liver transplantation (Todo et al. 1991), and as rescue therapy for failing primary and secondary liver allografts (Fung et al. 1991). Encouraging early results in heart (Armitage et al. 1991) and lung (Griffith et al. 1994) transplant recipients have also been reported. Graft survival rates in kidney transplant patients have been similar to those obtained with cyclosporine (Shapiro et al. 1991), while FK506 has been found to be capable of reversing ongoing acute rejection in cyclosporine-treated patients even when antilymphocyte preparations have been ineffective (Jordan et al. 1994).

The adverse effects of FK506 are similar to those of cyclosporine and include nephrotoxicity, neurotoxicity, gastrointestinal disturbances, and glucose intolerance. On the other hand, hypertension, gingival hyperplasia, and hirsutism are infrequently noted in FK506-treated patients.

RS-61443

Mycophenolate mofetil (RS-61443) is a potent inhibitor of de novo guanine nucleotide synthesis that selectively blocks both T and B lymphocyte proliferation, and inhibits antibody formation and the generation of cytotoxic T cells

(Platz et al. 1991). In animal models it has been shown to prolong islet, heart, and kidney allograft survival, reverse ongoing rejection, and induce strain-specific tolerance (Morris et al. 1990). Phase I trials in human kidney and heart recipients have documented its safety, efficacy, and pharmacokinetic profile. An oral dose range of 100 to 3500 mg/day was utilized in combination with cyclosporine and prednisone to treat 48 patients receiving primary cadaveric transplants (Sollinger et al. 1992). Though no reductions in rejection rates were seen in patients receiving less than 1000 mg/day, a recent US trial noted rejection rates to be reduced from 60% to 17% with daily doses of 2 to 3.5 g (Deierhoi et al. 1993). A recent phase I trial using RS-61443 in heart transplant recipients noted it to be less myelosuppressive and at least as equipotent as azathioprine (Ensley et al. 1993). Nephrotoxicity and bone marrow suppression have not been reported; however, gastrointestinal, genitourinary, and viral infections are commonly seen with RS-61443.

Rapamycin

Rapamycin (RPM) is a macrolide antibiotic that is structurally related to FK506. Although its precise mechanism of action is not completely understood, RPM inhibits a broad range of proliferative responses and appears to effectively block transduction of cytokine signals that trigger lymphocyte proliferation and differentiation (Sehgal and Bansbach 1993). While FK506 and RPM bind to the same immunophilin, this binding does not mediate RPM's immunosuppressive activity. A marked synergism between RPM and cyclosporine potentially offers an opportunity to reduce doses of each agent, if used in combination.

The ability of RPM to prevent chronic rejection and halt the progression of preexisting graft vascular disease distinguishes it from other new agents under development. RPM monotherapy has been shown to suppress acute allograft rejection in an number of animal heart and kidney transplant models (Calne et al. 1989; Morris and Meiser 1989). In early 1994, RPM was evaluated in several Phase I studies designed to profile its pharmacokinetics and maximal tolerated dose after a single intravenous injection. Though results of these studies have not been published yet, phase II studies are planned.

Brequinar sodium

Brequinar sodium (BQR) is a new immunosuppressive agent that acts by inhibiting the de novo pathway of pyrimidine synthesis (Makowka et al. 1992). Though BQR was originally developed as an antimetabolite for the treatment of cancer and psoriasis, it has the ability to suppress T and B cell-mediated immune responses. In initial studies BQR was highly effective in preventing rejection of rat vascularized organ grafts (Cramer et al. 1992).

Because of the dependence of lymphocytes on de novo pyrimidine synthesis, BQR has a selective effect on these cells compared to other proliferating cells (Kahan et al. 1993). The inhibition of B cell proliferation and subsequent antibody production means that BQR has a unique role in the management of highly sensitized patients. It may also become a novel agent in xenotransplantation.

Human phase I and II studies investigating the safety and pharmacokinetics of BQR in stable liver and kidney transplant recipients receiving cyclosporine A and prednisone immunosuppression began in 1992 (Sher et al. 1993). These protocols were divided into two components: single doses of BQR and multiple alternate day doses of BQR. Treatment was not associated with serious toxicities. Patients reported headache, diarrhea, and pain of mild to moderate degree. We await the results of ongoing phase II trials for this important new drug.

15-Deoxyspergualin

15-Deoxyspergualin (15-DS) is a guanidine derivative first described as an antineoplastic agent and later found to be immunosuppressive (Dickneite, Schorlemmer, and Sedlacek 1987). 15-DS blocks proliferative responses of lymphocytes and may exert some anti-B cell activity in humoral immunity. There may be beneficial effects of 15-DS in combination with other agents such as FK506 and cyclosporine. In human renal transplantation, 15-DS reversed acute rejection episodes in 81.4% of cases when used alone and in 94.4% of cases when used in combination with steroids (Amemiya et al. 1993). When DS-15 was added to quadruple immunosuppression strategies, it significantly reduced rejection within the first month and successfully reversed OKT3 resistant rejection (Koyama et al. 1991). Anemia and leukopenia appear to be the major side effects noted with this agent.

Organ transplantation

Intestinal transplantation

The short bowel syndrome (SBS) that results from loss of significant sections of small bowel remains a routinely difficult management problem. Total parenteral nutrition (TPN) is used. Currently more than 10 000 patients are registered in the North American Home Parenteral and Enteral Nutrition (HPEN) registry and 5393 patients receive TPN. TPN is expensive ($US 80 000 dollars/year), limits lifestyles, and requires long-term venous access. In children this poses a special problem because of their higher nutritional requirements, and the long-term risk of liver damage and other complications of TPN.

In stark contrast to the recent success of other transplanted organs, most small bowel transplants (SBTx) in humans fail due to rejection and/or the inability to control infection, particularly cytomegalovirus (CMV). In fact, all attempts at SBTx prior to the introduction of cyclosporine were uniformly unsuccessful ((Alican et al. 1971; Fortner et al. 1972). From March 1987 to July 1990, the European experience with SBTx included 15 transplantations performed in 12 patients under cyclosporine immunosuppression (Schroeder, Goulet, and Lear 1990). Four of those grafts are still functioning, with patients free from TPN.

From May 1990 to April 1993, the University of Pittsburgh Medical Center performed 45 intestinal transplants (23 adults and 22 pediatric) including two unsuccessful attempts (Todo et al. 1993). They performed three types of transplantation procedures. Isolated small bowel grafts ($n = 15$) were given to patients with intestinal failure only, combined liver and intestinal grafts ($n = 21$) were performed in patients with failure of both organs, and multivisceral grafts ($n = 6$) involving the entire mesenteric venous system of celiac axis were utilized in patients with thrombotic problems. All of the recipients were given FK506 immunosuppression and followed for a minimum of two months. The large bowel was included in the graft of 13 patients. Overall 1-year patient and graft survival were 82% and 73%, respectively. As of 1996, 32 patients were alive with a follow-up ranging from 2 months to 3 years, and 25 recipients were not dependent on TPN. Despite these encouraging results from this experienced group, recurrent and prolonged hospitalizations, a high incidence of infectious and lymphoproliferative complications, and the ever-present issue of monitoring for rejection will need to be overcome before SBTx becomes a routine clinical procedure.

Pancreas and islet cell transplantation

The discovery of insulin by Banting and Best in 1922 succeeded in replacing a uniformly fatal disease with that of a chronic illness for many patients with diabetes. Over the last 70 years, despite tremendous advances in medicine, the basic treatment of diabetes has not changed. More than 50% of diabetics surviving for more than 20 years will develop multiorgan involvement (i.e., neuropathy, retinopathy, nephropathy) related to the degree to which hyperglycemia is controlled. Although precise control of blood glucose will prevent these devastating complications, to date no perfect insulin delivery system has been developed. With the dramatic improvement in survival of diabetic patients who have undergone renal transplantation (Basadonna et al. 1993), a growing interest in both whole-organ pancreatic and islet cell transplantation has developed as a means of ameliorating the secondary complications of diabetes and improving quality of life by rendering such patients free from daily insulin injections.

In the last 27 years, the majority of pancreas transplants have been carried out simultaneously with renal transplantation in uremic diabetics. Pivotal work at the University of Minnesota, however, has explored a number of unique approaches, including pancreas transplantation alone in a large number of nonuremic diabetics (Sutherland et al. 1988), living related segmental pancreas transplants in combination with living renal donation from nondiabetic twins to their diabetic twin counterparts (Sutherland et al. 1984), and islet transplantation (Gores, Najarian, and Sutherland 1992).

Although the long-term goal of pancreas transplantation is to ameliorate secondary complications of diabetes, to date the main benefit for patients has been an improvement in day to day quality of life that accompanies insulin independence. Prevention of these complications would necessitate trans-plantation, with all its potential side effects, at a very early stage in the evolution of diabetes, which is not a practical issue at this time. Simultaneous pancreas-kidney transplantation with bladder drainage offers optimal graft survival because kidney graft rejection can be used as a marker of pancreas rejection (Sollinger, Cook, and Kamps 1984). In addition, graft survival rates are significantly higher when recipients are closely matched with respect to human leukocyte antigens (So et al. 1991).

Islet cell transplantation offers the possibility of insulin independence without the need for major surgery. This has been an extremely difficult endeavor, however, and sustained insulin independence was not achieved until 1992 despite its introduction as early as 1974 (Najarian et al. 1977). Earlier patients were only transiently insulin free or required insulin continuously following islet transplantation (Sutherland et al. 1980). Critical problems have been islet purification, where to place the islets (intraportal versus intra-abdominal), and diagnosis of rejection before islets have been irreversibly damaged. As of 31 December 1993, a total of 215 islet cell transplantations have been performed in 30 institutions worldwide (International Islet Transplant Registry 1994). In the 1990 to 1992 era, only 6 of 55 adult patients receiving pooled islets from multiple donors and 2 of 25 patients receiving islets from a single donor had functioning grafts and insulin independence at 1 year. Despite these poor results, many groups are pursuing strategies such as immunoalteration and immunoisolation with the belief that immunologic as well as surgical advantages will occur with islet cell transplantation.

Central themes in transplantation

Tolerance induction

Tolerance to nonself antigens has been a central albeit elusive goal in clinical organ transplantation. The induction of donor-specific tolerance, in which the immune system of the recipient is reeducated to see the donor as part of "self", will ultimately offer preservation of recipient immunocompetence and indefinite prolongation of allograft survival. To date, true tolerance without immunosuppression has occurred only sporadically in humans. Laboratory and clinical investigations during the last few years have identified at least three pathways for tolerance: clonal deletion, clonal anergy, and the induction of suppressor pathways.

Tolerance is an active process requiring early immune recognition of specific antigens (Schwartz 1989). In addition, rejection appears to be important for long-lasting tolerance to occur. Although immunosuppressive drugs administered at specific times following transplantation can induce tolerance, too much immunosuppression will prevent its development. The presence of antigen-specific downregulatory cells that suppress mixed lymphocyte culture reactions (MLR) appear to be necessary for tolerance induction in humans. The precise origin of these regulatory cells remains to be determined. Veto cells, dendritic cells, and natural suppressor cells have been identified in various immunosuppressive regimens and could be candidates for regulatory cells.

In animal models, recent studies suggest that the thymus is actively involved in regulatory pathways that permit tolerance to occur (Ramsdell and Fowlkes 1990). In fact, virtual abrogation of MLR and cell-mediated lympholysis, with preservation of third party responsiveness across major histocompatibility barriers, is seen in mice following total lymphoid irradiation and transplantation of allogenic thymus (Waer et al. 1990).

The unique properties of bone marrow to induce donor-specific tolerance and chimerism was first reported by Billingham, Brent, and Medawar in 1953. Since then, tolerance has been achieved in a number of animal species including humans. Lethal irradiation of recipient animals followed by reconstitution with allogenic bone marrow also leads to a lymphohematopoietic chimeric state that is tolerant to donor-specific antigens. Though these mixed allogenic chimeras display tolerance to host and donor skin grafts, they remain fully reactive to third-party skin grafts (Sachs 1990).

Although initial preparative techniques have involved lethal conditioning approaches that are unacceptable in humans, recent animal models have achieved nonlethal myeloablation by such techniques as low dose total lymphoid irradiation, monoclonal antibodies plus nonlethal irradiation, or cyclophosphamide (Cobbold et al. 1986). Particularly important was that resistance to graft-versus-host disease (GVHD) was observed in these models, even if the bone marrow had not been depleted of mature T cells.

The clinical use of bone marrow to prolong solid organ allograft survival has already begun. Two patients receiving HLA identical bone marrow allografts for cancer developed post-bone marrow transplant renal failure and were given transplanted kidneys from the same bone marrow donors

(Sayegh et al. 1991). Both patients have experienced rejection-free allograft survival without immunosuppression, except for low dose steroids for GVHD prophylaxis. The pioneering study of Barber and colleagues reported prolongation of renal allograft survival when inpatients who were administered cadaveric donor bone marrow 10 days following renal transplantation, in conjunction with induction, using Minnesota anti-lymphoblast globulin and cyclophosphamide. Baseline immunosuppression included cyclosporine, azathioprine, or cyclophosphamide and steroids (Barber et al. 1991). Though survival in the group receiving bone marrow was superior (85% versus 67%), the overall number and/or severity of rejection episodes was not significantly different (0.8 per patient) between the two groups. Though all patients displayed third-party reactivity, bone marrow patients were less reactive in MLC to their kidney donors than were control patients. Seventeen of 57 bone marrow patients were able to be withdrawn from steroids. However, the level of donor-specific responses and MLC did not correlate with the number and severity of rejection episodes nor with the ability to withdraw steroids in the bone marrow group. Barber et al. concluded "the most feasible method for the induction of functional allograft tolerance in mature hosts would appear to be the use of a form of profound immunosuppression followed by the administration of donor antigen." On the other hand, a recent randomized controlled trial (Rolles et al. 1994), showed no benefit from donor-specific bone marrow transfusion in patients undergoing liver transplantation. Immunosuppression was maintained with cyclosporine only following a 10-day induction with polyclonal anti-thymocyte globulin. Although the same dose of bone marrow cells was administered (2×10^8 to 3×10^8 cells/kg body weight) following induction, baseline immunosuppressive protocols differed between these two studies. The discrepancy between these pivotal studies requires explanation and may be related to differences in critical timing of bone marrow infusions with respect to the administration of anti-lymphoblast globulin, or to the timing of immunological monitoring.

Chimerism

It has been proposed that "successful engraftment of all whole organ transplants requires an exchange of cells of lymphocyte–macrophage lineage between the organ and the recipient" (Starzl et al. 1992a). The mixing of host cells with those of donor genome has been termed "chimerism." Bone marrow-derived dendritic cells are believed to be the predominant cells involved in the two-way migratory pathway between organ to recipient or recipient to organ. This process has been demonstrated in all organ transplants to a greater or lesser degree. In fact, the high density and quality of migratory cells to and from the allograft in liver transplant recipients is felt to be the basis for the "immunologic privilege" observed in this unique organ

(Starzl et al. 1992b). In addition, tolerance in humans has been associated with microchimerism in every instance where it has been carefully evaluated. The first evidence supporting the concept of chimerism in solid organ recipients (Kashiwagi et al. 1969) came in the late 1960s from karyotyping in female recipients of livers from cadaveric male donors. These studies demonstrated that characteristic Barr bodies of recipient origin had replaced donor Kupffer cells, while blood vessel endothelium and hepatocytes retained the male donor sex. Until recently the significance of this phenomenon remained elusive. In 1991, successfully transplanted intestinal allografts were shown to be chimeric (Murase et al. 1991b). In these pivotal studies, epithelium of the bowel was identified as that of donor while all lymphoreticular infiltrating the lamina propria were found to be from the recipient. Similar observations have now been extended to kidney (McDaniel et al. 1994) and thoracic organ recipients (Demetris, Murase, and Starzl 1992). In addition, the finding that migratory cells from liver allografts could influence metabolic functions at remote sites further confirmed the presence of chimerism (Starzl et al. 1993). This remarkable observation that donor-derived cells could transfer enzymatic activity to cells in the myocardium of children undergoing liver transplantation for glycogen storage and Gaucher's disease underscores the importance of chimerism in alleviating certain metabolic deficiencies.

Chimerism may simply represent a histological curiosity at this point. More exciting, however, is the possibility that chimerism invites a new avenue of research in the areas of transplantation and tolerance induction (Fontes at al. 1994). The ultimate understanding of this phenomenon may then allow for permanent graft acceptance without the need for lifetime immunosuppression.

References

Alexander, J. W. and Vaughan, W. K. (1991). The use of marginal donors for organ transplantation: the influence of donor age on outcome. *Transplantation*, **51**, 135–41.

Alican, F., Hardy, J. D., Cayirli, M. et al. (1971). Intestinal transplantation laboratory experience and report of a clinical case. *Am J Surg*, **121**, 150–9.

Amemiya, H., Taguchi, Y., Fukao, K. et al. (1993). Establishment of rejection therapy with deoxyspergualin by multicentral controlled clinical studies in renal recipients. *Transplant Proc*, **25**, 730–3.

Armitage, J. M., Kormos, R. L., Griffith, B. P. et al. (1991). A clinical trial of FK506 as primary and rescue immunosuppression in cardiac transplantation. *Transplant Proc*, **23**, 1149.

Banting, F. G. and Best, C. (1922). The internal secretion of the pancreas. *J Lab Clin Med*, **7**, 251–66.

Barber, W. H., Mankin, J. A., Laskow, D. A. et al. (1991). Long-term results of a controlled prospective study with transfusion of donor-specific bone marrow in 57 cadaveric renal allograft recipients. *Transplantation*, **51**, 71–5.

Basadonna, G. P., Matas, A. J., Gillingham, K. J. et al. (1993). Kidney transplantation in patients with type I diabetes: 26 years of experience at the University of Minnesota. In *Clinical Transplants – 1992*, 8th edn, ed. P. I. Terasaki, pp. 227–35. Los Angeles: UCLA Tissue Typing Laboratory.

Billingham, R. E., Brent, L., and Medawar, P. B. (1953). "Actively acquired tolerance" of foreign cells. *Nature*, **173**, 603–6.

Calne, R.Y. (1970). Organ transplantation between widely disparate species. *Transplant Proc*, **2**, 550–6.

Calne, R. Y., Collier, D. S., Lim, S. et al. (1989). Rapamycin for immunosuppression in organ allografting. *Lancet*, **2**, 227.

Cobbold, S. P., Martin, G., Qin, S., and Waldmann, H. (1986). Monoclonal antibodies to promote marrow engraftment and tissue graft tolerance. *Nature*, **323**, 164–6.

Cohen, B. and Wight, C. (1993). The shortage of donor organs: the European experience. *Xeno*, **1**, 21–2.

Cramer, D. V., Chapman, F. A., Jaffee, B. D. et al. (1992). The prolongation of concordant hamster-to-rat cardiac xenografts by Brequinar sodium. *Transplantation*, **54**, 403–8.

Deierhoi, M. H., Kauffman, R. S., Hudson, S.L. et al. (1993). Experience with mycophenolate mofetil (RS 61443) in renal transplantation at a single center. *Ann Surg*, **217**, 476–82, (discussion 482–4).

Demetris, A. J., Murase, N., and Starzl, T. E. (1992). Donor dendritic cells and after liver and heart allotransplantation under short-term immunosuppression. *Lancet*, **339**, 1610.

Dickneite, G., Schorlemmer, H. U., and Sedlacek, H. H. (1987). Decrease of mononuclear phagocyte cell functions and prolongation of graft survival in experimental transplantation by 15-deoxyspergualin. *Int J Immunopharmac*, **9**, 559–65.

Ensley, R. D., Bristow, M. R., Olsen, S. L. et al. (1993). The use of mycophenolate mofetil (RS-61443) in human heart transplant recipients. *Transplantation*, **56**, 75–82.

Financial Incentives (1991). Controversies in organ donation. Paper presented at the National Kidney Foundation Consensus Conference: New Orleans, Louisiana.

Fontes, P., Rao, A. S., Demetris, A. J. et al. (1994). Bone marrow augmentation of donor-cell chimerism in kidney, liver, heart, and pancreas islet transplantation. *Lancet*, **344**, 151–5.

Fortner, J. G., Sichuk, G., Litwin, S. D., and Beattie, E. J. (1972). Immunological responses to an intestinal allograft with HLA-identical donor-recipient. *Transplantation*, **14**, 531–5.

Fung, J. J., Todo, S., Tzakis, A. et al. (1991). Conversion of liver allograft recipients from cyclosporine to FK506-based immunosuppression: benefits and pitfalls. *Transplant Proc*, **23**, 14–21.

Gaber, A. O., Hall, G., and Britt, L. G. (1990a). An assessment of the impact of required request legislation on the availability of cadaver organs for transplantation. *Transplant Proc*, **22**, 318–19.

Gaber, A. O., Hall, G., Phillips, D. C., Tolley, E. A., and Britt, L. G. (1990b). Survey of attitudes of health care professionals towards organ donation. *Transplant Proc*, **22**, 313–15.

Gores, P. F., Najarian, J. S., and Sutherland, D. E. R. (1992). Clinical islet allotransplantation: the University of Minnesota experience. In *Pancreatic Islet Cell Transplantation*, ed. C. Ricordi, pp. 423–33. R. G. Landes: Texas.

Griffith, B. P., Bando, K., Hardesty, R. L. et al. (1994). A prospective randomized trial of FK506 versus cyclosporine after human pulmonary transplantation. *Transplantation*, **57**, 848–51.

International Islet Transplant Registry (1994). In *Newsletter* No. **5**, vol. 4 (No. 1, March), eds. B.J. Herhg, C. Geier, A.O. Schultz, R.G. Bretzel, and K. Federlin. Department of Medicine, Justus-Liebig-University of Giessen: Giessen.

Johansson, A. and Moller, E. (1990). Evidence that the immunosuppressive effects of FK506 and cyclosporine are identical. *Transplantation*, **50**, 1001–7.

Jordan, M. L., Shapiro, R., Vivas, C. A. et al. (1994). FK506 ''rescue'' for resistant rejection of renal allografts under primary cyclosporine immunosuppression. *Transplantation*, **57**, 860–5.

Kahan, B. D., Tejpal, N., Gibbons-Stubbers, S. et al. (1993). The synergistic interactions in vitro and in vivo of brequinar sodium with cyclosporine or rapamycin alone and in triple combination. *Transplantation*, **55**, 894–900.

Kashiwagi, N., Porter, K. A., Penn, I., Brettchneider, L., and Starzl, T.E. (1969). Studies of homograft sex and of gamma globulin phenotypes after orthotopic homotransplantation of the human liver. *Surg Forum*, **20**, 374–6.

Koyama, I., Amemiya, H., Taguchi, Y. et al. (1991). Prophylactic use of deoxyspergualin in a quadruple immunosuppressive protocol in renal-transplantation. *Transplant Proc*, **23**, 1096–8.

Kusserow, R. P. (1991). *The Distribution of Organs for Transplantation: Expectations and Practices*. Office of Inspector General, Department of Health and Human Services: Washington, DC.

Makowka, L., Chapman, F. A., Jaffee, B. D. et al. (1992). Inhibition of the pyrimidine biosynthetic pathway prolongs cardiac allograft survival in rats. *J Heart Lung Transplant*, in press.

Makowka, L., Wu, G. D., Hoffman, A. et al. 1993. Abstract: Immunohistopathologic lesions associated with the rejection of a pig-to-human liver xenograft. In *Proceedings of Second International Congress on Xenotransplantation*, **32**, 26–29 September, Cambridge, UK.

McDaniel, D. O., Nathan, J., Hulvey, K. et al. (1994). Peripheral blood chimerism in renal allograft recipients transfused with donor bone marrow. *Transplantation*, **57**, 852–6.

Morris, R. E., Hoyt, E. G., Murphy, M. P. et al. (1990). Mycophenolic acid morpholinoethylester (RS-61443) is a new immunosuppressant that prevents and halts heart allograft rejection by selective inhibition of T- and B-cell purine synthesis. *Transplant Proc*, **22**, 1659.

Morris, R. E. and Meiser, B. M. (1989). Identification of a new pharmacologic action for an old compound. *Med Sci Res*, **17**, 877–8.

Murase, N., Demetris, A. J., Matsuzaki, T. et al. (1991a). Long survival in rats after multivisceral versus isolated small bowel allotransplantation under FK506. *Surgery*, **110**, 87–98.

Murase, N., Kim, D. G., Todo, S., Cramer, D. V., Fung, J. J., and Starzl, T. E. (1990). Suppression of allograft rejection with FK506: 1. Prolonged cardiac and liver survival in rats following short-course therapy. *Transplantation*, **50**, 186–9.

Murase, N., Demetris, A. J., Woo, J. et al. (1991b). Lymphocyte traffic and graft-versus-host disease after fully allogeneic small bowel transplantation. *Transplant Proc*, **23**, 3246–7.

Najarian, J. S., Sutherland, D. E. R., Matas, A. J., Steffes, M. W., Simmons, R. L., and Goetz, F. C. (1977). Human islet transplantation a preliminary report. *Transplant Proc*, **9**, 233–6.

Nathan, H. M., Jarrell, B. E., Broznik, B. et al. (1991). Estimation and characterization of the potential renal organ donor pool in Pennsylvania: report of the Pennsylvania Statewide Donor Study. *Transplantation*, **51**, 142–9.

Peters, T. G. (1991). Life or death: the issue of payment in cadaveric organ donation. *JAMA*, **265**, 1302–5.

Platz, K. P., Sollinger, H. W., Hullett, D. A., Eckhoff, D. E., Eugui, E. M., and Allison, A. C. (1991). RS-61443 – a new, potent, immunosuppressive agent. *Transplantation*, **51**, 27–31.

Ramsdell, F. and Fowlkes, B. J. (1990). Clonal deletion versus clonal anergy: the role of the thymus in inducing self-tolerance. *Science*, **248**, 1342–8.

Reemstma, K., McCracken, B. H., Schlegel, D. H. et al. (1964). Renal heterotransplantation in man. *Ann Surg*, **160**, 384–410.

Roels, L., Vanrenterghem, Y., Waer, M., Gruwez, J., and Michielsen, P. (1990). Effect of a presumed consent law on organ retrieval in Belgium. *Transplant Proc*, **22**, 2078–9.

Rolles, K., Burroughs, A. K., Davidson, B. R., Karatapanis, S., Prentice, H. G., and Hamon, M. D. (1994). Donor-specific bone marrow infusion after orthotopic liver transplantation. *Lancet*, **343**, 263–5.

Sachs, D. H. (1990). Antigen-specific transplantation tolerance. *Clin Transplant*, **4**, 78.

Sayegh, M. H., Fine, N. A., Smith, J. L. et al. (1991). Immunologic tolerance to renal allografts after bone marrow transplants from same donors. *Ann Intern Med*, **114**, 954–5.

Schroeder, P., Goulet, O., and Lear, P. A. (1990). Small bowel transplantation: European experience. *Lancet*, **336**, 110–11.

Schwartz, R. H. (1989). Acquisition of immunologic self-tolerance. *Cell*, **57**, 1073–81.

Sehgal, S. N. and Bansbach, C. C. (1993). Rapamycin: in vitro profile of a new immunosuppressive macrolide. *Ann NY Acad Sci*, **685**, 58–67.

Shapiro, R., Jordan, M., Fung, J. et al. (1991). Kidney transplantation under FK506 immunosuppression. *Transplant Proc*, **23**, 920–3.

Sher, L. S., Eiras-Hreha, G., Komhauser, D. M. et al. (1993). Abstract: Safety and pharmacokinetics (PK) of brequinar sodium (BQR) in liver allograft recipients on cyclosporine (CYA) and steroids. *Hepatology*, **18**, 746.

So, S. K. S., Moudry-Munns, K. C., Gillingham, K. J., Minford, E. J., and Sutherland, D. E. R. (1991). Short-term and long-term effects of HLA matching in cadaveric pancreas transplantation. *Transplant Proc*, **23**, 1634–6.

Sollinger, H. W., Cook, K., and Kamps, D. (1984). Clinical and experimental experience with pancreaticocystostomy for exocrine pancreatic drainage in pancreas transplantation. *Transplant Proc*, **16**, 749–51.

Sollinger, H. W., Deierhoi, M. H., Belzer, F. O. et al. (1992). RS-61443 – a phase I clinical trial and pilot rescue study. *Transplantation*, **53**, 428–32.

Spital, A. and Kittur, D. S. (1990). Barriers to organ donation among housestaff physicians. *Transplant Proc*, **22**, 2414–16.

Squifflet, J. P., Pirson, Y., Poncelet, A., Gianello, P., and Alexandre, G. P. J. (1990). Unrelated living donor kidney-transplantation. *Transplant Int*, **3**, 32–5.

Starzl, T. E., Demetris, A. J., Murase, N., Ildstad, S., Ricordi, C., and Trucco, M. (1992a). Cell migration, chimerism and graft acceptance. *Lancet*, **339**, 1579–82.

Starzl, T. E., Demetris, A. J., Trucco, M. et al. (1992b). Systemic chimerism in human female recipients of male livers. *Lancet*, **340**, 876–7.

Starzl, T. E., Demetris, A. J., Trucco, M. et al. (1993). Chimerism after liver transplantation for type IV glycogen storage disease and type I Gaucher's disease. *N Engl J Med*, **328**, 745–9.

Starzl, T. E., Fung, J., Tzakis, A. et al. (1993). Baboon to human liver transplantation. *Lancet*, **341**, 65–71.

Sutherland, D. E. R., Kendall, D. M., Moudry, K. C. et al. (1988). Pancreas transplantation in nonuremic, type I diabetic recipients. *Surgery*, **104**, 453–64.

Sutherland, D. E. R., Matas, A. J., Goetz, F. C., and Najarian, J. S. (1980). Transplantation of dispersed pancreatic islet cell tissue in humans: autografts and allografts. *Diabetes*, **29**, 31–44.

Sutherland, D. E. R., Sibley, R. K., Xu, X. Z. et al. (1984). Twin-to-twin pancreas transplantation: reversal and reenactment of the pathogenesis of type I diabetes. *Trans Assoc Am Physicians*, **97**, 80–7.

Thomson, A. W. (1990). FK-506: profile of an important new immunosuppressant. *Transplant Rev*, **4**, 1.

Todo, S., Fung, J. J., Tzakis, A. et al. (1991). One hundred and ten consecutive primary orthotopic liver transplants under FK506 in adults. *Transplant Proc*, **23**, 1397–402.

Todo, S., Tzakis, A., Reyes, J. et al. (1993). Clinical intestinal transplantation: three-year experience. Abstract presented at the Third International Symposium on Small Bowel Transplantation, Paris, 3–6 November.

UNOS (1991). *Annual Report of the US Scientific Registry of Transplant Recipients and the Organ Procurement and Transplantation Network*, UNOS, Appendixes F, G, and H. (1991).

Varty, K., Veitch, P. S., Morgan, J. D. T., Kehinde, E. O., and Bell, P. R. F. (1993). Abstract presented at the British Transplantation Society Meeting, October.

Waer, M., Palathumpat, V., Sobis, H. et al. (1990). Induction of transplantation tolerance in mice across major histocompatibility barrier by using allogeneic thymus transplantation and total lymphoid irradiation. *J Immunol*, **145**, 499–504.

Index